Clinical Pain Management

This book is dedicated to our patients, their families and all people suffering with pain.

Clinical Pain Management: A Practical Guide

EDITED BY

Mary E. Lynch

MD, FRCPC
President Canadian Pain Society
Professor Psychiatry, Anesthesiology and Pharmacology
Dalhousie University
Director Pain Management Unit
QEII Health Sciences Centre

Kenneth D. Craig

PhD
Professor Emeritus
University of British Columbia
Department of Psychology

Philip W.H. Peng

MBBS, FRCPC
Director, Anesthesia Chronic Pain Program
University Health Network and Mount Sinai Hospital
Wasser Pain Management Center, Mount Sinai Hospital
Associate Professor
University of Toronto

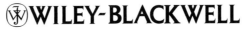

A John Wiley & Sons, Ltd., Publication

Library of Congress Cataloging-in-Publication Data
Clinical pain management : a practical guide / edited by Mary E. Lynch, Kenneth D. Craig, Philip W.H. Peng.
     p. ; cm.
   Includes bibliographical references.
   ISBN 978-1-4443-3069-4
   1. Pain.   2. Pain–Treatment.   I. Lynch, Mary E.   II. Craig, Kenneth D.,
1937-   III. Peng, Philip W. H.
   [DNLM: 1. Pain–therapy.   2. Palliative Care–methods. WL 704 C6415 2011]
     RB127.C593 2011
     616'.0472–dc22
                                          2010024524
ISBN: 978-1-4443-3069-4

A catalogue record for this book is available from the British Library.

This book is published in the following electronic formats: ePDF 9781444329728; Wiley Online Library 9781444329711; ePub 9781444329735

Set in 8/12 pt Stone Serif by Toppan Best-set Premedia Limited
Printed and bound in Malaysia by Vivar Prinitng Sdn Bhd

01   2011

Contents

Contents

List of contributors

Lene Baad-Hansen Associate Professor, Department of Clinical Oral Physiology, Aarhus University, Aarhus, Denmark

Cathrine Baastrup MScPharm, Danish Pain Research Center, Aarhus University Hospital, Aarhus, Denmark

Misha Bačkonja MD, Professor, Department of Neurology, University of Wisconsin, Madison, USA

Diaa Bahgat MD, Instructor, Department of Neurological Surgery, Oregon Health & Science University, Portland, USA

Allan I. Basbaum PhD FRS, Department of Anatomy, University of California at San Francisco, San Francisco, USA

Fabrizio Benedetti MD, Professor of Physiology and Neuroscience, Department of Neuroscience, University of Torino Medical School, Torino, Italy; National Institute of Neuroscience, Torino, Italy

Klaus Bielefeldt MD PhD, University of Pittsburgh Medical Center, Division of Gastroenterology, Pittsburgh, USA

Sharon Bishop BNurs MHlthSci, Clinical Nurse Specialist, Department of Neurosurgery, Regina General Hospital, Regina, Canada

Eduardo Bruera MD, Professor and Chair, Department of Palliative Care and Rehabilitation Medicine Unit 008, University of Texas M.D. Anderson Cancer Center, Houston, USA

Kim J. Burchiel MD FACS, Professor and Chair, Department of Neurological Surgery, Oregon Health and Science University, Portland, USA

Chantel C. Burkitt BA, Department of Educational Psychology, University of Minnesota, Minneapolis, USA

Eugene J. Carragee MD, Professor and Vice Chairman, Department of Orthopedic Surgery, Stanford University School of Medicine, Redwood City, USA

Daniel J. Cavanaugh PhD, Department of Anatomy, University of California at San Francisco, San Francisco, USA

Stéphanie Chevalier PhD, McGill Nutrition & Food Science Centre, McGill University Health Centre, Montreal, Canada

Alexander J. Clark MD FRCPC, Professor of Anesthesia, Dalhousie University, Halifax, Nova Scotia, Canada

Alexis Codrington PhD, Alan Edwards Pain Management Unit, McGill University Health Centre, Montreal, Canada

Beverly Collett FRCA FFPMRCA, Consultant in Pain Medicine, University Hospitals of Leicester, Leicester, UK

Kenneth D. Craig PhD, Professor Emeritus, Department of Psychology, University of British Columbia, Vancouver, Canada

Gilbert J. Fanciullo MD MS, Professor of Anesthesiology, Dartmouth Medical School, Lebanon, NH, USA; Director, Head of Pain Medicine, Department of Anesthesiology, Dartmouth-Hitchcock Medical Center, Lebanon, NH, USA

Perry G. Fine MD, Professor of Anesthesiology, Pain Research Center, School of Medicine, University of Utah, Salt Lake City, USA

Nanna Brix Finnerup MD PhD, Associate Professor, Danish Pain Research Center, Aarhus University Hospital, Aarhus, Denmark

Mary-Ann Fitzcharles MB ChB FRCP(C), Montreal General Hospital Pain Center, Montreal General Hospital, McGill University, Montreal, Canada; Division of Rheumatology, McGill University, Montreal, Canada

Gerald F. Gebhart PhD, Professor and Director, Center for Pain Research, Department of Anesthesiology, University of Pittsurgh, Pittsburgh, USA

Stephen Gibson PhD, Deputy Director, National Ageing Research Institute, Caulfield Pain Management Center, Royal Melbourne Hospital, Melbourne, Australia

Padma Gulur MD, Department of Anesthesia, Critical Care and Pain Medicine, Massachusetts General Hospital, and Harvard Medical School, Boston, USA

Maija Haanpää MD PhD, Chief Neurologist, Rehabilitation Orton, Helsinki, Finland; and Pian Consultant, Department of Neurosurgery, Helsinki University Hospital, Helsinki, Finland

Heather D. Hadjistavropoulos PhD, Professor, Department of Psychology, University of Regina, Regina, Canada

Thomas Hadjistavropoulos PhD ABPP, Professor, Department of Psychology and Center on Aging and Health, University of Regina, Regina, Canada

Winfried Häuser MD, Associate Professor, Department Internal Medicine I and Interdisciplinary Center of Pain Medicine, Klinikum Saarbrücken, Germany

Peter Henningsen MD, Professor, Department of Psychosomatic Medicine and Psychotherapy, Technische Universität München, München, Germany

Fred M. Howard MD MPH, Professor of Obstetrics & Gynecology, University of Rochester School of Medicine, Rochester, USA

David Hui MD MSc FRCPC, Palliative Oncology Fellow, Department of Palliative Care & Rehabilitation Medicine Unit 1414, University of Texas M.D. Anderson Cancer Center, Houston, USA

Gordon Irving MB BS FFA(SA) MSc MMed, Clinical Assistant Professor, University of Washington Medical School, Seattle, USA

Robert N. Jamison PhD, Associate Professor, Departments of Anesthesia and Psychiatry, Brigham and Women's Hospital, Harvard Medical School, Chestnut Hill, USA

Troels Staehelin Jensen MD PhD, Professor, Danish Pain Research Center, Aarhus University Hospital, Aarhus, Denmark; Department of Neurology, Aarhus University Hospital, Aarhus, Denmark

Roman D. Jovey MD, Medical Director, CPM Centers for Pain Management; Physician Director, Addictions and Concurrent Disorders Center, Credit Valley Hospital, Mississauga, Canada

Joel Katz PhD, Department of Psychology, York University, Toronto, Canada; Department of Anesthesia and Pain Management, Toronto General Hospital, Toronto, Canada; Department of Anesthesia, University of Toronto, Toronto, Canada

Jeffrey L. Koh MD, Professor, Anesthesiology and Perioperative Medicine, Oregon Health & Science University, Portland, USA

Krishna Kumar MB MS FRCS(C) FACS, Clinical Professor of Neurosurgery, University of Saskatchewan; Medical Office Wing, Regina General Hospital, Regina, Canada

Sandra M. LeFort Professor, School of Nursing, Memorial University of Newfoundland, St. John's, Canada

Mary Lynch MD FRCPC, President Elect Canadian Pain Society; Professor Anesthesia, Psychiatry and Pharmacology, Dalhousie University, Haifax, Nova Scotia, Canada; Director, Pain Management Unit, Queen Elizabeth II Health Sciences Center, Halifax, Nova Scotia, Canada

Anjali Martinez MD, Assistant Professor, Obstetrics and Gynecology, George Washington University, Washington DC, USA

Michael McGillion RN PhD, Assistant Professor, Lawrence S. Bloomberg Faculty of Nursing, University of Toronto, Toronto, Canada

Patrick J. McGrath OC PhD FRSC FCAHS, Vice President Research, IWK Health Center; Professor of Psychology, Pediatrics and Psychiatry, Canada Research Chair, Dalhousie University, Halifax, Nova Scotia, Canada

Ronald Melzack Professor Emeritus, Department of Psychology, McGill University, Montreal, Canada

Harold Merskey DM FRCPC, Professor Emeritus of Psychiatry, University of Western Ontario, London, Canada

Tim F. Oberlander MD FRCPC, Professor, Pediatrics, University of British Columbia, Vancouver, Canada; R. Howard Webster Professor in Early Child Development, University of British Columbia, Vancouver, Canada; Complex Pain Service, BC Children's Hospital, Vancouver, Canada

M. Gabrielle Pagé Department of Psychology, York University, Toronto, Canada

Tonya M. Palermo PhD, Associate Professor, Anesthesiology, Pediatrics and Psychiatry, Seattle Children's Hospital, University of Washington School of Medicine, Seattle, USA

Don Young Park MD, Clinical Instructor, Department of Orthopedic Surgery, Stanford University School of Medicine, Redwood City, USA

Philip W.H. Peng MBBS FRCPC, Director, Anesthesia Chronic Pain Program, University Health Network and Mount Sinai Hospital, Toronto, Canada; Associate Professor, University of Toronto, Toronto Western Hospital, Toronto, Canada

Antonella Pollo MD, Assistant Professor, Department of Neuroscience, University of Torino Faculty of Pharmacy, Torino, Italy; National Institute of Neuroscience, Torino, Italy

James P. Rathmell MD, Chief, Division of Pain Medicine, Department of Anesthesia, Critical Care and Pain Medicine, Massachusetts General Hospital, Boston, USA; Associate Professor, Department of Anesthesia, Harvard Medical School, Boston, USA

Jana Sawynok PhD, Professor, Department of Pharmacology, Dalhousie University, Halifax, Nova Scotia, Canada

Marcus Schiltenwolf MD, Professor, Universität Heidelberg, Stiftung Orthopädische Universitätsklinik, Heidelberg, Germany

Barry J. Sessle Professor and Canada Research Chair, Faculties of Dentistry and Medicine, University of Toronto, Toronto, Canada

Yoram Shir MD, Director Alan Edwards Pain Management Unit, McGill University Health Centre, Montreal, Canada

Christine Short MD FRCPC, Assistant Professor, Dalhousie University, Halifax, Nova Scotia, Canada; Department of Medicine, Division of Physical Medicine and Rehabilitation, Halifax, Nova Scotia, Canada; Department of Surgery, Division of Neurosurgery, Queen Elizabeth II Health Science Center, Halifax, Nova Scotia, Canada

Stephen D. Silberstein MD, Professor of Neurology, Jefferson Medical College, Thomas Jefferson University, Philadelphia, USA

Maureen J. Simmonds PhD PT, Professor and Director, School of Physical and Occupational Therapy, Associate Dean, (Rehabilitation), Faculty of Medicine, McGill University, Montreal, Canada

Blair H. Smith MD MEd FRCGP FRCP Edin, Professor of Primary Care Medicine, University of Aberdeen, Scotland, UK

Dawn A. Sparks DO, Assistant Professor of Anesthesiology, Pain and Pediatrics, Dartmouth Medical School, Hanover, NH; Pain Clinic, Dartmouth-Hitchcock Medical Center, and Pediatric Pain Specialist, Children's Hospital at Dartmouth (CHad), Lebanon, NH, USA

Boris Specktor MD, Center for Pain Medicine, Massachusetts General Hospital, Boston, USA; Assistant Professor, Department of Anesthesiology, Emory University School of Medicine, Atlanta, USA

Pam Squire MD CCFP CPE, Assistant Clinical Professor, University of British Columbia, Vancouver, Canada

Michael Stanton-Hicks MBBS DrMed FRCA ABPM FIPP, Pain Management Department, Center for Neurological Restoration, Cleveland, USA; Consulting Staff, Children's Hospital CCF Shaker Campus, Pediatric Pain Rehabilitation Program, Cleveland Clinic, Cleveland, USA; Chair, Department of Palliative Care & Rehabilitation Medicine, University of Texas, Houston, USA

Jennifer N. Stinson RN-EC PhD CPNP, Scientist, Child Health Evaluative Sciences, and Department of Anesthesia and Pain Medicine, The Hospital for Sick Children, Toronto, Canada; Assistant Professor, Lawrence S. Bloomberg Faculty of Nursing, University of Toronto, Toronto, Canada

Michael J.L. Sullivan PhD, Professor, Department of Psychology, McGill University, Montreal, Canada

Peter Svensson Professor and Chairman, Department of Clinical Oral Physiology, Aarhus University, Aarhus, Denmark; Department of Maxillofacial Surgery, Aarhus University Hospital, Aarhus, Denmark

Frank J. Symons PhD, Associate Professor, Department of Educational Psychology, Center for Neurobehavioral Development, University of Minnesota, Minneapolis, USA

Brian R. Theodore PhD, Department of
Anesthesiology & Pain Medicine, University of
Washington, Seattle, USA

Rolf-Detlef Treede MD, Medical Faculty
Mannheim, University of Heidelberg,
Mannheim, Germany

Dennis C. Turk PhD, Department of
Anesthesiology & Pain Medicine, University of
Washington, Seattle, USA

Judith Versloot PhD, Faculty of Dentistry,
Toronto, Canada

Ashwin Viswanthan MD, Instructor, Department
of Neurological Surgery, Oregon Health &
Science University, Portland, USA

David Walk MD, Associate Professor, Department
of Neurology, University of Minnesota,
Minneapolis, USA

Mark A. Ware MBBS MRCP(UK) MSc, Assistant
Professor, Departments of Anesthesia, Family
Medicine, Pharmacology and Therapeutics,
McGill University, Montreal, Canada

C. Peter N. Watson MD FRCP(C), Department of
Medicine, University of Toronto, Toronto,
Canada

Karen Webber MN RN, Associate Professor,
School of Nursing, Memorial University of
Newfoundland, St. John's, Canada

Timothy H. Wideman PT, Department of
Psychology, McGill University, Montreal,
Canada

Amanda C. de C. Williams Reader in Clinical
Health Psychology, University College London,
London, UK

Lonnie K. Zeltzer MD, Director of Pediatric Pain
Program, Mattel Children's Hospital at UCLA,
Los Angeles, USA; Professor of Pediatric
Anesthesiology, Psychiatry and Biobehavioral
Sciences, David Geffen School of Medicine,
UCLA, Los Angeles, USA

Foreword

This excellent guide to clinical pain management covers every important facet of the field of pain. It describes recent advances in diagnosing and managing clinical pain states and presents procedures and strategies to combat a wide range of chronic pains. Unfortunately, many people suffer various forms of pain even though we have the knowledge to help them, but our educational systems have failed. This book is a valuable contribution to the field of pain by providing up-to-date knowledge that will stimulate a new generation of health professionals who are dedicated to abolishing pain.

Despite the impressive advances and optimistic outlook, many chronic pains remain intractable. Some people who suffer chronic headaches, backaches, fibromyalgia, pelvic pain and other forms of chronic pain are helped by several therapies that are now available, but most are not. For example, we have excellent new drugs for some kinds of neuropathic pains, but not for all. The continued suffering by millions of people indicates we still have a long way to go.

The field of pain has recently undergone a major revolution. Historically, pain has been simply a sensation produced by injury or disease. We now possess a much broader concept of pain that includes the emotional, cognitive and sensory dimensions of pain experience, as well as an impressive array of new approaches to pain management. Chronic pain is now a major challenge to medicine, psychology, and all the other health sciences and professions. Every aspect of life, from birth to dying, has characteristic pain problems. Genetics, until recently, was rarely considered relevant to understanding pain, yet sophisticated laboratory studies and clinical observations have established genetic predispositions related to pain as an essential component of the field. The study of pain therefore now incorporates research in epidemiology and medical genetics.

Clinical Pain Management: A Practical Guide highlights a mission for all of us: to provide relief of all pain, pain in children and the elderly, and for any kind of severe pain that can be helped by sensible administration of drugs and other pain therapies. We must also teach patients to communicate about their pain, and inform them that they have a right to freedom from pain. If we can pursue these goals together – as members of the full range of scientific and health professions – we can hope to meet the goal we all strive for: to help our fellow human beings who suffer pain.

Ronald Melzack
McGill University
Montreal, Quebec, Canada
2010

The editors would like to thank Ms. Sara Whynot for considerable assistance with every phase of the manuscript.

Part 1

Basic Understanding of Pain Medicine

Chapter 1

The challenge of pain: a multidimensional phenomenon

Mary Lynch[1], Kenneth D. Craig[2] & Philip W.H. Peng[3]

[1] Dalhousie University, Pain Management Unit, Queen Elizabeth II Health Sciences Centre, Halifax, Nova Scotia
[2] Department of Psychology, University of British Columbia, Vancouver, Canada
[3] Department of Anesthesia, Wasser Pain Management Center, Mount Sinai Hospital, University of Toronto, Ontario, Canada

Pain is one of the most challenging problems in medicine and biology. It is a challenge to the sufferer who must often learn to live with pain for which no therapy has been found. It is a challenge to the physician or other health professional who seeks every possible means to help the suffering patient. It is a challenge to the scientist who tries to understand the biological mechanisms that can cause such terrible suffering. It is also a challenge to society, which must find the medical, scientific and financial resources to relieve or prevent pain and suffering as much as possible. (Melzack & Wall *The Challenge of Pain*, 1982)

Introduction

The International Association for the Study of Pain (IASP) taxonomy defines pain as "an unpleasant sensory and emotional experience associated with actual or potential tissue damage or described in terms of such damage" [1]. Pain is divided into two broad categories: acute pain, which is associated

Clinical Pain Management: A Practical Guide, 1st edition.
Edited by Mary E. Lynch, Kenneth D. Craig and Philip W.H. Peng.
© 2011 Blackwell Publishing Ltd.

with ongoing tissue damage, and chronic pain, which is generally taken to be pain that has persisted for longer periods of time. Many injuries and diseases are capable of instigating acute pain with sources including mechanical tissue damage, inflammation and tissue ischemia. Similarly, chronic pain can be associated with other chronic diseases, terminal illness, or may persist after illness or injury. The point at which chronic pain can be diagnosed may vary with the injury or condition that initiated it; however, for most conditions, pain persisting beyond 3 months is reasonably described as a chronic pain condition. In some cases one can identify a persistent pain condition much earlier, for example, in the case of post-herpetic neuralgia subsequent to an attack of shingles, if pain persists beyond rash healing it indicates a persistent or chronic pain condition is present.

Exponential growth in pain research in the past four decades has increased our understanding regarding underlying mechanisms of the causes of chronic pain, now understood to involve a neural response to tissue injury. In other words, peripheral and central events related to disease or injury can trigger long-lasting changes in peripheral nerves, spinal cord and brain such that the system becomes sensitized and capable of spontaneous activity or of responding to non-noxious stimuli as if painful. By such means, pain can persist beyond the point where normal healing takes place and is often associated with abnormal sensory findings. In consequence, the scientific advances are providing a biological basis for understanding the experience and disabling impact of persistent pain. Table 1.1 presents definitions of pain terms relevant to chronic pain.

Traditionally, clinicians have conceptualized chronic pain as a symptom of disease or injury. Treatment was focused on addressing the underlying cause with the expectation that the pain would then resolve. It was thought that the pain itself could not kill. We now know that the opposite is true. Pain persists beyond injury and there is mounting evidence that "pain can kill." In addition to contributing to ongoing suffering, disability and diminished life quality, it has been demonstrated that uncontrolled pain compromises immune function, promotes tumor growth and can compromise healing with an increase in morbidity and mortality following surgery [2,3], as well as a decrease in the quality of recovery [4]. Clinical studies suggest that prolonged untreated pain suffered early in life may have long-lasting effects on the individual patterns of stress hormone responses. These effects may extend to persistent changes in nociceptive processing with implications for pain experienced later in life [5]. Chronic pain is associated with the poorest health-related quality of life when compared with other chronic diseases such as emphysema, heart failure or depression and has been found to double the risk of death by suicide compared to controls [6]. Often chronic pain causes more suffering and disability than the injury or illness that caused it in the first place [7]. The condition has major implications not only for those directly suffering, but also family and loved ones become enmeshed in the suffering person's challenges, the work place suffers through loss of productive employees, the community is deprived of active citizens and the economic costs of caring for those suffering from chronic pain are dramatic.

Chronic pain is an escalating public health problem which remains neglected. Alarming figures demonstrate that more than 50% of patients still suffer severe intolerable pain after surgery and trauma [8]. Inadequately treated acute pain puts people at higher risk of developing chronic pain. For example, intensity of acute postoperative pain correlates with the development of persistent postoperative pain, which is now known to be a major and under-recognized health problem. The prevalence of chronic pain subsequent to surgery has been found in 10–50% of patients following many commonly performed surgical procedures and in 2–10% this pain can be severe [9].

The epidemiology of chronic pain has been examined in high-quality surveys of general populations from several countries which have demon-

Table 1.1 Definitions of pain terms.

Allodynia	Pain due to a stimulus that does not normally provoke pain
Anesthesia dolorosa	Pain in a region that is anesthetic dolorosa
Dysesthesia	An unpleasant abnormal sensation, whether spontaneous or evoked
Hyperalgesia	An increased response to a stimulus that is normally painful
Hyperpathia	A painful syndrome characterized by an abnormally painful reaction to a stimulus, especially a repetitive stimulus as well as an increased threshold
Neuropathic	Pain initiated or caused by a primary pain lesion or dysfunction in the nervous system
Nociceptor	A receptor preferentially sensitive to a noxious stimulus or to a stimulus that would become noxious if prolonged
Pain	An unpleasant sensory and emotional experience associated with actual or potential tissue damage or described in terms of such damage
Paresthesia	An abnormal sensation, whether spontaneous or evoked (use dysesthesia when the abnormal sensation is unpleasant)

Source: Based on Merskey H, Bogduk N, eds. (1994) *Classification of Chronic Pain, Descriptions of Chronic Pain Syndromes and Definitions of Pain Terms*, 2nd edn. Task Force on Taxonomy, IASP Press, Seattle.

strated that the prevalence of chronic pain is at least 18–20% [10–12]. These rates will increase with the aging of the population. In addition to the human suffering inflicted by pain there is also a large economic toll. Pain accounts for over 20% of doctor visits and 10% of drug sales and costs developed countries $1 trillion each year [13].

Chronic pain has many characteristics of a disease epidemic that is silent yet growing; hence addressing it is imperative. It must be recognized as a multidimensional phenomenon involving biopsychosocial aspects. Daniel Carr, in a recent *IASP Clinical Updates*, expressed it most succinctly: "The remarkable restorative capacity of the body after common injury ... is turned upside down (and) hyperalgesia, disuse atrophy, contractures, immobility, fear-avoidance, helplessness, depression, anxiety, catastrophizing, social isolation, and stigmatization are the norm" [14].

Such is the experience and challenge of chronic pain and it is up to current and future generations of clinicians to relieve or prevent pain and suffering as much as possible. The challenges must be confronted at biological, psychological and social levels. Not only is a better understanding needed, but reforms of caregiving systems that address medical, psychological and health service delivery must be undertaken.

References

1 Merskey H, Bogduk N. (1994) *Classification of Chronic Pain*. IASP Press, Seattle.
2 Liebeskind JC. (1991) Pain can kill. *Pain* **44**:3–4.
3 Page GG. (2005) Acute pain and immune impairment. *IASP Pain Clinical Updates* **XIII (March 2005)**:1–4.
4 Wu CL, Rowlingson AJ, Partin AW *et al.* (2005) Correlation of postoperative pain to quality of recovery in the immediate postoperative period. *Reg Anesth Pain Med* **30**:516–22.
5 Finley GA, Franck LS, Grunau RE *et al.* (2005) Why children's pain matters. *IASP Pain Clinical Updates* **XIII(4)**:1–6.
6 Tang N, Crane C. (2006) Suicidality in chronic pain: review of the prevalence, risk factors and psychological links. *Psychol Med* **36**:575–86.
7 Melzack R, Wall PD. (1988) *The Challenge of Pain*. Penguin Books, London.
8 Bond M, Breivik H, Niv D. (2004) Global day against pain, new declaration. http://www.painreliefhumanright.com
9 Kehlet H, Jensen TS, Woolf CJ. (2006) Persistent postsurgical pain: risk factors and prevention. *Lancet* **367**:1618–25.
10 Lynch ME, Schopflocher D, Taenzer P *et al.* (2009) Research funding for pain in Canada. *Pain Res Manag* **14(2)**:113–15.
11 Blyth FM, March LM, Brnabic AJ *et al.* (2001) Chronic pain in Australia: a prevalence study. *Pain* **89(2–3)**:127–34.
12 Eriksen J, Jensen MK, Sjogren P *et al.* (2003) Epidemiology of chronic non-malignant pain in Denmark. *Pain* **106(3)**:221–8.
13 Max MB, Stewart WF. (2008) The molecular epidemiology of pain: a new discipline for drug discovery. *Nat Rev Drug Discov* **7**:647–58.
14 Carr DB. (2009) What does pain hurt? *IASP Pain Clinical Updates* **XVII(3)**:1–6.

Chapter 2

Epidemiology and economics of chronic and recurrent pain

Dennis C. Turk & Brian R. Theodore

Department of Anesthesiology & Pain Medicine, University of Washington, Seattle, USA

Introduction

Pain is among the most common symptoms leading patients to consult a physician in the USA [1]. Data from the National Health Interview Survey [2] indicates that during the 3 months prior to the inventory 15% of adults had experienced a migraine or severe headache, 15% had experienced pain in the neck area, 27% in the lower back and 4% in the jaw. Extrapolating to the adult US population these percentages would translate to 31,066,000 for migraine, 28,401,000 head neck pain, 52,325,000 for low back pain and 9,535,000 for jaw pain. The National Center for Health Statistics estimates that about 25% of the US population has chronic or recurrent pain, and 40% state that the pain has a moderate or severe degrading impact on their lives [3].

Chronic and recurrent pain has not only significant health consequences, but also personal, economic and societal implications. It impacts on quality of life, productivity, healthcare utilization and has both direct and indirect costs. This chapter provides a summary of the prevalence of some of the most common chronic and recur-

Clinical Pain Management: A Practical Guide, 1st edition.
Edited by Mary E. Lynch, Kenneth D. Craig and Philip W.H. Peng.
© 2011 Blackwell Publishing Ltd.

rent pain disorders and describes their economic impact.

Epidemiology of chronic and recurrent pain

In a review of 15 epidemiological studies from industrialized nations, Verhaak *et al.* [4] noted that the point prevalence for chronic non-cancer pain (CNCP) in an adult population ranges 2–40%, with a median of 15%. Similar rates were reported from studies documenting the prevalence of CNCP in epidemiological studies conducted in lower income nations, with a point prevalence of approximately 18% [5]. The adolescent population also reports a prevalence ranging 1–15% [6]. As noted in these reviews, the wide range in the prevalence rate of CNCP is influenced by various factors, including the population sampled (e.g. community vs. primary care), the definition of CNCP by duration (e.g. >1 month, >3 months, >6 months), the type of methodology used in the epidemiological study (e.g. mail-in survey, telephone survey, physical exam), the phrasing of questions included, the focus on the various parts of the body being surveyed and response rates.

Musculoskeletal pain

Among musculoskeletal locations, the most commonly afflicted region is the lower back.

Epidemiological surveys in the USA report a prevalence rate of 25% for low back pain any time during a 3-month period [3], 19% prevalence rate for chronic low back pain during a 12-month period [7] and a lifetime prevalence rate of 29.5% [7]. Similar findings have been reported in other industrialized nations, with prevalence rates for chronic low back pain ranging 13–28% [6]. Over 13 million Americans are permanently disabled by back pain [8]. Low back pain is also the most common of chronic pain conditions reported by adolescents, with prevalence rates ranging 8–44% [6]. Recent reports based on data contained in a large national survey estimated that 46.4 million Americans (21% of the population) had self-reported doctor-diagnosed arthritis [9] and 30.1 million have had neck pain in the past 3 months [10]. The US Centers for Disease Control and Prevention noted that arthritis and other chronic rheumatic conditions (excluding low back) are projected to affect approximately 13% of the US population by year 2010, with an increase to 20% by the year 2030 [11].

Chronic widespread pain

In addition to site-specific chronic pain conditions, there are also consistent prevalence rates reported for chronic widespread pain (CWP), ranging 10–14%, in both adults and adolescents [6]. In conjunction with having a diagnosis of CWP, the development of the American College of Rheumatology (ACR) criteria for fibromyalgia syndrome also saw an increase in cases observed in clinical settings [6]. Prevalence rates of fibromyalgia syndrome reported in other industrialized nations range 0.7–4% [6].

Headache

According to the National Headache Foundation more than 45 million Americans experience chronic headaches [12]. Migraine alone affects 18% of women and 6% of men in the USA and has an estimated worldwide prevalence of approximately 10% [13].

Factors associated with chronic and recurrent pain

Overview of the biopsychosocial model

Recurrent and CNCP are not medical conditions that can be solely pinpointed to specific tissue pathology. For the vast majority of patients with back pain, headache and fibromyalgia no objective pathology is detectable. The biopsychosocial model of pain elaborates on the complex interplay of physical, psychological, social and environmental factors that exacerbate and perpetuate the pain condition [14]. For painful conditions that persist beyond the usual period of healing, the development of a pain–stress cycle may result in anger and distress at the situation. A prolonged state of the pain–stress cycle often results in the development of comorbid psychopathology. Individuals with chronic pain are at risk for adopting the sick-role and engaging in maladaptive behaviors that perpetuate the pain–stress cycle, resulting in both physical and psychological deconditioning.

Demographic factors

The most commonly identified demographic factors that have significant associations with CNCP are age, sex and socioeconomic status [6]. Older age is significantly associated with increased prevalence of CNCP. This increasing trend for prevalence with age was noted among patients with shoulder pain, low back pain, arthritis and other joint disorders, and CWP. Several factors [6] may account for the observed increase in prevalence among older adults, including degenerative processes and recurrent episodes of pain.

There are also pronounced differences in the prevalence rate of various CNCP disorders between males and females. Marked increases in prevalence rates have been observed among females for CNCP disorders such as shoulder pain, low back pain, arthritis, CWP pain, as well as migraine. This sex difference persists even when other factors such as age are accounted for. Several hypotheses may explain these sex differences, and include a difference between the sexes in hormones, body focus, evaluation and appraisal of symptoms, increased sensitivity or lower thresholds among females, differences in symptom reporting and healthcare-seeking behaviors, and differential exposure to risk factors (e.g. childbearing) [6].

Increased prevalence of CNCP has also been observed among individuals with lower socioeconomic status, which includes dimensions such as household income, employment status, occupational class and level of education. Specifically, the strongest associations with CNCP were observed for lower level of education, lower household income and unemployment [6]. However, socioeconomic status may not be a direct risk factor for CNCP, but significantly associated with underlying psychosocial factors consequent to the onset of pain [6].

Psychopathology as a predisposing factor

There is some evidence that underlying psychological factors may predispose an individual to develop CNCP, specifically emotional distress. These psychological predispositions may shape the response of an individual during the onset of a pain. A comprehensive review of the link between chronic pain and psychological comorbidity revealed a bidirectional relationship between pain and psychopathology. For example, in a community-based sample in the UK, asymptomatic individuals with higher elevations on anxiety and depressive measures were 2.4 times more likely to develop subsequent low back pain. Similar findings were noted in the First National Health and Nutrition Examination [15], where patients who had depression but not pain were 2.1 times more likely to develop CNCP when assessed again 8 years later. Psychological factors have been shown to be better predictors of back pain and related disability than physical pathology [16,17]. Furthermore, a study on the relationship between migraine and psychological disorders, based on a prospective cohort followed for 1 year, indicated a substantial link between major depression and later onset of migraines [18].

However, the relationship between CNCP and psychopathology is reciprocal; initial pain also predicted later onset of major psychological disorders

with approximately the same magnitude. Such comorbid psychopathology may pose as barriers to recovery, negatively impacting on the prognosis of the painful condition, and thus contributing to the overall prevalence rate of CNCP observed during population surveys.

Occupational factors

Several population-based prospective studies have confirmed occupational-related stressors as a risk factor for CNCP. These factors included high job demands, low requirement for learning new skills and repetitive work. Furthermore, they were associated with later onset of persistent pain, independent of occupational class, shift work, working hours and job satisfaction levels. The association between these stressors and onset of pain was more pronounced among individuals with relatively lower levels of education. In addition, a study conducted by the World Health Organization included a cohort from 14 nations with a 12-month follow-up [19]. The strongest predictor for development of chronic pain was occupational role disability at baseline, due to an injury. Risk of CNCP was 3.6 times greater among those with occupational role disability, and it was a stronger predictor than the presence of initial anxiety or major depressive disorders.

Role of disability compensation

The complex and often adversarial nature of the medicolegal system associated with disability compensation may result in contributing barriers to recovery. In examining this area one will often read of "secondary gain". Secondary gain refers to the notion that a contributing factor to disability may be a patient's wish to avoid work. There has been significant controversy in this area, and unfortunately several studies that have received widespread attention in the media were later found to have problems methodologically. Thus one must be very cautious in reading and interpreting studies in this area.

More recently it has been found that the prevalence rate of fibromyalgia syndrome has been reported to be equivalent in a non-litigious population with no disability compensation, relative to populations that had a disability compensation system in place and associated litigation [20]. Therefore, it is possible that the increased incidences of "secondary gain" related to litigation observed in some studies were mediated by the stress of being involved in potentially protracted legal battles. Furthermore, as reviewed in an earlier section on the prevalence rate of CNCP, similarities in the range of prevalence rates have been observed across nations with differing systems of disability compensation and healthcare structures. As noted in a review of "secondary gain" concepts in the literature, there is inconsistent evidence for the isolation of the effect of disability compensation and litigation as a secondary factor that perpetuates the chronic pain condition [21]. At present it is reasonable to conclude that medico-legal and compensation-related conflict and activities may cause additional stress that must be addressed in the overall management plan for each patient.

Economic impact of chronic pain

The economic impact of healthcare in general has been serious enough to have spurred debates about healthcare reforms aimed at managing costs. In addition, there have been calls for legislative reforms to contain the costs of healthcare and to make these costs manageable for all stakeholders. The effect of CNCP is certainly one of the drivers of healthcare costs. For example, in a review of costs documented by a US State Workers' Compensation system, a small minority of patients with chronic low back pain (7%) were responsible for approximately 75% of the annual costs incurred [22]. According to the National Headache Foundation [12], chronic headaches account for losses of $50 billion a year to absenteeism and medical expenses and an excess of $4 billion spent on over-the-counter medications alone.

In considering the economic impact of CNCP, we differentiate direct costs incurred through healthcare utilization, and indirect costs that are the financial consequences of the often debilitating nature of CNCP and recurrent pain. Finally, current estimates are provided for the total costs of illness associated with CNCP disorders.

Direct costs

CNCP is associated with a high utilization rate of healthcare services. In the USA, approximately 17% of patients in primary care settings report persistent pain [23]. This subset of patients is also among the highest utilizers of healthcare services. For example, the presence of CNCP was shown to be associated with a twofold increase in the number of primary care visits and hospitalizations, and also a fivefold increase in the number of visits to emergency rooms. In a review of cost data obtained from a large US Workers' Compensation database, the overall direct costs associated with healthcare utilization increased exponentially as a function of disability duration [24]. Specifically, the cost-per-claim for patients disabled for more than 18 months due to musculoskeletal injuries was $67,612. In contrast, patients disabled for 4–8 months and 11–18 months in duration incurred total medical costs-per-claim of $21,356 and $33,750, respectively. Among the biggest cost drivers for the direct costs associated with healthcare utilization are the costs associated with pharmaceuticals and surgeries.

The cost of pharmaceuticals for pain management amounts to $13.8 billion annually for prescription analgesics and an additional $2.6 billion for non-prescription analgesics [25,26], and these costs are increasing annually. Opioids are the most common class of medication prescribed by physicians in the USA [25,26]. The annual cost estimate for just one type of opioid alone (Oxycontin) is approximately $6,903 per patient [27]. Overall pharmaceutical costs per claim in a Workers' Compensation setting reveal exponential increases as a function of disability duration due to CNCP. The cost-per-claim for patients disabled for more than 18 months due to musculoskeletal injuries is $11,818. In contrast, patients disabled for 4–8 months and 11–18 months in duration incurred pharmaceutical costs-per-claim of $2,270 and $4,284, respectively [24].

Similar variations in costs are noted for surgical procedures often used to treat CNCP. The most current estimates of surgical costs are available from the US Centers for Medicare and Medicaid Services (CMS) (Table 2.1). These surgical costs range $5,708–23,555 per surgery, with lumbar fusions being the costliest of these surgical procedures for common musculoskeletal disorders. The costs reported by CMS are a conservative estimate, and may not necessarily reflect the true costs billed which vary by geographic region. Taking lumbar fusion as an example, the most recent estimate for the annual frequency of lumbar fusion surgery for

Table 2.1 Estimated costs of specific musculoskeletal surgeries based on reimbursement schedule of the Center of Medicare and Medicaid Services (CMS). The costs reported by CMS are a conservative estimate, and may not necessarily reflect the true costs billed which vary by geographic region.

Type of surgery	Cost per surgery
Major arm and shoulder surgeries – with complications or pre-existing conditions	$7,182
Two or more hip, knee or ankle surgeries	$19,418
Replacement of hip, knee, or ankle or reattachment of thigh, foot or ankle	$11,916
Repair of previous hip or knee replacement	$15,552
Lumbar fusion – with complications or pre-existing conditions	$23,555
Lumbar fusion	$18,094
Cervical fusion – with complications or pre-existing conditions	$16,706
Cervical fusion	$10,853
Spine surgeries (excl. fusion) – with complications or pre-existing conditions	$8,786
Spine surgeries (excl. fusion)	$5,708

Source: CMS Health Care Consumer Initiatives (http://www.cms.hhs.gov/HealthCareConInit/02_Hospital.asp).

degenerative conditions is 122,316 cases during year 2001 [28]. Therefore, costs of lumbar fusions alone amount to approximately $2.9 billion annually. Pharmaceutical and surgical costs, while substantial, are only two aspects of the variety of costs incurred by CNCP patients. Other direct costs that substantially add to the total cost of illness over the lifetime of CNCP include costs associated with physician visits, diagnostic and imaging, injection therapeutics, hospital admissions, physical therapy, complementary and alternative medicine (e.g. chiropractic, acupuncture), psychological services, comprehensive pain management programs and medical and case management services. In addition to these direct costs associated with healthcare utilization, there are substantial indirect costs incurred from the resulting disability due to CNCP.

Indirect costs

Indirect costs incurred due to CNCP include disability compensation, lost productivity, legal fees associated with litigation for injuries, lost tax revenue, reduction in quality of life and any additional healthcare costs associated with comorbid medical and psychological disorders consequent to CNCP. Projected annual estimates for some of these indirect costs due to back pain alone, range $18.9–71 billion in disability compensation, $6.9 billion in lost productivity due to disability and $7 billion in legal fees [27]. Back pain cases have been estimated to result in approximately 149 million lost work days at an estimated cost of $14 billion [29]. The estimated annual lost productive work time cost from arthritis in the US workforce was $7.11 billion, with 65.7% of the cost attributed to the 38% of workers with pain exacerbations [30]. Lost productive time from common pain conditions among workers cost an estimated $61.2 billion per year. The majority (76.6%) of the lost productive time was explained by reduced performance while at work, and not work absence [31]. The total cost of lost productive time in the US workforce due to arthritis, back pain and other musculoskeletal pain from August 2001 to July

2002 was estimated at approximately $40 billion, including $10 billion for absenteeism and $30 billion for employees who were at work but impaired by pain ("presenteeism") [31].

On a per-patient basis, using estimates from a Workers' Compensation setting for chronic musculoskeletal disorders ($\geq$ 4 months' duration), the average cost of disability compensation ranges $7,328–36,790 [24]. Similarly, the estimated productivity losses, based on pre-injury earnings, ranges $12,547–73,075 [24]. Both estimates have a range that depends on the duration of disability, from 4–8 months at the lower limit to > 18 months for the upper limit.

Total cost of illness

Estimates for the total cost (both direct and indirect) of chronic pain exceed $150 billion annually [32]. On a per-patient basis, as estimated using costs available from the Workers' Compensation setting, total cost of illness per patient ranges $70,486–208,030 depending on duration of disability [24]. Table 2.2 summarizes the total cost of illness due to CNCP, while delineating the associated major direct and indirect costs.

Conclusions

The estimated population prevalence of CNCP varies from 2% to 40%. This wide range is a result of several factors (e.g. the population sampled, definition of CNCP by duration, body parts targeted, sampling methodology, phrasing of survey items and the survey response rate). Overall, the perpetuation of chronic painful disorders may exceed a total annual cost of $150 billion, which includes direct costs associated with healthcare utilization as well as indirect costs associated with disability compensation losses in productivity, lost tax revenue and out of pocket expenses. Therefore, CNCP and recurrent pain have a significant impact on society, resulting in poorer quality of life for those afflicted, imposing substantially on the costs of healthcare, and exacting societal costs in terms of disability compensation and productivity losses. However, these figures do not reflect the incalculable suffering experienced by patients and their significant others.

Table 2.2 Estimated total cost of illness due to chronic non-cancer pain.

Type of cost	Per-patient cost estimate[*]	Annual cost estimate
Total cost of illness	$70,486–208,030	$150 billion
Direct costs	$21,356–67,612	n.a.
Pharmaceuticals	$2,270–11,818	$16.4 billion
Surgeries	$5,708–23,555[†]	$2.9 billion[†]
Indirect costs		
Disability compensation	$7,328–36,790	$18.9–71 billion
Productivity losses	$12,547–73,075	$6.9 billion

n.a. – No data available.
* Based on a US Workers' Compensation population.
[†] Costs per surgery based on US Centers for Medicare and Medicaid Services (CMS) estimates for musculoskeletal surgeries.
[†] Estimated cost of lumbar fusions only.

References

1 Hing E, Cherry DK, Woodwell DA. (2006) National Ambulatory Medical Care Survey: 2004 Summary. In: *Advance Data from Vital Health Statistics: no. 374.* National Center for Health Statistics, Hyattsville, MD.

2 Lethbridge-Cejku M, Vickerie J. (2005) Summary health statistics for US adults: National Health Interview Survey, 2003. National Center for Health Statistics. *Vital Health Stat 10* **225**.

3 National Center for Health Statistics. (2006) *Health, United States, 2006 with Chartbook on Trends in the Health of Americans.* National Center for Health Statistics, Hyattsville, MD.

4 Verhaak PF, Kerssens JJ, Dekker J *et al.* (1998) Prevalence of chronic benign pain disorder among adults: a review of the literature. *Pain* **77(3)**:231–9.

5 Volinn E. (1997) The epidemiology of low back pain in the rest of the world: a review of surveys

in low- and middle-income countries. *Spine (Phila Pa 1976)* **22(15)**:1747–54.

6 McBeth J, Jones K. (2007) Epidemiology of chronic musculoskeletal pain. *Best Pract Res Clin Rheumatol* **21(3)**:403–25.

7 Von Korff M, Crane P, Lane M *et al.* (2005) Chronic spinal pain and physical-mental comorbidity in the United States: results from the national comorbidity survey replication. *Pain* **113(3)**:331–9.

8 Holbrook JL. (1996) *The Frequency of Occurence, Impact and Cost of Selected Musculoskeletal Conditions in the United States.* American Academy of Orthopedic Surgery, Park Ridge, IL.

9 Helmick CG, Felson DT, Lawrence RC *et al.* (2008) Estimates of the prevalence of arthritis and other rheumatic conditions in the United States. Part I. *Arthritis Rheum* **58(1)**:15–25.

10 Lawrence RC, Felson DT, Helmick CG *et al.* (2008) Estimates of the prevalence of arthritis and other rheumatic conditions in the United States. Part II. *Arthritis Rheum* **58(1)**: 26–35.

11 Centers for Disease Control and Prevention. (2003) Public health and aging: projected prevalence of self-reported arthiritis or chronic joint symptoms among persons aged ≥65 years – United States, 2005–2030. *MMWR Morb Mortal Wkly Rep* **52(21)**:489–91.

12 National Headache Foundation. (2005) National Headache Foundation: Fact Sheet.

13 Sheffield RE. (1998) Migraine prevalence: a literature review. *Headache* **38(8)**:595–601.

14 Turk DC, Monarch ES. (2002) Biopsychosocial perspective on chronic pain. In: Turk DC, Gatchel RJ, eds. *Psychological Approaches to Pain Management: A Practitioner's Handbook*, 2nd edn. Guilford, New York. pp. 3–29.

15 Magni G, Caldieron C, Rigatti-Luchini S *et al.* (1990) Chronic musculoskeletal pain and depressive symptoms in the general population: an analysis of the 1st National Health and Nutrition Examination Survey data. *Pain* **43(3)**:299–307.

16 Carragee EJ, Alamin TF, Miller JL *et al.* (2005) Discographic, MRI and psychosocial determinants of low back pain disability and remission:

a prospective study in subjects with benign persistent back pain. *Spine J* **5(1)**:24–35.

17 Jarvik JG, Hollingworth W, Heagerty PJ *et al.* (2005) Three-year incidence of low back pain in an initially asymptomatic cohort: clinical and imaging risk factors. *Spine (Phila Pa 1976)* **30(13)**:1541–8; discussion 1549.

18 Breslau N, Davis GC. (1992) Migraine, major depression and panic disorder: a prospective epidemiologic study of young adults. *Cephalalgia* **12(2)**:85–90.

19 Gureje O, Simon GE, Von Korff M. (2001) A cross-national study of the course of persistent pain in primary care. *Pain* **92(1–2)**: 195–200.

20 White LA, Robinson RL, Yu AP *et al.* (2009) Comparison of health care use and costs in newly diagnosed and established patients with fibromyalgia. *J Pain* **10(9)**:976–83.

21 Fishbain DA, Rosomoff HL, Cutler RB *et al.* (1995) Secondary gain concept: a review of the scientific evidence. *Clin J Pain* **11(1)**:6–21.

22 Hashemi L, Webster BS, Clancy EA *et al.* (1997) Length of disability and cost of workers' compensation low back pain claims. *J Occup Environ Med* **39(10)**:937–45.

23 Gureje O, Von Korff M, Simon GE *et al.* (1998) Persistent pain and well-being: a World Health Organization Study in Primary Care. *JAMA* **280(2)**:147–51.

24 Theodore BR. (2009) Cost-effectiveness of early versus delayed functional restoration for chronic disabling occupational musculoskeletal disorders. *Dissertation Abstracts International* **B 70/05** (Publication Number: AAT 3356104).

25 Stagnitti MN. (2006) The top five therapeutic classes of outpatient prescription drugs ranked by total expense for adults age 18 and older in the US civilian non-institutionalized population, 2004. Statistical Brief 154. Agency for Healthcare Research and Quality.

26 Anonymous. (2007) Top generics based on retail dollar sales. *Chain Drug Rev* **29**:62.

27 Turk DC, Swanson K. (2007) Efficacy and cost-effectiveness of treatments for chronic pain: An analysis and evidence-based synthesis. In: Schatman M, Cooper A, eds. *Multidisciplinary*

Chronic Pain Management: A Guidebook for Program Development and Excellence of Treatment. Informa Healthcare, New York. pp. 15–38.

28 Deyo RA, Gray DT, Kreuter W *et al.* (2005) United States trends in lumbar fusion surgery for degenerative conditions. *Spine (Phila Pa 1976)* **30(12)**:1441–5; discussion 1446–7.

29 Guo HR, Tanaka S, Halperin WE *et al.* (1999) Back pain prevalence in US industry and estimates of lost workdays. *Am J Public Health* **89(7)**:1029–35.

30 Ricci JA, Stewart WF, Chee E *et al.* (2005) Pain exacerbation as a major source of lost productive time in US workers with arthritis. *Arthritis Rheum* **53(5)**:673–81.

31 Stewart WF, Ricci JA, Chee E *et al.* (2003) Lost productive time and cost due to common pain conditions in the US workforce. *JAMA* **290(18)**:2443–54.

32 United States Bureau of the Census. (1996) *Statistical Abstracts of the United States.* United States Bureau of the Census; Washington, DC.

Chapter 3

Basic mechanisms and pathophysiology

Daniel J. Cavanaugh & Allan I. Basbaum

Department of Anatomy, University of California at San Francisco

Introduction

The ability to experience pain is essential for survival and wellbeing. The pathological consequences of the inability to experience pain are particularly well-illustrated by the extensive injuries experienced by children with congenital indifference to pain [1–3]. The pain system, including afferent fibers (nociceptors) that respond to injury, and the circuits engaged by these afferents, not only generates reflex withdrawal to injury, but also provides a protective function following tissue or nerve injury. In these situations, neurons in the pain pathway become sensitized such that normally innocuous stimuli are perceived as painful (allodynia), and normally painful stimuli are perceived as more painful (hyperalgesia). The sensitization process is presumably an adaptive response in that it promotes protective guarding of an injured area. In some cases, however, sensitization can be long-lasting, leading to the establishment of chronic pain syndromes that outlive their usefulness, persisting well after the acute injury has resolved. In these pathological, often debilitating conditions, aberrant plasticity in the pain pathway establishes a maladaptive condition in which pain no longer serves as an acute warning system.

The ability to prevent or treat such conditions is critically dependent upon a comprehensive understanding of the basic mechanisms through which pain signals are generated by nociceptors and how this information is transmitted to the central nervous system (CNS). In this chapter, we focus on the molecules and cell types that underlie normal pain sensation, with specific emphasis on the nociceptor and on second order neurons in the spinal cord. We also discuss how these processes are altered following tissue or nerve injury and in persistent pain states.

Primary afferent neurons

The detection of somatosensory stimuli is initiated by primary sensory neurons that have their cell bodies in the trigeminal and dorsal root ganglia. These pseudo-unipolar neurons extend an efferent branch that innervates peripheral target tissues, and a central afferent branch that targets the spinal cord dorsal horn or medullary nucleus caudalis (for trigeminal afferents). Primary afferents that innervate somatic tissue are traditionally categorized into three classes: Aβ, Aδ and C fibers, based on diameter, degree of myelination and conduction velocity [4]. These physiological differences are associated with distinct functional contributions to somatosensation. Thus, the largest diameter cell

Clinical Pain Management: A Practical Guide, 1st edition.
Edited by Mary E. Lynch, Kenneth D. Craig and Philip W.H. Peng.

bodies give rise to myelinated Aβ fibers that rapidly conduct nerve impulses and detect innocuous mechanical stimulation. In contrast, noxious thermal, mechanical and chemical stimuli are detected by medium diameter, thinly myelinated Aδ fibers, and by small diameter, unmyelinated C fibers. These latter two groups constitute the nociceptors, and represent a dedicated system for the detection of stimuli capable of causing tissue damage, as they are only excited when stimulus intensities reach the noxious range [4]. The Aδ nociceptors mediate the fast, pricking sensation of "first pain," and the C fibers convey information leading to the sustained, burning quality of "second pain" [5].

Nociceptor subtypes

Electrophysiologic studies have identified two main classes of Aδ nociceptor. The first type is readily activated by intense mechanical stimulation. These cells are relatively unresponsive to short duration, noxious heat stimulation, but respond more robustly to extended periods of heat stimulation. The second class is insensitive to mechanical stimulation but is robustly activated by heat. Aδ nociceptors are further characterized by the expression of several molecular markers [6]. Consistent with their myelination status, they express the neurofilament, N52, a marker of myelinated fibers. Subsets of Aδ nociceptors additionally express the neuropeptide, calcitonin gene-related peptide (CGRP), the TRPV2 ion channel and the δ subtype of opioid receptor [7].

The majority of C-fiber nociceptors show polymodal response properties: they are activated by multiple modalities of painful stimuli, including thermal, chemical and mechanical. Although much rarer, modality-specific (e.g. exclusively heat-responsive) C fibers also exist. C-fiber nociceptors are traditionally subdivided, based on their neurochemical identity, into two broad classes: peptidergic nociceptors express the neuropeptides substance P (SP) and CGRP; non-peptidergic nociceptors lack neuropeptides and bind the lectin IB4 [5]. Importantly, recent evidence suggests that these molecularly defined C-fiber subtypes make

functionally distinct contributions to the detection of noxious stimuli of different modalities [8]. Additional nociceptor characteristics are presented in Table 3.1.

Nociceptors and noxious stimulus detection

The peripheral terminal of the nociceptor is specialized to detect and transduce noxious stimuli [9]. This process depends on the presence of specific ion channels and receptors at the peripheral terminal. Among these are the acid-sensing ion channels (ASICs), purinergic P2X receptors, voltage-gated sodium, calcium and potassium channels, and the transient receptor potential (TRP) family of ion channels [9]. Notably, many of these molecules are uniquely or preferentially expressed in nociceptors, compared to other parts of the nervous system.

Molecular mechanisms of nociception: thermal, mechanical and chemical

The activation thresholds of several peripheral receptors closely match the psychophysical demarcation between the perception of innocuous and noxious thermal stimuli. For example, the heat pain threshold in humans, which rests around 43°C, matches the activation threshold for the sensory ion channel, TRPV1, and mice lacking TRPV1 exhibit deficits in cellular and behavioral responses to noxious heat [10]. Similarly, a related ion channel, TRPM8, is excited by temperatures below 25°C, and mice lacking this receptor show a drastic reduction in their responses to a range of cool and cold temperatures, including some in the noxious range [11]. In addition, several other receptors contribute to the detection of noxious thermal stimuli, including the TRPV3 and TRPV4 ion channels.

Several candidate receptors have been proposed to underlie the transduction of noxious mechanical stimuli, including members of the degenerin/epithelial Na+ channel (DEG/ENaC) families, and members of the TRP family (e.g. TRPV2, TRPV4 and TRPA1). To date, however, gene knockout studies

Table 3.1 Nociceptor subtypes and characteristics.

Type	Cell body diameter	Myelination/ conduction velocity	Activating stimuli	Molecular markers	Functional aspects
Aδ	Medium	Thinly myelinated ~2–10 m/s	**Type I** Intense mechanical or extended heat **Type II** Primarily heat*	Neurofilament N52 CGRP TRPV2 ion channels δ-opioid receptor	
C	Small	Unmyelinated ~1.0 m/s	**Polymodal** (predominant) noxious thermal, chemical and mechanical Modality-specific: heat cold mechanical **Others** Mechanically insensitive or "sleeping nociceptors"† Cooling (non-nociceptive) Pleasant touch (non-nociceptive)‡	**Peptidergic** Substance P CGRP NGF receptor (trkA) μ opioid receptor **Non-peptidergic** Glycoconjugates that bind lectin IB4 GDNF receptor (c-Ret) ATP sensitive P2X$_3$ receptor Mrgpr family of receptors (G-protein coupled) δ opioid receptor	Loss of peptidergic afferents eliminates heat pain sensitivity Loss of non-peptidergic afferents reduces mechanical pain sensitivity

CGRP, calcitonin gene-related peptide; GDNF, glial-derived neurotrophic actor; NGF, nerve growth factor.

* Also called mechanically insensitive afferents (MIAs) or "sleeping nociceptors," which respond to mechanical stimuli only after tissue injury [6].

† May be especially relevant for injury-induced sensitization; may account for up to 30% of all C fibers.

‡ Expresses VGLUT3 subtype vesicular glutamate transporter and contributes to injury-induced mechanical hypersensitivity [8].

in mice have failed to unequivocally support an essential function for these molecules in mechanotransduction [5]. Because mechanical hypersensitivity is a major clinical problem, identification of key molecular transducers remains a major challenge.

Finally, noxious chemical stimuli activate a range of receptors found in nociceptor terminals. Among these are the ASICs and the ATP-responsive purinergic receptors, which may be especially relevant in the setting of tissue injury, where pH changes and ATP release are common. Some TRP channels (e.g. TRPV1) are also regulated by pH, and many are targets of plant-derived irritants, including capsaicin (TRPV1), menthol (TRPM8) and the

pungent ingredients in mustard and garlic plants (TRPA1). TRPA1 also responds to a host of environmental irritants [5,12]. Finally, it is certain that there are endogenous chemical mediators that activate the different TRP channel subtypes. These mediators may be especially critical in the setting of injury to visceral tissue, the afferent innervation of which is not accessible to exogenous chemical or intense thermal stimuli.

Conduction of nociceptive signals

Nociceptors express a panoply of voltage-gated ion channel subtypes. Among these are the sensory neuron-specific sodium channels Nav1.8 and

1.9, which, along with the more ubiquitously expressed sodium channel Nav1.7, contribute to the generation and transduction of action potentials in nociceptors [1]. A pivotal role for Nav1.7 in nociception has been demonstrated by the report that loss-of-function mutations of this channel in humans lead to the inability to detect painful stimuli, while gain-of-function mutations lead to disorders characterized by intense burning pain [1,2]. The KCNQ type of potassium channel is also critical as it determines the repolarization time of nociceptors.

Once an action potential invades the central terminal of a nociceptor, neurotransmitter release is evoked via the activation of N-, P/Q-, and T-type voltage-gated calcium channels. Although glutamate is the predominant, if not the obligatory, excitatory neurotransmitter in all nociceptors, peptidergic neurons additionally release SP and CGRP [4]. Specific receptors for these neurotransmitters, including N-methyl-D-aspartic acid (NMDA) and α-amino-3-hydroxy-5-methyl-4-isoxazolepropionic acid (AMPA) receptors for glutamate, neurokinin 1 receptors for SP, and CGRP receptors, are located in appropriate regions of the spinal cord dorsal horn, and mediate the postsynaptic response to primary afferent activation [13].

Organization of the "pain system"

The afferent terminal

Nociceptors not only transmit pain messages, centrally to the spinal cord, but also release a variety of molecules from their peripheral terminals. These molecules (e.g. the neuropeptides SP and CGRP) influence the local tissue environment by acting on blood vessels and other cells to cause vasodilatation and plasma extravasation, key features of neurogenic inflammation. Neurogenic inflammation alters the extracellular milieu of the peripheral terminals of nociceptors, which can sensitize the nociceptor to subsequent stimulation.

The biochemical complexity of nociceptor subtypes is paralleled by their distinct peripheral innervation patterns. For example, some markers delineate populations of nociceptors whose peripheral innervation is restricted to particular tissues. Thus, nociceptors that express the Mrgprd subtype of G-protein coupled receptor innervate skin, but not visceral organs [14].

Central projections of nociceptors

The central branches of primary afferents terminate in the dorsal horn of the spinal cord, which is classically divided into five parallel laminae, based on cytoarchitectural grounds [13]. Neurons in lamina III and IV are innervated by myelinated fibers that respond to innocuous touch. In contrast, neurons in laminae I, II and V receive inputs from nociceptive afferents and are therefore important relays in the transmission of pain-related information, both locally and via projection neurons of laminae I and V, which target the brain [13].

The remarkable stratification of spinal cord inputs is further demonstrated by the distinct projection patterns of Aδ and C-fiber nociceptors (Figure 3.1). Lamina I spinal cord neurons are innervated by both Aδ and C fibers. Consistent with this input, the majority of neurons in lamina I are selectively activated by noxious stimuli, and are thus referred to as nociceptive-specific neurons. Lamina I also contains so-called wide dynamic range (WDR) neurons, which receive convergent input from nociceptors and non-nociceptive fibers. Lamina I also contains neurons that appear to encode selectively innocuous sensations such as cooling, itch and sensual touch [15]. Although most lamina I neurons are interneurons that are engaged in local dorsal horn circuits, a small but critical number (~10%) are projection neurons that directly access pain processing centers in the brain [13].

Lamina II predominantly contains nociresponsive interneurons and can be further subdivided into outer (IIo) and inner (IIi) regions, which receive inputs from peptidergic and non-peptidergic afferents, respectively. The most ventral part of lamina II is characterized by a group of excitatory interneurons that express the gamma

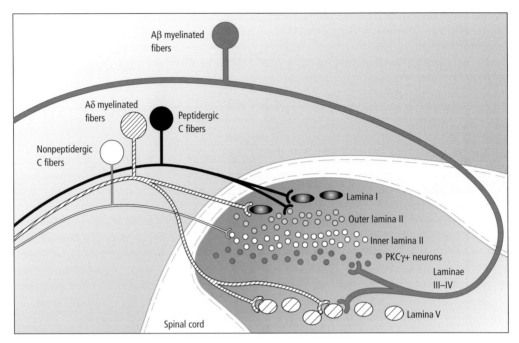

Figure 3.1 Primary afferent connections with the spinal cord dorsal horn. There is a very precise laminar organization of the spinal cord dorsal horn; subsets of primary afferents target spinal cord neurons within discrete laminae. The most superficial laminae (I and outer lamina II) are the target of unmyelinated peptidergic C (black) and myelinated Aδ nociceptors (striped). Lamina I contains large projections neurons (black ovals), while outer lamina II is exclusively made up of interneurons (light gray circles). The unmyelinated non-peptidergic nociceptors (white) target interneurons (white circles) in the inner part of lamina II. Ventral to this band of non-peptidergic inputs, protein kinase C gamma (PKCγ) expressing interneurons (dark gray circles) are targeted by myelinated Aβ fibers (gray) that carry innocuous information. A second set of projection neurons within lamina V (striped ovals) receives convergent input from Aδ and Aβ fibers, as well as indirect polysynaptic input from C fibers. Reprinted from Basbaum *et al.* [5], with permission from Elsevier.

isoform of protein kinase C (PKCγ). In contrast to the predominant nociceptor input to the dorsalmost part of lamina II, the PKCγ neurons are targeted by myelinated non-nociceptive afferents and by low threshold C mechanoreceptors, and participate in the process of nerve-injury induced persistent pain [16–18].

Although some lamina V neurons are nociceptive-specific, most are WDR neurons that receive convergent innocuous and noxious monosynaptic inputs from Aβ and δ fibers, respectively, and indirect polysynaptic input from C fibers. As in lamina I, a portion of neurons of lamina V are projection neurons that carry information to the brain [13].

Ascending pain pathways

Projection neurons in laminae I and V are at the origin of multiple ascending pathways. Among these are the spinothalamic and spinoreticular tracts, which project to various brain regions implicated in pain processing, including the thalamus, periaqueductal gray (PAG), parabrachial region, reticular formation of the medulla, hypothalamus and amygdala [19]. From these areas, nociceptive information is transferred to brain regions involved in sensory-discriminatory (somatosensory cortex) and affective-motivational (insula and anterior cingulate cortex) aspects of pain sensation, as well as to areas that are involved in descending modulation of spinal cord neurons that transmit pain messages to the brain (rostral ventromedial medulla; RVM) [19].

Sensitization and persistent pain

In the setting of injury, two often complementary and contemporaneous mechanisms underlie the process of sensitization that leads to allodynia and hyperalgesia. The first involves peripheral sensitization, of the nociceptor itself, and the second, central sensitization, results from sensitization of downstream CNS neurons in the pain pathway [5,20].

Peripheral sensitization

In addition to directly activating nociceptors, tissue injury evokes the release of pro-inflammatory mediators from primary afferent neurons and from non-neuronal cells. Among these mediators are neurotransmitters (serotonin, glutamate), peptides (SP, CGRP, bradykinin), ATP, protons, lipids (prostaglandins, thromboxanes, leukotrienes, endocannabinoids), chemokines and cytokines (interleukin-1β, interleukin-6 and tumor necrosis factor α [TNFα]) and neurotrophins (nerve growth factor [NGF], artemin, neurterin, GDNF, glial-derived neurotrophic actor [GDNF]), which act on receptors expressed by the peripheral terminal of the nociceptor to increase responsiveness to subsequent stimulation. This enhancement often occurs via the activation of second messenger signaling cascades that directly sensitize sensory channels [4]. For example, inflammation causes the release of bradykinin and prostaglandin E2, which decreases the threshold for heat activation of TRPV1 via second messengers, such as protein kinase C [20].

Central sensitization

As a result of the increased peripheral activation associated with tissue or nerve injury, neurons in the dorsal horn of the spinal cord and brain undergo long-term changes, a process known as central sensitization [20]. Central sensitization shares many properties with other forms of long-term plasticity observed in the CNS [20]. In the spinal cord, this form of plasticity is characterized by significant changes in the firing properties of neurons: decreased activation thresholds, increased receptive field size and increased spontaneous activity.

A variety of mechanisms have been proposed to underlie the development of central sensitization (Figure 3.2). The most well-studied involves activation of the NMDA subtype of glutamate receptor, a process that is functionally similar to the neuronal plasticity implicated in memory formation. Acute stimulation of nociceptors evokes the release of glutamate from primary afferent terminals. The glutamate activates calcium-impermeable AMPA and kainate receptors, but fails to activate NMDA receptors. However, following sustained release of glutamate, such as in the setting of persistent tissue or nerve injury, the postsynaptic spinal cord neurons are sufficiently depolarized to engage calcium-permeable NMDA receptors. Calcium influx through these channels leads to long-term molecular changes in spinal cord neurons, thereby strengthening synaptic connections between these neurons and nociceptors, and enhancing the central effects of subsequent nociceptive (and even non-noxious) inputs [20].

Loss of inhibitory control is also a major contributor to central sensitization. Inhibitory interneurons are densely distributed throughout the spinal cord dorsal horn, and these neurons regulate the transmission of noxious information by dampening excitatory inputs and preventing overactivation of nociceptive circuits. Following injury, however, there is a decrease in inhibitory inputs to superficial spinal cord neurons, which enhances spinal cord output in response to painful stimuli, and can additionally unmask inputs from non-nociceptive primary afferents [21,22]. There is evidence that disinhibition can result from a shift in the effect of normally inhibitory transmitters, e.g. gamma-aminobutyric acid (GABA) and glycine, such that they now excite, rather than inhibit, postsynaptic neurons, or because of alterations of inhibitory receptors on spinal cord neurons, making them less responsive to inhibitory transmitters

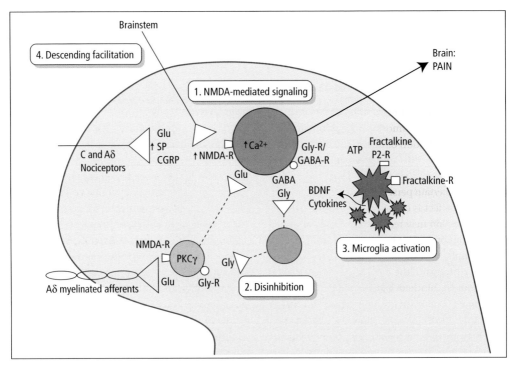

Figure 3.2 Mechanisms of central sensitization. (1) N-methyl-D-aspartic acid (NMDA) receptor-mediated signaling. After intense stimulation, sustained release of glutamate from C and Aδ nociceptors activates normally silent NMDA receptors located on postsynaptic spinal cord neurons. As a consequence, calcium enters, leading to a host of calcium-dependent signaling pathways and the triggering of long-term molecular and structural changes in spinal cord neurons, thus increasing their excitability. (2) Disinhibition. Under normal conditions, inhibitory interneurons (light gray circles) modulate pain transmission by continuously releasing GABA and/or glycine (Gly) to decrease the excitability and activity of lamina I output neurons. However, in the setting of injury, this inhibition can be reduced, resulting in hyperalgesia. Additionally, disinhibition can enable non-nociceptive myelinated Aβ primary afferents to engage the pain transmission circuitry, such that normally innocuous stimuli are now perceived as painful. This occurs, in part, through the disinhibition of excitatory PKCγ-expressing interneurons. (3) Microglial activation. Peripheral nerve injury also evokes the release of factors, such as ATP and fractalkine, which stimulate microglial cells by binding to receptors located on the microglia. In particular, activation of purinergic P2-R receptors (for ATP) and CX3CR1 (for fractalkine), promotes the release of the neurotrophin, brain-derived neurotrophic factor (BDNF) and cytokines, such as TNFα, interleukin-1β and interleukin-6. These factors contribute to central sensitization through an action on neurons in the spinal cord dorsal horn. (4) Descending facilitation. The brainstem contains neurons that facilitate the processing of pain signals at the level of the spinal cord. Under certain persistent pain conditions, these facilitatory neurons become sensitized, thus increasing excitatory tone in the dorsal horn. Adapted from Basbaum et al. [5], with permission from Elsevier.

[23,24]. Frank loss of inhibitory interneurons secondary to a massive injury has also been reported [22], although the magnitude of the loss is debated.

Central sensitization also involves interactions among microglia, astrocytes and spinal cord neurons. In response to soluble factors released from the terminals of injured primary afferent fibers, microglia are activated and accumulate in the superficial dorsal horn. In turn, the microglia release a host of pathophysiologic signaling molecules, including interleukin-1β, interleukin-6, TNFα, fractalkine and brain-derived neurotrophic factor (BDNF), which enhance central sensitization and therefore contribute to persistent pain states [25]. Astrocytes are also induced in the spinal cord following injury. Although their contribution to central sensitization is less clear, astrocytes appear to be more critical for the maintenance rather than the induction of persistent pain [25].

Finally, sensitization of the pain pathway also results from changes in the brainstem. In addition to their more commonly recognized role in descending inhibition of pain processing, neurons of the midbrain PAG and RVM can facilitate the processing of pain signals at the level of the spinal cord. Under certain persistent pain conditions, this facilitatory effect is enhanced. In fact, the persistence of the pain may require sustained facilitatory inputs from brainstem neurons to the spinal cord. For example, in a model of nerve injury-induced (neuropathic) pain, the resulting mechanical allodynia can be blocked by injections of lidocaine into the RVM [26]. Sensitization of the supraspinal facilitatory circuits likely occurs via mechanisms similar to those involved in sensitization of spinal cord neurons. Thus, activation of NMDA receptors has been implicated in the sensitization of RVM neurons [26] and, very recently, a BDNF and microglial contribution to the process has been reported [27].

Analgesic targets

Our increased knowledge of the mechanisms that produce pain, in particular the process of sensitization, has identified a number of novel targets for the treatment of pain. In addition, we have come to better understand the mechanisms of action of traditional analgesics such as opioids and nonsteroidal anti-inflammatory drugs (NSAIDs). As with any pharmacotherapy, the goal is to treat pain while limiting the deleterious impact of drug binding at sites unrelated to the process of pain.

For this reason, targets enriched or exclusively expressed in elements of the pain pathway are of great interest; for example, the sensory-neuron specific sodium channels. Although it has proven difficult to design drugs selective for these channels (e.g. Nav 1.7 and 1.8), it is significant that tricyclic antidepressants, which effectively treat neuropathic pain (notably diabetic neuropathy

and post-herpetic neuralgia), are not only monoamine uptake inhibitors, but also excellent use-dependent sodium channel blockers. It is thus possible that their utility involves blockade of action potential generation and transmission in nociceptors. The importance of targeting nociceptors is further demonstrated by the recent approval of high dose topical capsaicin for neuropathic pain [28], an approach that likely produces a transient degeneration of nociceptor terminals. As many of the elements of the inflammatory milieu exert their effects via TRPV1 (e.g. in preclinical models of metastatic bone cancer), the development of TRPV1 antagonists for the treatment of pain is also being pursued extensively [29]. Finally, there is very encouraging evidence that targeting pro-inflammatory mediators such as NGF and TNFα with neutralizing antibodies are effective in the treatment of chronic inflammatory pain conditions such as arthritis [5].

Other classes of analgesic do not specifically target the nociceptor, but act at different levels of the pain transmission pathway. These agents include the opioids (e.g. morphine), but also a variety of calcium channel blockers, notably ziconotide, a cone snail derived toxin that targets N-type calcium channels [30]. Also included in these more general agents are anticonvulsants (e.g. gabapentin and pregabalin), which constitute the first line therapy for neuropathic pain. Although the target of gabapentin and pregabalin is unquestionably the α2δ subunit of calcium channels, the mechanism of action of these compounds remains a mystery [31]. Given the prominent role of NMDA receptors in the development of central sensitization, this channel remains very attractive target. As NMDA receptors are ubiquitously expressed throughout the nervous system, however, the potential for adverse side effects of NMDA receptor antagonists is high.

Finally, new approaches are being developed to prevent the contribution of glial cells to chronic pain. Thus, glial modulators, which directly affect glial cell function, and purinergic drugs, which prevent the glial activation by ATP, are candidate drugs for the treatment of neuropathic pain [25]. Despite the challenges, the future of pharmacologic management of pain is encouraging. As more details of nociception and the process of sensitization are uncovered, there is no question that the opportunities for drug development will continue to grow.

References

1 Dib-Hajj SD, Black JA, Waxman SG. (2009) Voltage-gated sodium channels: therapeutic targets for pain. *Pain Med* **10**:1260–9.

2 Cox JJ, Reimann F, Nicholas AK *et al.* (2006) An SCN9A channelopathy causes congenital inability to experience pain. *Nature* **444**:894–8.

3 Indo Y, Tsuruta M, Hayashida Y *et al.* (1996) Mutations in the TRKA/NGF receptor gene in patients with congenital insensitivity to pain with anhidrosis. *Nat Genet* **13**:485–8.

4 Julius D, Basbaum AI. (2001) Molecular mechanisms of nociception. *Nature* **413**:203–10.

5 Basbaum AI, Bautista DM, Scherrer G *et al.* (2009) Cellular and molecular mechanism of pain. *Cell* **139**:267–84.

6 Meyer RA, Ringkamp MR, Campbell JN *et al.* (2006) Peripheral mechanisms of cutaneous nociception. In: McMahon SB, Koltzenburg M, eds. *Textbook of Pain*, 5th edn. Elsevier, Maryland Heights, MO. pp. 3–34.

7 Scherrer G, Imamachi N, Cao YQ *et al.* (2009) Dissociation of the opioid receptor mechanisms that control mechanical and heat pain. *Cell* **137**:1148–59.

8 Cavanaugh DJ, Lee H, Lo L *et al.* (2009) Distinct subsets of unmyelinated primary sensory fibers mediate behavioral responses to noxious thermal and mechanical stimuli. *Proc Natl Acad Sci U S A* **106**:9075–80.

9 Woolf CJ, Ma Q. (2007) Nociceptors: noxious stimulus detectors. *Neuron* **55**:353–64.

10 Caterina MJ, Leffler A, Malmberg AB *et al.* (2000) Impaired nociception and pain sensation in mice lacking the capsaicin receptor. *Science* **288**:306–13.

11 Bautista DM, Siemens J, Glazer JM *et al.* (2007) The menthol receptor TRPM8 is the principal detector of environmental cold. *Nature* **448**:204–8.

12 Bautista DM, Jordt SE, Nikai T *et al.* (2006) TRPA1 mediates the inflammatory actions of environmental irritants and proalgesic agents. *Cell* **124**:1269–82.

13 Todd AJ, Koerber HR. (2006) Neuroanatomical substrates of spinal nociception. In: McMahon SB, Koltzenburg M, eds. *Textbook of Pain*, 5th edn. Elsevier, Maryland Heights, MO. pp. 73–90.

14 Zylka MJ, Rice FL, Anderson DJ. (2005) Topographically distinct epidermal nociceptive circuits revealed by axonal tracers targeted to Mrgprd. *Neuron* **45**:17–25.

15 Craig AD. (2003) A new view of pain as a homeostatic emotion. *Trends Neurosci* **26**:303–7.

16 Seal RP, Wang X, Guan Y *et al.* (2009) Injury-induced mechanical hypersensitivity requires C-low threshold mechanoreceptors. *Nature* **462**:651–5.

17 Neumann S, Braz JM, Skinner K *et al.* (2008) Innocuous, not noxious, input activates PKCgamma interneurons of the spinal dorsal horn via myelinated afferent fibers. *J Neursci* **28**:7936–44.

18 Malmberg AB, Chen C, Tonegawa S *et al.* (1997) Preserved acute pain and reduced neuropathic pain in mice lacking PKCγ. *Science* **278**:279–83.

19 Almeida TF, Roizenblatt S, Tufik S. (2004) Afferent pain pathways: a neuroanatomical review. *Brain Res* **1000**:40–56.

20 Ji R-R, Kohno T, Moore KA *et al.* (2003) Central sensitization and LTP: do pain and memory share similar mechanisms? *Trends Neurosci* **26**:696–705.

21 Miraucourt LS, Dallel R, Voisin DL. (2007) Glycine inhibitory dysfunction turns touch into pain through PKCgamma interneurons. *PLoS One* **2**:e116.

22 Moore KA, Kohno T, Karchewski LA *et al.* (2002) Partial peripheral nerve injury promotes a selective loss of GABAergic inhibition in the superficial dorsal horn of the spinal cord. *J Neurosci* **22**:6724–31.

23 Harvey RJ, Depner UB, Wassle H *et al.* (2004) GlyR alpha3: an essential target for spinal PGE2-mediated inflammatory pain sensitization. *Science* **304**:884–7.

24 Coull JA, Boundreau D, Bachand K *et al.* (2003) Trans-synaptic shift in anion gradient in spinal lamina I neurons as a mechanism of neuropathic pain. *Nature* **424**:938–42.

25 Milligan ED, Watkins LR. (2009) Pathological and protective roles of glia in chronic pain. *Nat Rev Neurosci* **10**:23–36.

26 Porreca F, Ossipov MH, Gebhart GF. (2002) Chronic pain and medullary descending facilitation. *Trends Neurosci* **25**:319–25.

27 Guo W, Robbins MT, Wei F *et al.* (2006) Supraspinal brain-derived neurotrophic factor signaling: a novel mechanisms for descending pain facilitation. *J Neurosci* **26**:126–37.

28 Noto C, Pappagallo M, Szallasi A. (2009) NGX-4010, a high-concentration capsaicin dermal patch for lasting relief of peripheral neuropathic pain. *Curr Opin Investig Drugs* **10**:702–10.

29 Honore P, Chandran P, Hernandez G *et al.* (2009) Repeated dosing of ABT-102, a potent and selective TRPV1 antagonist, enhances TRPV1-mediated analgesic activity in rodents, but attenuates antagonist-induced hyperthermia. *Pain* **142**:27–35.

30 Basbaum AI. (2005) The future of pain therapy: something old, something new, something borrowed, and something blue. In: Merskey H, Loeser JD, Dubner R, eds. *The Paths of Pain.* IASP Press, Seattle. pp. 513–32.

31 Eroglu C, Allen NJ, Susman MW *et al.* (2009) Gabapentin receptor alpha2delta1 is a neuronal thrombospondin receptor responsible for excitatory CNS synaptogenesis. *Cell* **139**:380–92.

Chapter 4

Psychosocial perspectives on chronic pain

Kenneth D. Craig[1] & Judith Versloot[2]

[1] Department of Psychology, University of British Columbia, Vancouver, Canada
[2] Faculty of Dentistry, Toronto, Canada

Introduction

Understanding the central role of psychosocial determinants of pain and their impact on the challenges individual patients confront is crucial to optimal delivery of care. Those interested in caring for persons in pain must address the subjective experience of the suffering person. It is featured in the widely endorsed definition of pain: "An unpleasant sensory and emotional experience associated with actual or potential tissue damage, or described in terms of such damage" [1]. The definition carefully explains that tissue damage is associated with or described by the person as a feature of the experience, but it establishes that it is not necessarily the exclusive or sufficient cause, thereby pointing to important roles for psychosocial determinants.

Increasingly well-defined psychological factors should be considered when attempting to understand an individual's unique pattern of pain experience and expression. Perceptual processes, emotions and mood, thought patterns, stable personality characteristics and features of behavior

Clinical Pain Management: A Practical Guide, 1st edition.
Edited by Mary E. Lynch, Kenneth D. Craig and
Philip W.H. Peng.
© 2011 Blackwell Publishing Ltd.

have been implicated. Further, exploring how the individual's current life situation and history of personal and social experiences influence pain and pain-related disability may be crucial in delivery of care. Immediate work, family and other demands on the individual are likely to have central roles and should be considered in the broader contexts of socioeconomic status and ethnocultural and/or familial background. Appraisal of psychosocial determinants of pain typically leads to important targets and specific interventions for working with patients. This chapter describes fundamental psychosocial processes and their clinical relevance, with the chapters on psychological assessment (Chapter 10) and psychological interventions (Chapter 24) applying the perspective, among other chapters in this volume.

Modeling the network of biological, psychological and social determinants of pain

Biopsychosocial perspective

This chapter endorses the biopsychosocial model of health and illness that posits biological, psychological and social factors must be considered in understanding human health or illness, whether one is interested in being well-informed or caring for an individual [2]. Substantial evidence supports

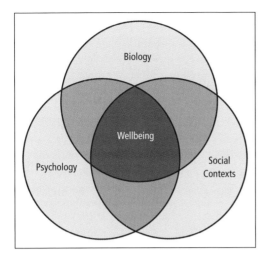

Figure 4.1 The biopsychosocial approach to human disease and injury. Optimal wellbeing arises through consideration of the whole person – biological, psychological and social factors are important when addressing an individual's pain and related disability.

the position [3,4], although attention to biological phenomena overwhelms the field; psychologically based approaches are often ignored by those with strong biomedical orientations, and social determinants of pain have received relatively minimal attention. Figure 4.1 illustrates dimensions of the model, signifying the importance of each component to the wellbeing of the person. It has been embraced by those arguing the necessity of multidisciplinary care for people suffering from chronic pain and calls for the integration of contributions from various healthcare practitioners, including medicine, nursing, physical therapy, psychology, social work and rehabilitation. Healthcare professionals who do not have competencies in all domains must engage in consultation to insure comprehensive care.

Social communication model of pain

This perspective provides a more detailed framework for describing the complex interactions among biological, psychological and social factors of pain (Figure 4.2) [5]. The model examines the typical temporal sequence: (a) the person experiences exposure to painful events; (b) pain is perceived; (c) the distress becomes manifest in pain expression; (d) pain may be inferred by an observer; and (e) observer decisions are made concerning delivery of care. Benevolent care is not the only possibility – indifference and malevolent exploitation are not unusual in human relationships, but less common in clinical settings. The model directs attention to both intrapersonal (biological and psychological) and interpersonal (social) determinants of the experience and its overt expression, as well as to the caregiver's perception and the process whereby decisions are made concerning delivery of care. Both intrapersonal and interpersonal determinants of each stage are important to an understanding of this dynamic temporal sequence.

Intrapersonal determinants concern the personal dispositions to experience or express pain, in the case of the patient. Similar dispositions govern assessment and the reactions of caregivers. For the person in pain, the dispositions are embodied in the biological substrates that support pain. These are plastic and dynamic. While inherited dispositions are important [6], the biological substrates of pain are changed by personal life experiences, including the individual's medical and social history. Any individual's personal history includes myriad formative personal, familial and ethnocultural influences. A parallel analysis is needed for caregiver dispositions during assessment and treatment. Their reactions are similarly constrained by biological systems and reflect informal and formal education and life experience.

Interpersonal determinants concern the impact of the immediate social context on the person at the time pain is experienced, expressed and thereafter. Patients often confront difficult work, family and other interpersonal challenges which influence pain, personal coping, pain-related disability and demands for healthcare. These are related to the substantial variability in how people experience pain and express their distress as well as in how observing people interpret and respond to those reactions. The social context and the manner in which those present treat the person in pain

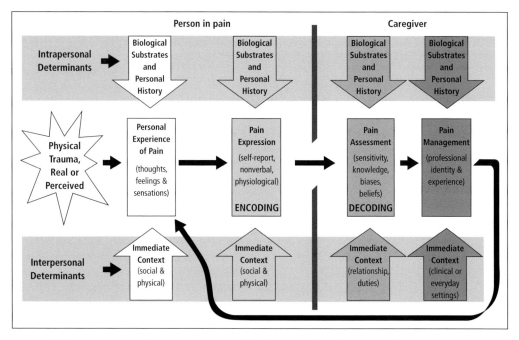

Figure 4.2 The social communication model of pain. This framework identifies biological, psychological features of pain through the sequence of events during typical injury and exacerbation of chronic pain, including reactions of caregivers, and identifies both intrapersonal and interpersonal determinants of the stages of the sequence.

have a potent impact on the individual's current and future status. Access to a clinician disposed and able to deliver effective interventions is a key feature of the patient's interpersonal context.

Clinicians serve as pivotal social agents who control services provided to individuals, with public health and institutional policies determining whether and which caregivers will be available. Their training and competence in delivering effective interventions are crucial determinants of whether the person in pain will receive relief from acute or chronic pain. Observations that pain is often ignored, poorly assessed, underestimated, not treated, inadequately treated or poorly treated draw attention to the necessity to include psychosocial factors in the care of people suffering from pain.

Psychological and social features of pain cannot be construed as less important than their biological counterparts. Early assessment and intervention of these dimensions can address primary problems, thereby enhancing the effectiveness of biological, psychological and socially based therapies and preventing long-term difficulties. A recent study emphasizes their importance, identifying psychosocial difficulties among a large number of patients referred to a tertiary care, hospital-based pain clinic [7]. Both psychosocial and biomedical issues were important in 51% of the patients. For an additional 20.9% of the patients, no medical factors could be established and painful experience and disability were attributed to psychological factors. Importantly, the pain of only 25.5% of the patients could be attributed directly to general medical conditions. Despite the tendency for patients seen in specialty clinics to have high levels of functional impairment and psychosocial difficulties, it is striking that only about 75% of the patients had detectable biomedical pathology and close to 72% had diagnosable psychological issues. The study emphasizes the importance of treating the whole person rather than focusing exclusively on physical pathology.

Psychosocial factors in best practice

The model depicted in Figure 4.2 encourages consideration of best clinical practice with respect to its numerous dimensions.

The person in pain

Pain experience

Clinical care must begin with careful attention to the subjective experience of the patient. Pain is typically assessed as a unidimensional construct, using self-report of numerical and verbal descriptor scales; however, the report is better conceptualized as an integration of multiple dimensions, inclusive of sensation, emotional distress and the thoughts of the person in pain [8]. Use of scales that differentiate sensory/discriminative, affective/motivational and cognitive parameters offers focused targets for different forms of intervention.

Intrapersonal determinants

Firmly entrenched beliefs concerning the importance of the pathophysiological factors in pain among healthcare practitioners, patients and the public ensure efforts to provide specific and accurate biomedical diagnoses. There also is general agreement that clear feedback to patients should be provided, whether a firm medical diagnosis is available or not. A careful and complete diagnosis reduces the likelihood that dissatisfied patients will seek further opinions and/or additional testing, which is often expensive, unnecessary and sometimes harmful [9,10]. Perseverating on medical diagnosis can trap patients in self-perpetuating roles as invalids as they seek medical care exclusively. Knowing a pathophysiological source of discomfort, with the potential for medical treatment to eliminate it can be very comforting, whereas discomfort from unknown sources with unknown futures can be very disturbing. To the disappointment of many patients and their physicians, tissue damage arising from injury and disease very often does not account for patient complaints [11]. Efforts to identify peripheral and central neuro-

physiological mechanisms responsible for dysfunctional central regulation and long-term persistence of chronic pain offer promising alternative explanations [12].

These can be construed as the biological substrates of specific psychological processes that increase the severity of painful experience and risk for persistence of pain-related disability. Assessment of personal, medical, family and social history often discloses the formative role of life history events. Several chapters in this book discuss excessive stress reactivity and emotional reactions (e.g. debilitating fear of pain or depression), destructive thinking (e.g. catastrophizing, passive coping), behavioral maladjustment (excessive avoidant behavior and inactivity) and deteriorating social relationships as risk factors for excessive pain and disability, including failure to respond to treatment.

Factors have been identified that protect against the debilitating impact of painful injury or disease and the development of disability. Key protective factors include:

1 A strong sense of self-efficacy, or confidence in one's ability to follow a course of action that will accomplish desired outcomes (e.g. control of pain) [4].
2 Effective use of cognitive, affective and behavioral coping skills, such as muscle relaxation, distraction, commitment to activity and an ability to redefine situations in less catastrophic ways [13].
3 A readiness or willingness to engage in active roles that are contradictory to lapsing into maladaptive patterns of thinking, feeling and behaving [4].
4 A capacity for accepting certain limitations or handicaps, thereby avoiding one's life being consumed by unsuccessful efforts to eliminate pain [14].
These processes not only describe resilience to pain and pain-related disability, but they represent reasonable objectives for therapeutic intervention.

Interpersonal determinants

Recognizing the impact of the immediate setting on pain experience is important in understanding variability in patient behavior. Demands for intense engagement in activities can diminish the experience of pain, as in the case of injured athletes or others in life-threatening situations. However, the social environment is often a major source of stress reactivity, with vocational, familial and other sources of social stress able to exacerbate pain. Dubin & King-Van Vack [15] observed dramatic increases in medical visits, use of analgesics and hospital admissions to coincide with major life events, including conflicts with employers, insurers and lawyers, and financial distress. Being compelled to abandon usual roles, such as a worker, family member or friend, also leads to deteriorating social relationships. Stress and strain in interactions with others, lapsing into the role of the sick person or invalid, and social isolation are common problems for people with chronic pain.

Pain expression

Pain and other features of subjective experience must be inferred through overt manifestations. Various actions, including self-report, qualities of speech and other vocalizations, facial expression, body activity and escape or avoidance behavior, and evidence of physiological activity may signal pain and associated psychological states to others.

Intrapersonal determinants

Painful expression is governed by both automatic (reflexive, unintentional) and controlled (intentional, purposive) neuroregulatory processes [16,17]. Automatic expressions of pain (e.g. reflexive escape, facial grimaces, guarded posture) represent the immediate biological reaction to sudden tissue insult or exacerbation of chronic pain. In contrast, controlled expression reflects the complex features of painful experience as processed through higher levels of executive control, including memory, problem solving and planning as modulating influences. Non-verbal expression and self-report typically are recognized as different categories of pain response with different sources. Self-report can be a valid estimate of pain in the competent well-motivated person, but the clinician must recognize that self-report can be biased by the individual's perception of their best interests and

requires a high level of linguistic and social competency. Non-verbal expression typically adds context and meaning to self-report and usually is perceived as less amenable to conscious control than verbal report. It is noteworthy to add that non-verbal expression is not invariably reflexive but is subject to misrepresentation and can confound spontaneous with socially predicated expression [18].

Interpersonal determinants

Self-report and non-verbal expressions typically are only modestly correlated, with contextual factors determining the magnitude of the relationship. Pain expression is modulated contingent upon the audience. If the audience is comprised of those who are close and sympathetic, more expressive behavior can be expected; if the audience is comprised of strangers or enemies, expression of painful distress is likely to be diminished or very carefully controlled. This influence is not always straightforward. A study in patients with rheumatoid arthritis found that when the support of a spouse is perceived as satisfying, a reduction in pain expression and an increase in the use of adaptive coping strategies results. When patients became disappointed in their support, efforts to engage in adaptive ways of coping became derailed [19]. Thus, the expression of pain is best recognized as an integrated product of somatosensory events, life history and sensitivity to the immediate context.

Particularly problematic is the potential for exaggerated or suppressed pain expression under purposive control in the interests of intentionally manipulating audiences. Both self-report and non-verbal expression can be deliberately controlled, as evident in both children [20] and adults [18], and clinicians may be challenged to identify circumstances in which pain is deliberately misrepresented [21].

Caregivers

Pain assessment

Clinicians confront a considerable challenge in understanding expressions of painful distress.

While manifestations can be highly objective (what the person says, what they write on paper, reproducible video recordings of non-verbal activity), their relationship to subjective experience may not be so clear. Added to the behavioral mix of information would be information concerning events leading to injury or disease, evidence of tissue damage and biomedical status, and general understanding of the individual's history and life status. From all this, clinicians infer subjective states and are disposed to attributing causes to the actions.

Intrapersonal determinants

Clinicians are variable in their sensitivity, knowledge and biases. Some features of the response to pain in other people appear biologically prepared or hard-wired, whereas others demand cognitive interpretation. Witnessing another's immediate reaction to painful events is capable of instigating a "visceral" or "gut level" emotional experience. In parallel, the observer will be challenged to attach meaning and understand the event. In this manner, the "bottom-up" external sources of information come to be subjected to "top-down" influences, as the observer appraises the situation and applies knowledge, beliefs, expectancies, attitudes and biases to achieve understanding [22]. It is not surprising that estimates of pain in others frequently underestimate self-report [23–25]. The challenge for the observer is heightened when only self-report or other controlled expressions of pain are available. Given the potential for suppressing or enhancing pain expression, concerns regarding credibility often develop [26]. Systematic use of assessment strategies, including structured interviews and objective psychometric scales (Chapter 10), tend to minimize personal bias.

Interpersonal determinants

Professional identity, training experiences, clinical setting, peer influences and many other social and contextual factors can be expected to have an impact on judgments of pain in others. The evidence indicates clinicians and others tend to be "good enough" rather than "perfectly accurate" in estimating the pain of others [27]. Perfect empathy for another's pain is improbable, given the pain will have distinct sensory components related to injury or disease, although the emotional impact of witnessing others in pain can lead to "vicarious traumatization." Work on burn units, emergency and intensive care units can be difficult and clinicians come to use cognitive social strategies to minimize personal distress, thereby increasing the likelihood of delivering objective professional care to people experiencing high levels of distress. Similarly, clinicians tend to be cognizant that patients realize they must provide a convincing case for delivery of care services to them. The challenge is particularly demanding for patients with chronic pain. Werner & Malerud [28] provided accounts of women with medically unexplained pain encountering skepticism, lack of comprehension, rejection, being blamed for their condition and experiencing feelings of being ignored or belittled. Clearly, these are situations to be avoided.

Pain management

Intrapersonal determinants

Decisions concerning whether or not to deliver care follow from an assessment of patient needs and inevitably reflect practitioner training and individual differences in personal background and experience in clinical settings. Given the diversity of causes potentially implicated in any given person's painful condition and disability, the full range of biomedical, psychological and social interventions must be considered. This book provides a compendium of treatment options available to practitioners with different backgrounds and competencies for understanding specific clinical states and special populations.

Interpersonal determinants

Given the importance of public and institutional policy to the delivery of care, availability and accessibility of care for any given individual will reflect the nature of the healthcare system in particular jurisdictions, and policies and practices concerning assessment and delivery of pain management in a given setting. The importance of facilitative policies cannot be underestimated and it is conceivable that more can be done to enhance quality of care for people suffering from pain through efforts to change policies than efforts to improve service delivery on the part of any given practitioner [29–31].

Conclusions

The biopsychosocial perspective and the Social Communication Model of Pain provide a useful framework for consideration of best practice in delivery of care to patients.

References

1 International Association for the Study of Pain. (1979) Pain terms: a list with definitions and notes on usage. *Pain* **6**:147.

2 Engel GL. (1977) The need for a new medical model: a challenge for biomedicine. *Science* **196(4286)**:129–36.

3 Gatchel RJ, Peng YB, Peters ML *et al*. (2007) The biopsychosocial approach to chronic pain: scientific advances and future directions. *Psychol Bull* **133(4)**:581–624.

4 Turk DC, Okifuji A. (2002) Psychological factors in chronic pain: evolution and revolution. *J Consult Clin Psychol* **70(3)**:678–90.

5 Craig KD. (2009) The social communication model of pain. *Can Psychol* **50(1)**:22–32.

6 Mogil JS. (2009) Are we getting anywhere in human pain genetics? *Pain* **146(3)**:231–2.

7 Mailis-Gagnon A, Yegneswaran B, Lakha SF *et al*. (2007) Pain characteristics and demographics of patients attending a university-affiliated pain clinic in Toronto, Ontario. *Pain Res Manag* **12(2)**:93–9.

8 Melzack R, Katz J. (2005) Pain assessment in adult patients. In: McMahon SB, Koltzenburg M, eds. *Melzack and Wall's Textbook of Pain*, 5th edn. Churchill-Livingstone. pp. 291–304.

9 Carragee EJ, Don AS, Hurwitz EL *et al*. (2009) Does discography cause accelerated progression of degeneration changes in the lumbar disc: a ten-year matched cohort study. *Spine* **34(21)**:2338–45.

10 Hadler NM. (2003) MRI for regional back pain: need for less imaging, better understanding. *JAMA* **289(21)**:2863–5.

11 Mayer EA, Bushnell MC, eds. (2009) *Functional Pain Syndromes: Presentation and Pathophysiology*. IASP Press, Seattle, WA.

12 Tracey I, Bushnell MC. (2009) How neuroimaging studies have challenged us to rethink: is chronic pain a disease? *J Pain* **10(11)**:1113–20.

13 Morley S, Eccleston C, Williams A. (1999) Systematic review and meta-analysis of randomized controlled trials of cognitive behaviour therapy and behaviour therapy for chronic pain in adults, excluding headache. *Pain* **80(1–2)**:1–13.

14 McCracken LM, Eccleston C. (2005) A prospective study of acceptance of pain and patient functioning with chronic pain. *Pain* **118(1–2)**:164–9.

15 Dubin R, King-Van Vlack C. (in press) The trajectory of chronic pain: can a community-based exercise/education program soften the ride? *Pain Res Manag*

16 Craig KD, Versloot J, Goubert L *et al*. (2010) Perceiving others in pain: automatic and controlled mechanisms. *J Pain* **11(2)**:101–8.

17 Hadjistavropoulos T, Craig KD. (2002) A theoretical framework for understanding self-report and observational measures of pain: a communications model. *Behav Res Ther* **40(5)**:551–70.

18 Hill ML, Craig KD. (2002) Detecting deception in pain expressions: the structure of genuine and deceptive facial displays. *Pain* **98(1)**:135–44.

19 Holtzman S, Newth S, Delongis A. (2004) The role of social support in coping with daily pain among patients with rheumatoid arthritis. *J Health Psychol* **9(5)**:677–95.

20 Larochette AC, Chambers CT, Craig KD. (2006) Genuine, suppressed and faked facial expressions of pain in children. *Pain* **126(1–3)**:64–71.

21 Craig KD, Badali MA. (2004) Introduction to the special series on pain deception and malingering. *Clin J Pain* **20(6)**:377–82.

22 Goubert L, Craig KD, Vervoort T *et al.* (2005) Facing others in pain: the effects of empathy. *Pain* **118(3)**:286–8.

23 Chambers CT, Reid GJ, Craig KD *et al.* (1998) Agreement between child and parent reports of pain. *Clin J Pain* **14(4)**:336–42.

24 Prkachin KM, Solomon PA, Ross AJ. (2007) The underestimation of pain among health-care providers. *Can J Nurs Res* **39(2)**:88–106.

25 Kappesser J, Williams AC, Prkachin KM. (2006) Testing two accounts of pain underestimation. *Pain* **124(1–2)**:109–16.

26 Craig KD, Stanford EA, Fairbairn NS *et al.* (2006). Emergent pain language communication competence in infants and children. *Enfance* **58(1)**:52–71.

27 Goubert L, Craig KD, Buysse A. (2009) Perceiving others in pain: experimental and clinical evidence on the role of empathy. In: Decety J, Ickes WJ, eds. *The Social Neuroscience of Empathy*. MIT Press, Cambridge, MA. pp. 153–66.

28 Werner A, Malterud K. (2003) It is hard work behaving as a credible patient: encounters between women with chronic pain and their doctors. *Soc Sci Med* **57(8)**:1409–19.

29 Blyth FM, Macfarlane GJ, Nicholas MK. (2007) The contribution of psychosocial factors to the development of chronic pain: the key to better outcomes for patients. *Pain* **129(1–2)**:8–11.

30 McGrath PJ, Finley GA, eds. (2003) *Pediatric Pain: Biological and Social Context*. IASP Press, Seattle, WA.

31 Rashiq S, Schopflocher D, Taenzer P *et al.* eds. (2008) *Chronic Pain: A Health Policy Perspective*. Wiley-VCH, Weinheim.

Chapter 5

Identification of risk and protective factors in the transition from acute to chronic post surgical pain

Joel Katz[1,2,3] & M. Gabrielle Pagé[1]

[1] Department of Psychology, York University, Toronto, Canada
[2] Department of Anesthesia and Pain Management, Toronto General Hospital, Toronto, Canada
[3] Department of Anesthesia, University of Toronto, Toronto, Canada

Introduction

All chronic pains were, at one time, acute. Yet not all acute pain becomes chronic. Some pains develop spontaneously. Others arise as the result of surgery, accident or illness. Regardless of the cause, most people recover and do not go on to develop long-term pain. Nevertheless, there is obvious interest in determining the factors responsible for the transition of acute pain to chronic intractable pathological pain. Identification of such causal risk factors is the first step in developing effective treatments to prevent and manage pain. In this chapter we focus on the transition of acute to chronic pain after surgery. For several reasons, the study of pain after surgery can serve as a model for the transition to chronicity for other types of pain:

1 Chronic postsurgical pain (CPSP) develops in an alarming proportion of patients.

2 Research into the transition from acute to chronic pain has already revealed specific risk factors associated with patients who develop CPSP.

3 Elective surgery is unique in that the timing and nature of the physical injury are known in advance. This facilitates identification of risk and protective factors that predict the course of recovery.

4 There is a growing body of literature examining preventive efforts to minimize the development of CPSP.

The aim of this chapter is to provide an overview of CPSP. We review literature on the epidemiology of CPSP, define the concept of a risk factor and the requirements for determining causality, describe the surgical, psychosocial, social-environmental and patient-related factors that confer a greater risk of developing CPSP, and review the rationale and evidence for a preventive analgesic approach to surgery designed to reduce the incidence and intensity of CPSP.

Definition and epidemiology of CPSP

Macrae & Davies [1] propose the following four-point definition of CPSP:

1 Pain develops after surgery;

2 Pain has been present for at least 2 months;

3 Other causes for the pain have been ruled out;

4 The possibility that the pain is a continuation of a pre-existing problem should be ruled out.

Clinical Pain Management: A Practical Guide, 1st edition.
Edited by Mary E. Lynch, Kenneth D. Craig and Philip W.H. Peng.
© 2011 Blackwell Publishing Ltd.

Table 5.1 Incidence/prevalence of chronic postsurgical pain (CPSP) following various surgical procedures.

Surgical procedure	Follow-up time after surgery and incidence of CPSP

Modified radical mastectomy (MRM) or breast conserving surgery (BCT) with axillary clearance	*1 year after surgery*
	Breast region
	  MRM, 17%
	  BCT, 33%
	Ipsilateral arm
	  MRM, 13%
	  BCT, 23%

Hernia repair	*1 year after surgery*
	Inguinal pain, 56.6%
	Ejaculation pain, 18.3%
	Pain in:
	  testes, 39.7%
	  shaft, 5.4%
	  glans, 4.5%
	  thigh, 11.6%
	5 years
	Groin pain, 19–29%
	Severe or very severe groin pain, 1.8%
	Testicular pain, 16.1%
	6.5 years
	Chronic inguinal pain, 8.1%

Thoracotomy	*1–1.5 years after surgery* Post-thoracotomy pain, 39–52% Pain described as dull, aching or burning pain of moderate intensity, 52% Severe pain, 0–5%
C-section	*1 year after surgery* Abdominal scar pain, 12.3%
Amputation	*6 months to 2 years after surgery* Phantom limb pain, 59–78.8% Stump pain, 21–57%
Open cholecystectomy	*1 year after surgery* Pain, 26%
Sternotomy for cardiac surgery	*1 year after surgery* Post-sternotomy pain, 11–28% With pain intensity ≥30/100, 13%
Hip replacement	*12–18 months (prevalence)* Chronic hip pain, 28.1% Pain limited activities to a moderate, severe or very severe degree, 12.1%

Although most patients who undergo major surgery do not go on to develop CPSP, the incidence of CPSP following certain surgical procedures is unacceptably high (Table 5.1) [2]. The 1-year incidence of CPSP is variable and surgery-specific, ranging from a low of approximately 10–15% following modified radical mastectomy to a high of 61–70% for thoracotomy and amputation. More generally, the 1-year CPSP incidence has been estimated to be between 1.5% and 10%. We know next to nothing about CPSP beyond the 1 year mark. Pain persists in 8.1–19% of patients up to 6 years after hernia repair, with severe or very severe pain occurring in 1.8%. Two years after amputation, approximately 60% and 21–57% of amputees report phantom limb pain and stump pain, respectively. These statistics are alarming in light of the total number of patients worldwide who undergo surgery each year. That almost 25% of patients referred to chronic pain treatment centers have CPSP is a reflection of the intractability of the problem.

Understanding risk and attributing causality to outcomes

An important goal of epidemiological and clinical research is to identify the necessary and sufficient conditions under which specific health-related outcomes arise. Typically, this is achieved over the course of many years involving progressively more sophisticated research designs from observation and description through to experimental manipulation. Initially, an understanding is developed through careful observation of the conditions under which the phenomenon occurs. The next stage typically involves prediction: specifying in advance the situations under which the phenomenon occurs and the factors that reliably predict its occurrence. The final stage involves prevention and control, which requires detailed knowledge of the mechanisms that give rise to the phenomenon and specialized tools to facilitate or inhibit its occurrence. In the field of CPSP, the process of moving from understanding through prediction to control is linked to the concept of risk and to identifying the (risk and protective) factors that place an individual at greater or lesser probability of developing CPSP.

A risk factor is defined as a "measurable characterization of each subject in a specified population that precedes the outcome of interest and can be used to divide the population into … high-risk and … low-risk groups" [3]. Merely identifying a risk factor, however, does not provide information about risk estimation, and this is particularly relevant for studies with large sample sizes. Risk estimation should be based on the relative potency of a risk factor. Tools to evaluate the potency of a risk

factor include odds ratio, risk ratio and Cramer's V [4].

A relevant and often overlooked issue pertinent to the concept of risk is that of correlation versus causality, necessitating a distinction between the terms causal risk factor and correlated risk factor [3]. To meet the requirements for a risk factor, the observed variable must precede the outcome of interest. If the factor is measured at the same time as, or after, the outcome, then it may be a symptom or consequence of the outcome. As such, when the temporal criterion of precedence is not met, then the observed variable is simply a correlate of the measured outcome. Moreover, the temporal criterion of precedence is necessary, but not sufficient, to infer causality. Thus, even if a risk factor is shown to precede the development of the outcome, it does not imply causality and still may be a correlate. A risk and/or protective factor is determined to be causal only if its manipulation increases and/or decreases the risk associated with the measured outcome [3]. Determining the status of a given risk factor as causal or non-causal is essential to progress in understanding the development of CPSP and in prevention and treatment efforts; attempts to manipulate a non-causal risk factor (i.e. a correlate) will have no effect on the outcome (Figure 5.1). Demonstrating the causal role of specific risk factors for CPSP is time-consuming, expensive and requires an evidence base of many randomized controlled trials.

Factors associated with CPSP

Surgical factors

The following surgical factors are associated with a greater risk of developing CPSP: increased duration of surgery, low (vs. high) volume surgical unit, open (vs. laparoscopic) approach, pericostal (vs. intracostal) stitches for thoracotomy, conventional hernia repair and intraoperative nerve damage [2]. Whether the above factors are causally related to the development of CPSP is not yet known. However, these factors appear to be associated with greater surgical trauma and, in particular, they point to intraoperative nerve injury as a likely

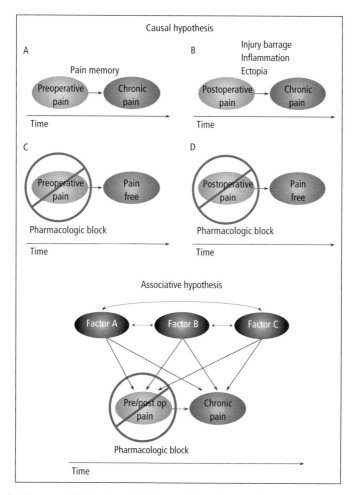

Figure 5.1 Figure depicting causal (top) and associative (bottom) hypotheses predicting the prevention and non-prevention of CPSP by pharmacologic blockade at various times throughout the perioperative period. Top. Transition to chronicity (A, B) may be prevented by pharmacologic blockade of preoperative pain (C) and/or acute postoperative pain (D) assuming the former causes the latter. Bottom. Transition to chronicity will not be prevented if pains are merely correlated and caused by one or more inter-related factors.

causal mechanism and the main factor in producing both acute and chronic neuropathic pain. Thus, one useful preventive measure that can be taken is to avoid intraoperative nerve damage. This is not possible for certain surgeries, such as limb amputation, that involve ligation and section of major nerve trunks. However, the practice of intentionally transecting nerves for surgical convenience can be avoided and doing so will reduce the incidence of CPSP.

Psychosocial factors

Research has only recently begun to examine psychosocial risk factors associated with the development of CPSP. Several risk factors CPSP or CPSP disability have been identified, including heightened preoperative state anxiety; greater preoperative catastrophizing; higher concurrent emotional numbing (a symptom of post-traumatic stress) at 6 and 12 months after thoracotomy; fear of surgery; an introverted personality; and "psychic vulnerability"; a construct similar to neuroticism. It remains to be established whether these factors are causally linked to the development of CPSP [2].

Social support and social environmental factors

A relationship between solicitous responding from significant others and the patient's chronic pain intensity and pain behaviors is explained by operant conditioning principles. The operant model proposes that in offering pain contingent help (e.g. taking over household jobs) in response to pain behaviors (e.g. guarding, limping) and verbal expressions of pain, well-intentioned spouses unwittingly negatively reinforce the patient's pain behaviors leading to an increase in their frequency of occurrence. The relevance to CPSP of social support in general, and solicitous responding in particular, has been reported in a 2-year prospective study of amputees with phantom limb pain. Greater social support and less spousal solicitousness 1 month after lower limb amputation has been reported to be associated with improvement in pain interference scores 2 years later [5].

Patient-related factors

Concurrent or past pain is the most consistent patient-related risk factor for the development CPSP [2]. The presence, intensity or duration of preoperative pain is a risk factor for the development of CPSP as is severity of acute postoperative pain in the days and weeks after surgery. No other individual difference factor is as consistently related to the development of future pain problems as is pain itself. Younger age and female gender are markers of CPSP but neither predicts CPSP as consistently or strongly as does pain itself. What is essential to determine, however, is the precise feature(s) of pain that is predictive. There are many possibilities for why pain predicts pain, including those that propose a causal or correlative role; however, the evidence to date has not advanced to the point where we can identify pain

as a causal risk factor. We propose the following non-mutually exclusive possibilities [2]:

1 Intraoperative nerve damage and the injury barrage that it produces.

2 Sensitization of nociceptors in the surgical field.

3 Early postoperative ectopic activity of injured afferent fibers and of somata of intact neurons in dorsal root ganglia neighboring those associated with damaged nerves.

4 Collateral sprouting from intact nociceptive A-delta afferents that are proximal to the field innervated by injured afferents.

5 Central sensitization induced by the surgery and maintained by peripheral input.

6 Structural changes in the CNS induced by perioperative nociceptive activity (e.g., loss of antinociceptive inhibitory interneurons in the spinal dorsal horn, centralization of pain and somatosensory pain "memories").

7 As yet unidentified pain genes that confer increased risk of developing intense acute pain and CPSP.

8 Consistent response bias over time. Some people report more intense pain than others and they would therefore do so immediately after surgery as well as in the long term.

9 Psychosocial factors, including greater emotional numbing, pain catastrophizing and less social support.

10 Social environmental factors, such as greater solicitous responding from significant others.

11 Publication bias in which studies that do not show a significant relationship between pain before and after surgery are not published.

Preventive analgesia

The current practice of treating pain only after it has become established is being replaced by a preventive approach that aims to block the transmission of the primary afferent injury discharge, the inflammatory response and ensuing ectopic activity. The idea is that acute postoperative pain is amplified by a state of central neural hyperexcitability induced by incision. This concept has been expanded to include the sensitizing effects of preoperative noxious inputs and pain, other noxious intraoperative stimuli as well as perioperative peripheral and central inflammatory mediators and ectopic neural activity.

However, as shown in Figure 5.1, it is critical to determine the precise mechanisms that underlie the relationship between pain at time one (e.g. preoperative pain or acute postoperative pain) and pain at time two (e.g. CPSP 1 year after surgery). The idea that pain is in some way etched into the CNS has been at the heart of efforts to halt the transition to chronicity by blocking noxious perioperative impulses from reaching the CNS using a preventive pharmacological approach. The assumption has been that pain or some aspect of it (e.g. the peripheral nociceptive barrage associated with surgery, central sensitization) is a causal risk factor for CPSP. However, if the relationship between acute postoperative pain and CPSP is merely correlative, and both are caused by one or more factors that themselves are inter-related, then no type or amount of blocking will prevent the development of CPSP (Figure 1, bottom panel).

The focus of preventive analgesia is on attenuating the impact of the peripheral nociceptive barrage associated with noxious preoperative, intraoperative and/or postoperative events and/or stimuli. The rationale is to capitalize on the combined effects of several analgesic agents, administered across the preoperative, intraoperative and postoperative periods, in reducing peripheral and central sensitization [6]. Recent reviews of the preventive analgesia literature indicate that, across a variety of classes of agents, preventive analgesia reduces acute postoperative pain, analgesic consumption, or both [6,7]. Although the in-hospital evidence favors a preventive approach, relatively few studies have been designed to examine the possibility that CPSP can be prevented or attenuated.

Table 5.2 describes the randomized controlled trials that have been conducted to evaluate the long-term efficacy of preventive analgesia to reduce the incidence and intensity of CPSP. The studies vary in several fundamental ways including sample size, patient population, nature and extent of surgery, analgesic agent, route and timing of administration relative to incision. Space limitations preclude a detailed discussion of the results; however, taken together, the results are equivocal. There is some evidence that CPSP can be minimized by an analgesic approach involving aggressive perioperative multimodal treatment, but other studies fail to show this benefit. A careful examination of these results raises several related issues that must be addressed:

1 Significant reductions in the incidence and/ or intensity of CPSP occur in some instances. However, a preventive analgesic approach does not work for everyone and, at present, we do not know for whom such an approach is effective. One possibility is that preoperative pain interferes with the effectiveness of preventive analgesia, perhaps because central sensitization has already been established.

2 We do not know the mechanism(s) by which CPSP is reduced when preventive analgesia is effective. The acute pain relieving effects can be attributed to the pharmacological action of the agents used preventively, but, by definition for studies that compare an active agent with a placebo control condition, preventive analgesia requires that the reduction in analgesic consumption and pain be observed at a point in time that exceeds the clinical duration of action of the target agent used preventively. The most common explanation for the prolonged effect is that the agent(s) prevented (obtunded) peripheral and/or central sensitization and thereby reduced long-term pain. However, there really is very little evidence that this is in fact the case.

3 Pain is a complex perceptual experience that encompasses several domains (e.g. sensory-discriminative, affective-aversive and cognitive-evaluative). However, the main outcome measures in most clinical trials are pain intensity, presence or absence of pain and analgesic use. Assessment of additional domains of functioning [8] may help to shed light on the predictors of severe acute postoperative pain, the processes involved in recovery from surgery and the risk factors for developing CPSP.

Table 5.2 Summary of randomized controlled trials of preventive analgesia designed to reduce the risk of developing CPSP.

Type of surgery	Agent(s) used preventively and duration of treatment	Follow-up time after surgery and outcome
Major digestive surgery [9]	Patients received three agents (local anesthesic, opioid, α_2-adrenergic agonist) by the intravenous route (Group 1) vs. epidural route (Group 3) before surgery and immediately after recovery for 72 hours, vs. the intravenous route followed the epidural route (Group 2) vs. the epidural route followed by the intravenous route (Group 4)	*6 and 12 month follow-ups* Incidence of CPSP in Group 1 at the 6 (48%) and 12 (28%) month follow-ups was significantly greater than the zero incidence in Groups 3 and 4 at both time points
Thyroidectomy [10]	A single preoperative dose of (1) gabapentin vs. (2) placebo	*6 month follow-up* Incidence of CPSP was significantly lower gabapentin (4.3%) vs. placebo (29.2%) treated patients
Major abdominal-gynecological surgery [11]	(1) Saline vs. (2) low dose alfentanil vs. (3) high dose alfentanil before and during surgery	*6 month follow-up* Significant differences were not found among the three groups in pain incidence (50% vs. 17% vs. 58%) or severity at rest, when sitting up or or coughing
Major abdominal-gynecological surgery [12]	(1) Preincisional epidural lidocaine and fentanyl followed by postincisional saline vs. (2) preincisional saline followed by postincisional epidural lidocaine and fentanyl vs. (3) standard treatment with a sham epidural	*3 week and 6 month follow-ups* Pain disability ratings at 3 weeks but not 6 months were significantly lower in the groups that received the active epidural compared with the standard treatment group
Iliac crest bone graft harvest surgery [13]	Multiple injections of bupivacaine and morphine vs. saline into the harvest site beginning 10 minutes after the start of surgery	*12 week follow-up* Incidence of harvest site pain was significantly lower in the treated patients (0%) than the saline control group (33%)
Iliac crest bone graft harvest surgery [14]	48-hour continuous infusion of bupivacaine vs. saline into the harvest site beginning at the time of wound closure after procurement of the graft	*4 year follow-up* CPSP was not present in any of the 9 bupivacaine treated patients but was in 7 of the 10 saline controls
Radical prostatectomy [15]	(1) Preoperative epidural bupivacaine, (2) preoperative epidural fentanyl, or (3) preoperative epidural saline. All patients received postoperative patient-controlled epidural analgesia with morphine and bupivacaine	*3.5, 5.5 and 9.5 week follow-ups* Activity scores at 3.5 weeks, but not later, were significantly higher in the two treatment groups than the saline treated controls. Pain incidence at 9.5, but not at 3.5 or 5.5, weeks after surgery was significantly lower in the groups that received the epidural agents before and during surgery compared with the control group
Radical prostatectomy [16]	(1) Preoperative vs (2) postincisional intravenous fentanyl plus low dose intravenous ketamine vs. (3) a standard treatment group receiving intraoperative intravenous fentanyl but not ketamine	*2 week and 6 month follow-ups* Significant differences were not found among the three groups in pain incidence, intensity, disability or mental health

Table 5.2 (*continued*)

Type of surgery	Agent(s) used preventively and duration of treatment	Follow-up time after surgery and outcome
Breast cancer surgery [17]	(1) Gabapentin, (2) mexiletine or (3) placebo capsules three times daily beginning the evening before surgery and continuing for 10 days after surgery	*3 month follow-up* No difference in the incidence or intensity of CPSP
Breast cancer surgery [18]	(1) Gabapentin or placebo before surgery and for 8 days after plus (2) transdermal EMLA cream or placebo on the day of surgery and for 3 days after, plus (3) intraoperative ropivacaine or placebo irrigation of the brachial plexus and intercostal spaces	*3 and 6 month follow ups* 3, but not 6, months after surgery, patients in the multimodal treatment group had a significantly lower incidence of axilla pain (14% vs. 45%), arm pain (23% vs. 59%) and analgesic use (0% vs. 23%) compared with the placebo control patients
Upper limb amputation [19]	Continuous brachial plexus anesthesia for 7 days with or without the NMDA receptor antagonist memantine	*4 weeks, 6 months and 1 year follow-ups* At 4 weeks and 6 months, but not at 1 year, the incidence and intensity of phantom limb pain in the memantine treated group was significantly lower than the control group
Lower limb amputation [20]	Continuous epidural morphine and bupivacaine administered 18 hours before, during surgery and for ~1 week after lower limb amputation. The control group received epidural saline before and throughout surgery followed by epidural morphine and bupivacaine for ~1 week after lower limb amputation	*3, 6 and 12 month follow-ups* Significant differences in phantom limb pain were not found between the treatment and control groups in intensity, opioid consumption or incidence at the 3 (82% vs. 50%), 6 (81% vs. 55%) or 12 (75% vs. 69%) month follow-ups

EMLA, eutectic mixture of local anesthetics.

Summary and conclusions

The transition of acute postoperative pain to CPSP is a complex and poorly understood process involving biological, psychological and social-environmental factors that interact across the three phases of the perioperative period (Figure 5.2). The noxious effects of surgery (e.g. arising from incision inflammation, nerve injury-induced ectopic activity, central sensitization), offset by the competing protective effects of preventive analgesia, interact with pre-existing and concurrent pain, psychological and emotional factors as well as the social environment to determine the nature, severity, frequency and duration of CPSP. Psychological management programs for other chronic pain problems have established efficacy, but prevention and treatment efforts for CPSP

have lagged behind in part because we have not yet identified causal risk factors. Further research is necessary to identify the causal risk factors for CPSP and develop the tools to ensure that all patients who undergo major surgery recover uneventfully. In the meantime there is good evidence to support that one should minimize nerve damage in the surgical field, and maximize pain control in the perioperative and postoperative periods. Preliminary data show that in certain cases perioperative multimodal preventive analgesia may reduce the incidence of CPSP. It is also probable that providing a caring environment, within which the patient's anxiety and fears regarding surgery and its impact are addressed, will provide additional benefit. However, until we know more about the source and nature of the psychological causal risk factors for CPSP

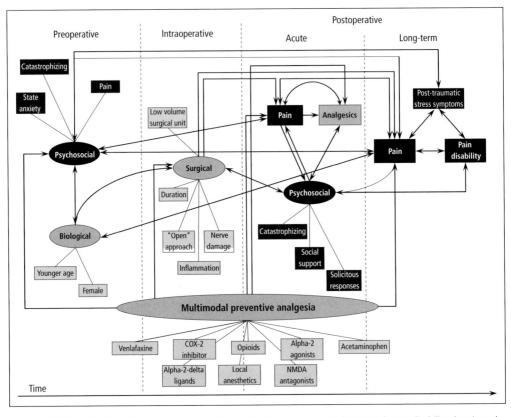

Figure 5.2 Schematic illustration of the processes involved in the development of CPSP and CPSP disability showing relationships (arrows) among preoperative, intraoperative and postoperative factors. Lines with double arrows between variables show associative relationships reported in the literature. Lines with a single arrow show causal relationships based on randomized controlled trials of preventive analgesia.

it is premature to make specific treatment recommendations.

References

1 Macrae WA, Davies HTO. (1999) Chronic postsurgical pain. In: Crombie IK, Linton S, Croft P *et al.* eds. *Epidemiology of Pain.* IASP Press, Seattle, WA. pp. 125–42.

2 Katz J, Selter Z. (2009) Transition from acute to chronic postsurgical pain: risk factors and protective factors. *Expert Rev Neurother* **9(5)**: 723–44.

3 Kraemer HC, Kazdin AE, Offord DR *et al.* (1997) Coming to terms with the terms of risk. *Arch Gen Psychiatry* **54**:337–43.

4 Kraemer HC, Kazdin A, Offord DR *et al.* (1999) Measuring the potency of risk factors for clinical or policy significance. *Psychol Methods* **4(3)**:257–71.

5 Hanley MA, Jensen MP, Ehde DM *et al.* (2004) Psychosocial predictors of long-term adjustment to lower-limb amputation and phantom limb pain. *Disabil Rehabil* **26(14–15)**:882–93.

6 Katz J, Clarke H. (2008) Preventive analgesia and beyond: current status, evidence, and future directions. In: Macintyre PE, Rowbotham DJ, Howard R, eds. *Clinical Pain Management: Acute Pain*, 2nd edn. Hodder Arnold, London. pp. 154–98.

7 McCartney CJ, Sinha A, Katz J. (2004) A qualitative systematic review of the role of N-methyl-

D-aspartate receptor antagonists in preventive analgesia. *Anesth Anal* **98(5)**:1385–400.

8 Dworkin RH, Turk DC, Farrar JT *et al.* (2005) Core outcome measures for chronic pain clinical trials: IMMPACT recommendations. *Pain* **113(1–2)**:9–19.

9 Lavand'homme P, De Kock M, Waterloos H. (2005) Intraoperative epidural analgesia combined with ketamine provides effective preventive analgesia in patients undergoing major digestive surgery. *Anesthesiology* **103(4)**:813–20.

10 Brogly N, Wattier JM, Andrieu G *et al.* (2008) Gabapentin attenuates late but not early post-operative pain after thyroidectomy with superficial cervical plexus block. *Anesth Anal* **107(5)**:1720–5.

11 Katz J, Clairoux M, Redahan C *et al.* (1996) High dose alfentanil pre-empts pain after abdominal hysterectomy. *Pain* **68(1)**:109–18.

12 Katz J, Cohen L. (2004) Preventive analgesia is associated with reduced pain disability 3 weeks but not 6 months after major gynecologic surgery by laparotomy. *Anesthesiology* **101(1)**: 169–74.

13 Gundes H, Kilickan L, Gurkan Y *et al.* (2000) Short- and long-term effects of regional application of morphine and bupivacaine on the iliac crest donor site. *Acta Orthop Belg* **66(4)**: 341–4.

14 Singh K, Phillips FM, Kuo E *et al.* (2007) A prospective, randomized, double-blind study of the efficacy of postoperative continuous local anesthetic infusion at the iliac crest bone graft site after posterior spinal arthrodesis: a minimum of 4-year follow-up. *Spine* **32(25)**: 2790–6.

15 Gottschalk A, Smith DS, Jobes DR *et al.* (1998) Preemptive epidural analgesia and recovery from radical prostatectomy: a randomized controlled trial. *JAMA* **279(14)**:1076–82.

16 Katz J, Schmid R, Snijdelaar DG *et al.* (2004) Preemptive analgesia using intravenous fentanyl plus low-dose ketamine for radical prostatectomy under general anesthesia does not produce short-term or long-term reductions in pain or analgesic use. *Pain* **110(3)**:707–18.

17 Fassoulaki A, Patris K, Sarantopoulos C *et al.* (2002) The analgesic effect of gabapentin and mexiletine after breast surgery for cancer. *Anesth Anal* **95(4)**:985–91.

18 Fassoulaki A, Triga A, Melemeni A *et al.* (2005) Multimodal analgesia with gabapentin and local anesthetics prevents acute and chronic pain after breast surgery for cancer. *Anesth Anal* **101(5)**:1427–32.

19 Schley M, Topfner S, Wiech K *et al.* (2007) Continuous brachial plexus blockade in combination with the NMDA receptor antagonist memantine prevents phantom pain in acute traumatic upper limb amputees. *Eur J Pain* **11(3)**:299–308.

20 Nikolajsen L, Ilkjaer S, Christensen JH *et al.* (1997) Randomised trial of epidural bupivacaine and morphine in prevention of stump and phantom pain in lower-limb amputation. *Lancet* **350(9088)**:1353–7.

Chapter 6

Placebo/nocebo: a two-sided coin in the clinician's hand

Antonella Pollo[1,3] & Fabrizio Benedetti[2,3]

[1] Department of Neuroscience, University of Torino Faculty of Pharmacy, Torino, Italy
[2] Department of Neuroscience, University of Torino Medical School, Torino, Italy
[3] National Institute of Neuroscience, Torino, Italy

Introduction

The use of placebos dates back to the origins of medicine itself. Much of the ongoing confusion about the term, still pervading both the society and the scientific community, probably derives from the shifting focus on its different aspects across the centuries, such as: an inert medication given more to please than to benefit, a deceiving expedient to trick the naive layman, a means to detect the mystifying patient, a tool to isolate specific drugs effects in the course of clinical trials and, finally, an additional therapeutic aid. Current neurobiological and pharmacological evidence has placed placebo effects at the intersection between expectation, hope, desire, anxiety and previous experience (conditioning), involving both patient and attending staff, and has provided scientific ground for their exploitation. Interest in the placebo's evil twin, the nocebo, is more recent. If a placebo is a sham treatment inducing a positive outcome, a nocebo is a sham treatment inducing a negative one. It could actually be the same inert substance (e.g. coupled to opposite verbal instruc-

tions to reverse the patient's expectations). As for placebos, the whole context surrounding the therapeutic act impacts on different psychological aspects to produce the end result. In modern clinical practice, ethical concerns have been raised about the legitimacy of placebo administration. Informed consent and patient deceit seem irreconcilable; still a more widespread awareness of the importance of the patient–provider interaction and the introduction of specific therapeutic protocols can represent a way to exploit placebo effects to the patient's advantage while at the same time avoiding nocebo effects.

In this chapter a brief overview on current knowledge of the biology of placebo and nocebo effects is outlined, followed by some suggestions for clinical application. Emphasis is on pain studies and pain treatment, but it should be remembered that placebo and nocebo effects have been described in many other clinical conditions, such as Parkinson's disease and depression; in different systems, like the endocrine and immune systems; and even outside the medical domain, as in sport performance. Indeed, they pervade our everyday life, at the conscious and unconscious level, affecting our evaluations and decisions.

The interested reader is referred to a number of reviews and books that address these topics in greater detail [1–6].

Clinical Pain Management: A Practical Guide, 1st edition.
Edited by Mary E. Lynch, Kenneth D. Craig and Philip W.H. Peng.
© 2011 Blackwell Publishing Ltd.

Before we begin: a few facts on placebo/nocebo

Q1: *Is the placebo effect the same as the placebo response?*

A. The two terms are often used synonymously. Technically, however, the placebo effect is that observed in the placebo arm of a clinical trial, which is produced by the placebo biological phenomenon in addition to other potential factors contributing to symptom amelioration, such as natural history, regression to the mean, biases, judgment errors. The placebo response, on the other hand, designates the biological phenomenon in isolation, as can best be studied in specifically designed experimental protocols.

Q2: *Is the placebo an inert treatment?*

A. Yes and no. The adjective "inert" correctly suggests that the substance or treatment is devoid of specific effects for the condition being treated. However, it cannot by definition be inert if it produces an effect. The solution to the conundrum can be found by shifting the attention from the treatment to the patient who receives it: it is in fact the symbolic meaning of the treatment, rather than the treatment itself, which by different mechanisms triggers active processes in the patient's brain, ultimately producing the placebo effect. The placebo need not be a "treatment" either. Its archetype is, of course, the sugar pill, but more subtle or more general factors work equally well. For example, the symbolic meaning can be ascribed to one or all aspects of the context surrounding the therapeutic act, and the simulation of a therapeutic situation can thus adequately replace the sugar pill.

Q3: *Is a nocebo effect the opposite of a placebo effect?*

A. Yes, the nocebo has been defined as negative placebo. As expectations of amelioration can lead to clinical improvement, expectations of worsening can result in negative outcome. The term nocebo (Latin "I shall harm") was originally introduced to designate noxious effects produced by a placebo (e.g. side effects of the drug the placebo is substituting for). In that case, however, the negative outcome is produced in spite of an expectation of benefit. True nocebo effects, on the other hand, are always the result of negative expectations, specific or generic (like a pessimistic attitude).

Proposed mechanisms of placebo/nocebo effects

Different explanatory mechanisms have been proposed for both placebo and nocebo effects, each supported by experimental evidence. They need not be mutually exclusive and can actually be at work simultaneously.

Classical conditioning

This theory posits the placebo/nocebo effect as the result of Pavlovian conditioning. In this process, the repeated co-occurrence of an unconditioned response to an unconditioned stimulus (e.g. salivation after the sight of food) with a conditioned stimulus (e.g. a bell ringing) induces a conditioned response (i.e. salivation that is induced by bell ringing alone). Likewise, aspects of the clinical setting (e.g. taste, color, shape of a tablet, as well as white coats or the peculiar hospital smell) can also act as conditioned stimuli, eliciting a therapeutic response in the absence of an active principle, just because they have been paired with it in the past. In the same way, the conditioned response can be a negative outcome, as in the case of nausea elicited by the sight of the environment where chemotherapy has been administered in the past. Classical conditioning seems to work best where unconscious processes are at play, as in placebo/nocebo effects involving endocrine or immune systems, but it has also been documented in clinical and experimental placebo analgesia and nocebo hyperalgesia.

Expectations

This theory conceives the placebo effect as the product of cognitive engagement, with the patient consciously foreseeing a positive or negative outcome, based on factors as diverse as verbal instructions, environmental clues, previous experience, emotional arousal and the interaction with care-providers. This anticipation of the future outcome in turn triggers internal changes resulting in specific experiences (e.g. analgesia or hyperalgesia). Desire, self-efficacy and self-reinforcing feedback all interact with expectation, potentiating its effects. Desire is the experiential dimension of wanting something to happen or wanting to avoid something happening [5], while self-efficacy is the belief to be able to manage the disease, performing the right actions to induce positive changes (e.g. to withstand and lessen pain). Self-reinforcing feedback is a positive loop whereby the subject attends selectively to signs of improvement, taking them as evidence that the placebo treatment has worked. This is also called the somatic focus (i.e. the degree to which individuals focus on their symptoms) [5]. A related proposed mechanism posits that anxiety reduction also has a role in placebo responses, because the subject interpretation of ambiguous sensations is changed from noxious and menacing to benign and unworthy of attention.

Embodiment

Central to the constructionist view of the placebo experience held by medical anthropologists is the concept of embodiment, which states that the human mind is strongly influenced and shaped by aspects of the body, such as the sensory systems and our interaction with the environment and the society. Thus, our experiences can not only be consciously stored as memories, but also imprinted straight onto our body, without involvement of any cognitive process. An example of how sociocultural experiences can impact on the individual's physiology is offered by trauma or stress, as in post-traumatic stress disorder (PTSD), where symptoms such as sleep disorders or frightening thoughts are the result of an implicit perception, the literal "incorporation" of a terrifying event in the external world, which bypassed conscious awareness. According to this view, the placebo effect is a positive effect of embodiment and the nocebo effect a negative one. Lived positive experiences can be channelled into objects or places, which then acquire potential to trigger healing responses. Importantly, this process needs not involve conscious expectation or conscious attribution of symbolic meaning to the object or place [7].

Performative efficacy

Therapeutic performances may have *per se* a convincing persuading effect; just by the ritual of the therapeutic act, a change in the body can be achieved. The performance inducing a placebo effect may be social, as in sham surgery in clinical trials with positive outcomes in the placebo arm, or in the case of a mother's kiss on a child's wound; or it may be internal, as for athletes mentally rehearsing before a competition. In this framework, a placebo effect could result from the internal act of imagining a specific change of state of the body. It is tempting to speculate that as mirror motor neurons fire when observing somebody perform a motor task (in the same way as they would when the individual performs the task himself), so could neural pathways activated by the internal performance of healing change, in turn facilitate healing itself. Central in the performative efficacy of the ritual is the patient–provider relationship, with factors such as empathy, prestige of the healer, gesture and recitation all contributing to the treatment success.

All these mechanisms may contribute to the final placebo/nocebo effect in varying proportion, or combine differently in specific cases. To some extent, some of them can influence one another, as for conditioning and expectation, which both represent a form of learning; thus, conditioning can bring about conscious expectations. Many forms of learning may take place, including social observational learning: observing beneficial effects in a demonstrator induced stronger analgesic placebo responses than those induced by verbal suggestions alone, and as potent as those induced by a conditioning procedure.

The importance of each mechanism can be different in placebo vs. nocebo effects. For example, it has been shown in healthy volunteers in a pain conditioning/expectation protocol that conditioning was more important than verbal instructions (inducing expectation) for placebo effects, while the opposite was true for nocebo effects.

Neurobiology of placebo analgesia

The last decade has witnessed the beginning of clarification of neurochemical and pharmacological details of placebo analgesia. In 1978, a pioneering study by Levine *et al.* [8] showed that the opiate antagonist naloxone was able to reduce the placebo response in dental postoperative pain. That was the first indication that endogenous opioids were involved in placebo analgesia. Subsequent experiments provided ever more compelling evidence that the secretion of endogenous opioids in the brain was the key event in placebo pain modulation. Placebo responders had levels of β-endorphin in the cerebrospinal fluid that were more than double those of non-responders; opioids released by a placebo procedure displayed the same side effects as exogenous opiates; naloxone-sensitive cardiac effects could be observed during placebo-induced expectation of analgesia. Indirect support also came from the placebo-potentiating role of the cholecystokinin (CCK) antagonist proglumide. In fact, the CCK system effects counteracted those of opioids, delineating a picture where the placebo effect seems to be under the opposing influence of facilitating opioids and inhibiting CCK. In some situations, however, a placebo effect can still occur after blockade of opioid mechanisms by naloxone, indicating that systems other than opioids are also implicated. For example, with a morphine conditioning and/or expectation-inducing protocol, naloxone was able to completely reverse placebo analgesia induced in experimental ischemic arm pain. Conversely, with the use of ketorolac (a non-opioid analgesic) in the same protocol, only a partial blockade could be observed. Almost nothing is currently known on these non-opioid systems, and further research is needed to clarify them (Fig. 6.1).

The advent of neuroimaging techniques and of their use for experimental purposes added anatomic and temporal details to the neurochemical information. The first positron emission tomography (PET) study to investigate placebo analgesia was conducted in 2002. It showed overlapping in the brain activation pattern generated by opioid-induced analgesia (by the μ-agonist remifentanil)

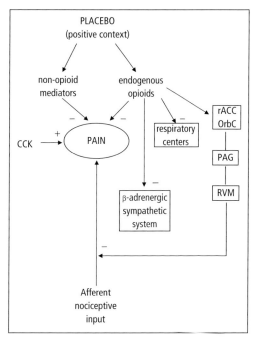

Figure 6.1 Cascade of events that may take place during a placebo procedure. Pain is inhibited by a descending inhibitory network involving the rostral anterior cingulate cortex (rACC), the orbitofrontal cortex (OrbC), the periacqueductal gray (PAG) and the rostral ventromedial medulla (RVM). Endogenous opioids inhibit pain through this descending network and/or other mechanisms. The respiratory centers may be inhibited by opioid mechanisms as well. The β-adrenergic sympathetic system is also inhibited during placebo analgesia. Non-opioid mechanisms are also involved. Cholecystokinin (CCK) counteracts the effects of the endogenous opioids, thus antagonizing placebo analgesia.

and by placebo-induced analgesia. Common activated areas included the rostral anterior cingulate cortex (rACC) and the orbitofrontal cortex. In the following years, in spite of some discrepancies likely explained by methodological and procedural differences, PET, functional magnetic resonance imaging (fMRI) and magnetoelectroencephalography (MEG) studies all suggested placebo activation of the descending pain control system, with modulation of activity in areas such as periaqueductal gray (PAG), the ventromedial medulla, the parabrachial nuclei, the ACC, the orbitofrontal cortex, the hypothalamus and the central nucleus of the amygdala. Notably, direct demonstration of endogenous opioid release was obtained through [¹¹C] carfentanil displacement by the activation of opioid neurotransmission, with the decrease in binding correlating with placebo reduction of pain intensity reports. Recently, naloxone was observed to block placebo-induced responses in pain modulatory cortical structures and in key structures of the descending pain control system [9] (for a review on neuroimaging studies see Zubieta & Stohler [6]).

Also of interest is the fact that knowledge of placebo analgesia can be gained by focusing on changes in brain activity that take place with modulation of expectation alone. In fact, expectation of benefit can induce a placebo effect even without the physical administration of a placebo. Because no placebo is actually given, these effects may be more appropriately called "placebo-like" effects. Thus, activity in pain areas following a constant painful stimulus can be modulated just by varying the subject's expectation of the level of stimulation: the higher the *expected* level of the stimulus, the stronger the activity in ACC and other areas implicated in the activation of the descending inhibitory pathway. Taken together, these studies show how the same result (i.e. the activation of the same receptors in the brain) can be obtained by a pharmacologic (drug) or a psychologic (placebo) means. A more comprehensive description of the studies mentioned here can be found in Zubieta & Stohler [6].

Neurobiology of nocebo hyperalgesia

Compared to placebo effect research, the investigation of the nocebo effect raises more ethical difficulties, especially in the clinical setting. However, in recent times a few experimental studies have begun to shed light on this phenomenon, focusing mainly on the model of nocebo hyperalgesia. In the protocols used, an inert treatment is given along with verbal suggestions of pain worsening, resulting in exacerbation of pain. It has been suggested that the anticipatory anxiety about the impending pain, brought about by negative expec-

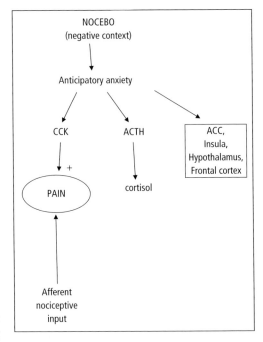

Figure 6.2 Events that may occur during a nocebo procedure. Nocebo induces anticipatory anxiety which, in turn, affects both the hypothalamus-pituitary-adrenal axis (adrenocorticotropic hormone [ACTH] and cortisol) and pain mechanisms. The link between anxiety and pain is represented by cholecystokinin (CCK), which has a facilitating effect on pain. Anticipatory anxiety about the impending pain also activates different brain regions that are involved in pain processing.

tations, triggers the activation of CCK, which in turn facilitates pain transmission and results in hyperalgesia. Accordingly, this hyperalgesia can be blocked by proglumide, a non-specific CCK-1 and CCK-2 antagonist, in a dose-dependent manner. The proglumide block is related specifically to nocebo/anxiety-induced hyperalgesia rather than to the more general process of nocebo-induced anxiety, as it is selectively exerted on nocebo hyperalgesia but not on the concurrent stress-induced hypothalamic-pituitary-adrenal axis hyperactivity (Fig. 6.2).

Proglumide also exhibited placebo-potentiating effects, raising the question of how the two endogenous systems, CCK and opioids, may interact in producing negative or positive outcomes. It can be speculated that the placebo/nocebo phenomenon is a continuum, with opioid and CCK-ergic systems acting as the mediators of opposing effects.

As for placebo analgesia, neuroimaging techniques have also brought important contributions to the knowledge of nocebo hyperalgesia. Here again, expectations without the physical administration of a nocebo treatment have been exploited ("nocebo-like" effects). Inducing negative expectations resulted in both amplified unpleasantness of innocuous stimuli as assessed by psychophysical pain measures (subject report) and increased fMRI responses in ACC, insula, hypothalamus, secondary somatosensory areas and prefrontal cortex. From these studies it appears that the circuitry underlying nocebo hyperalgesia largely involves, with opposite modulation, the same areas engaged by placebo analgesia [10–12].

The coin in the clinician's hand

What is the relevance of placebo/nocebo studies to clinical practice and how can patients benefit from the application of these research findings? It could be argued that today's ethical restrictions prevent the widespread use of placebos that was commonplace in ancient times. Still, its practice is common, and physicians surveyed in many countries reported using placebos to calm patients, avert requests for unnecessary medications or as a supplement treatment. But from what we know today, deception is not necessarily involved in the use of placebo. We have learned that anything inducing expectation of benefit (e.g. analgesia) can act as a placebo, positively impacting on the patient's (pain) brain circuitry. In fact, every real treatment administered in routine health care has two distinct components: the active constituent and the placebo (psychosocial) factor. Every effort should be made to enhance the latter to maximize the benefit of the therapeutic act. This behavior is perfectly acceptable and does not challenge ethical imperatives. Central in the psychosocial context is the patient–provider relationship, with empathy, perceived skill, correct attitudes and words, ceremony and encouragement all contributing to a positive outcome.

The reverse actions represent nocebos, and they may lessen the effectiveness of therapeutic agents. Although the harmful effect of natural situations such as the impact of negative diagnoses or the patient's disbelief in a therapy are sometimes difficult to circumvent, care should be given to at least eliminate negligence and minimize distrust. Of note, nocebo suggestions can be more powerful than placebo ones, as reversing the verbal instructions can turn a placebo analgesic response into a hyperalgesic nocebo one, in spite of previous placebo conditioning. Even a seemingly innocuous act such as communicating to the patient that a therapy is going to be interrupted can have a negative impact, as showed by the faster and larger intensity relapse of pain after open versus hidden interruption of morphine analgesic therapy.

Conclusions

Thus, the clinician has in his hand a coin with two sides: when the coin is tossed on the "plus" side the clinician has an extra tool to minimize the patient's distress. When tossed on the "minus" side, the clinician unwillingly minimizes drug efficacy. Although a positive doctor–patient relationship and good medical practice have long been known to affect the therapeutic outcome and the patient's quality of life, what is new today is that we are beginning to understand the underlying biological mechanisms. It is to be hoped that awareness and good knowledge of placebo/nocebo mechanisms will govern the physician's conduct, rather than the random toss of a coin.

References

1 Benedetti F. (2007) Placebo and endogenous mechanisms of analgesia. *Handb Exp Pharmacol* **177**:393–413.

2 Benedetti F. (2008) Mechanisms of placebo and placebo-related effects across diseases and treatments. *Annu Rev Pharmacol Toxicol* **48**: 33–60.

3 Benedetti F. (2008) *Placebo Effects: Understanding the Mechanisms in Health and Disease.* Oxford University Press, Oxford.

4 Enck P, Benedetti F, Schedlowski M. (2008) New insights into the placebo and nocebo responses. *Neuron* **59**:195–206.

5 Price DD, Finniss DG, Benedetti F. (2008) A comprehensive review of the placebo effects: recent advances and current thought. *Annu Rev Psychol* **59**:565–90.

6 Zubieta JK, Stohler CS. (2009) Neurobiological mechanisms of placebo responses. *Ann N Y Acad Sci* **1156**:198–210.

7 Thompson JJ, Ritenbaugh C, Nichter M. (2009) Reconsidering the placebo response from a broad anthropological perspective. *Cult Med Psychiatry* **33**:112–52.

8 Levine JD, Gordon NC, Fields HL. (1978) The mechanisms of placebo analgesia. *Lancet* **2**:654–7.

9 Eippert F, Bingel U, Schoell ED, Yacubian J *et al.* (2009) Activation of the opioidergic descending pain control system underlies placebo analgesia. *Neuron* **63**:533–43.

10 Benedetti F, Lanotte M, Lopiano L *et al.* (2007) When words are painful: unraveling the mechanisms of the nocebo effect. *Neuroscience* **147**: 260–71.

11 Colloca L, Benedetti F. (2007) Nocebo hyperalgesia: how anxiety is turned into pain. *Curr Opin Anaesthesiol* **20**:435–9.

12 Price DD, Craggs JG, Zhou QQ *et al.* (2009) Widespread hyperalgesia in irritable bowle syndrome is dynamically maintained by tonic visceral impulse input and placebo/nocebo factors: evidence from human psychophysics, animal models, and neuroimaging. *Neuroimage* **47**:995–1001.

Acknowledgments

This work was supported by a grant from Istituto San Paolo di Torino and from Regione Piemonte (Torino, Italy) and from the Volkswagen Foundation (Hannover, Germany).

Part 2

Assessment of Pain

Chapter 7

Clinical assessment in adult patients

Christine Short[1] & Mary Lynch[2]

[1] *Assistant Professor, Dalhousie University; Department of Medicine, Division of Physical Medicine and Rehabilitation; Department of Surgery, Division of Neurosurgery, Queen Elizabeth II Health Sciences Centre, Halifax, Nova Scotia*
[2] *Professor Anesthesia, Psychiatry, Pharmacology, Dalhousie University, Pain Management Unit, Queen Elizabeth II Health Sciences Center, Halifax, Nova Scotia*

Pain is what the patient says it is
(Ronald Melzack, 1975)

Introduction

There is no objective imaging study or laboratory test that can measure pain; however, we can objectively measure the manifestations of pain. One of the main ways we know if someone is in pain is from their verbal report or behavior. In some cases there is a limp or some other obvious manifestation of the pain, in many there is not; in most there will be an impact on the patient's ability to function. Carr *et al.* [1] have reviewed the importance of narrative in pain and the fact that narrative is particularly required in chronic pain because, given that there are no specific diagnostic tests for pain, words are often all the patient has [2]. Thus, the best clinical tools in pain assessment, in cognitively intact adults, are the clinician's capacity to listen to the patient as they tell their story, careful observation and a thorough physical assessment which includes a good neurosensory examination.

Clinical Pain Management: A Practical Guide, 1st edition.
Edited by Mary E. Lynch, Kenneth D. Craig and Philip W.H. Peng.
© 2011 Blackwell Publishing Ltd.

The history

It is best to start with an open-ended question, simply ask the patient to tell you about their pain. Make time for the patient to tell their story. Later you can fill in the gaps. Table 7.1 presents the key elements required in a full biopsychosocial history. In most cases, in order to obtain a full history and physical examination as well as communicating diagnosis and a suggested management, the clinician will need 90–120 minutes. We realize that this length of time will not be possible in all clinical contexts, so it is reasonable to obtain this information over several appointments, depending on the clinical setting. The important thing is that the initial assessment is not complete until you have obtained all of this information.

Patient expectations and goals

Within the first few minutes ask the patient about their expectations or goals. Patients may not be looking for complete relief and will often surprise you by saying they are looking for strategies to control or cope better with the pain. They may also present specific goals such as a wish to walk farther, play with their grandchildren or return to work, whether this be unpaid work within the home, or wage earning work outside of the home.

Table 7.1 Essential elements in the history and physical examination of the patient presenting with chronic pain.

Chief complaint and history of present illness	Exploring location, onset, quality, context, severity, duration, modifying factors, spontaneous/evoked aspects and associated signs and symptoms (sleep, appetite, energy, concentration, memory, mood, libido, suicidal ideation), previous treatment for pain (include complimentary therapies), previous consultations and investigations
Functional history	Impact of pain on level of function Mobility: bed mobility, transfers, wheelchair mobility, ambulation, driving, and devices required Activities of daily living: e.g. bathing, toileting, dressing, eating, hygiene and grooming Instrumental activities of daily living: e.g. meal preparation, laundry, telephone use, home maintenance, child or pet care Communication issues, sexual function
Past medical and surgical history	Specific conditions: cardiopulmonary, musculoskeletal, neurological and rheumatological Medications
Psychosocial history	Past psychiatric and addiction history Home environment and living circumstances, family and friends support system, vocational activities, finances, recreational activities, spirituality and litigation
Family history	
Review of systems	
General medical physical examination	Cardiac Pulmonary Gastrointestinal Genital/urinary and pelvic Lymphatics
General neurological and mental status examination	General appearance, behavior, flow of speech Orientation: most patients in an outpatient setting will be oriented to person, place and time, in an inpatient setting questions re orientation may be more important Affect: is affect congruent with the content of the interview? Attention and concentration Thought content: is it consistent with questions posed and the context of the pain interview or is there evidence of disorganized thought, delusional thinking? Is there any unusual behavior that might suggest a perceptual abnormality such as hallucinations
Cranial nerve	**1** Odor perception (smell) **2** Confrontation visual fields, fundi, visual acuity **3,4,6** External ocular movements, diplopia, nystagmus, pupil response **5** Jaw strength, corneal reflexes, facial sensation **7** Facial power **8** Auditory acuity (hearing) **9 &10** Dysarthria, dysphagia **11** Sternocleidomastoid and trapezius power **12** Tongue atrophy strength and fasiculations
Sensation	Light touch and pinprick Presence or absence of allodynia, hyperalgesia, cold and heat hypersensitivity

Table 7.1 (*continued*)

Motor	Strength (0 = total paraysis, 1 = flicker, 2 = movement with gravity eliminated, 3 = movement only against gravity, 4 = movement can be overcome by resistence, 5 = full power)
	Coordination
	Involuntary movements
	Tone/spasticity
Reflexes (roots)	Biceps C5–6, brachioradialis C6, triceps C7, knee L3–4, ankle S1
Musculoskeletal	
Inspection	Behavior ease of movement during the history and physical examination
	Physical symmetry, e.g. joint deformity
Palpation	Joint stability
	Range of motion (active and passive)
	Strength testing
	Bony/joint/muscles and soft tissues
	Include assessment of trigger points of myofascial pain and tender points of fibromyalgia

Psychological history

Given the importance of psychosocial determinants of pain and related disability, enquiry into these factors is imperative. Chapter 10 presents the details of this assessment. We provide brief observations here. When patients present with a chief complaint of chronic pain they are usually comfortable reviewing the details of the pain but some patients may experience discomfort with questions along psychological lines fearing that you are suggesting that the pain is psychologically caused. Starting with a focus on the physiological aspects of the pain will ease some of these fears. A statement like "Now that I have heard about the pain I would like to get to know more about how this pain is affecting you and what strategies you are using to get through each day with it." This places the questions about mood and anxiety in context for the patient. You can then move into questions regarding the impact the pain has had on sleep, appetite, energy, concentration, mood and sex drive. If the patient reports depression or significant irritability of mood, this is the time to ask about suicidal ideation. For example, you may ask "Has it ever gotten to the point where you feel that life might not be worth living? If yes, "Have you ever come close to acting on these thoughts?" "Can you tell me about it?" "What stopped you?"

"How do you feel now?" Tables 7.2 and 7.3 present a screening instrument for suicide risk. For survivors of trauma, whether this be domestic abuse, military exposure or industrial or motor vehicle accidents, it is also important to screen for post-traumatic stress disorder (PTSD).

Examples of questions to begin to explore anxiety or panic might include: "Do you feel that you suffer from excessive anxiety or worry?" "Do you have any physical symptoms associated with this like trembling, restlessness, increased heart rate, sweating, trouble breathing?"

Examples of questions to begin to explore for PTSD: "Have you re-experienced the accident (or other traumatic event) in any way such as recurrent distressing intrusive recollections or memories, dreams or nightmares or flashbacks?" "Do you avoid the site of the accident?" "Have you found yourself more vigilant, hyperaware or easily startled?"

The risk of substance abuse or chemical dependency should be explored, especially when prescription of opioid is considered. Details of this assessment can be found in Chapter 39.

The suggestions above are examples of ways to begin to explore for psychological pathology. If you find symptoms suggestive of a mood or anxiety disorder then further assessment and referral for psychological services may be required.

Table 7.2 Screening instrument for suicide risk. Five-step suicide assessment and triage.

Identify risk factors	Psychiatric diagnosis current or past	Mood disorders, psychosis, substance abuse, cluster B personality disorder[*]
	Key symptoms	Anhedonia, impulsivity, hopelessness, anxiety/panic, global insomnia, command hallucinations
	Suicidal behavior	Prior or aborted attempts, self-injurious behavior
	Family history	Suicide or attempts or Axis 1 psychiatric diagnoses requiring hospitalization[*]
	Precipitants or stressors	Events leading to humiliation, shame or despair, ongoing medical illness (especially CNS disorders, history of abuse or neglect, intoxication
	Access to firearms	
Protective factors (even if present may not counteract significant risk)	Internal	Ability to cope with stress, religious beliefs, frustration tolerance, no psychosis
	External	Responsibility to children or beloved pets, positive therapeutic relationship, social supports
Suicide inquiry[†]	Ideation	Past 48 hours, past month and worst ever
	Plan	Timing, location, lethality, availability, preparatory acts
	Behaviors	Past or aborted attempts, rehearsals vs. non-suicidal self-injurious action
	Intent	Extent to which patient expects to carry out the plan and believes the plan to be lethal
		Explore ambivalence: reasons to live vs. reasons to die
Risk level/intervention	Assessment of risk	Based on clinical judgment after reviewing above
	Reassess	If patient status or circumstances change
Document	Risk level and treatment plan to address or reduce current risk	Medications and other treatments, setting, contact with significant others, consultation, firearm instructions, follow-up plan

[*] See *Diagnostic and Statistical Manual for Mental Disorders* [11].
[†] Homicide enquiry should be conducted when indicated especially postpartum, character disordered paranoid males dealing with loss or humiliation.
Source: Table adapted from Suicide Assessment 5 Step Evaluation and Triage originally conceived by D. Jacobs MD and developed as a collaboration between Screening for Mental Health Inc. www.mentalhealthscreening.org and the Suicide Prevention Resource Centre www.sprc.org and drawing upon the American Psychiatric Association Practice Guidelines for the Assessment and Treatment of Patients with Suicidal Behavior, see also http://www.psychiatryonline.com/pracGuide/pracGuideTopic_14.aspx

Personal social vocational history

An individual who has grown up in an abusive or traumatic environment will be less likely to have learned healthy coping strategies to deal with experiences such as chronic pain and will require training in healthy strategies. Also, current social circumstances including shelter, financial stress, supports and dependants are critical when understanding what the patient is dealing with and are important in planning appropriate management.

Functional impact

Level of education, ability to function, current work or disability, losses caused by pain and the patient's perspective about the future must also be assessed. The interference items from the Brief Pain Inventory (BPI) [3] are helpful in beginning to

Table 7.3 Suicide risk levels.

Risk level	Risk/protective factor	Suicidality	Possible interventions
High	Psychiatric diagnosis with severe symptoms or acute precipitating event, protective factors not relevant	Potentially lethal suicide attempt or persistent ideation with strong intent or suicide rehearsal	Admission indicated Suicide precautions
Moderate	Multiple risk factors, few protective factors	Suicidal ideation with plan, but no intent or behavior	Admission may be necessary depending on risk factors, develop crises plan, give emergency crises numbers
Low	Modifiable risk factors, strong protective factors	Thoughts of death, no plan, intent or behavior	Outpatient referral, symptom reduction, give emergency crises numbers

assess functional impact and more detail regarding standardized measures are presented in Chapter 10.

Measurement of pain and screening instruments

For the measurement of pain intensity we have found the numerical rating scale easiest for patients, "On a 0 to 10 point scale, where 0 equals no pain and 10 indicates worst possible pain, how bad is your pain?" For pain quality the Short Form McGill Pain Questionnaire is excellent [4], for physical function and interference with function the BPI interference scale is highly regarded [3] and to assess health-related quality of life the SF-36 scale is widely used [5]. These are some of our favorite measures. For further detail, Chapter 4 provides a conceptual basis for psychosocial parameters of assessment and Chapter 10 provides a review of the many screening instruments available for measurement of pain, see also the chapter on pain assessment by Melzack & Katz in the *Textbook of Pain* [6]. For a discussion regarding measurement of core domains in the assessment of pain in clinical trials, see publications by the IMMPACT[1] group [7].

Physical examination

The goal of the physical examination is to confirm any suspicions you have obtained from the history as to possible sources or generators of pain. It is

[1] Initiative on Methods, Measurement and Pain Assessment in Clinical Trials (IMMPACT) see also www.immpact.org

important to identify reversible factors that are contributing to pain. It is this information that will provide the foundation upon which to build your treatment plan. A brief outline is presented in Table 7.1.

The time spent during the history and physical examination has many functions. One is to build the database you need for diagnosis and treatment. The other is to continue to build a relationship of trust with the patient. With this in mind, first and foremost put the patient at ease. We always let the patient know that some of the physical examination will be uncomfortable, but it may be necessary to cause some discomfort in order to find out where the sources of pain might be. Always reassure the patient to let you know if anything is too uncomfortable so that part of the examination can be adjusted or discontinued. Lastly, make sure at all times that the patient is draped/dressed appropriately for their comfort throughout the physical examination.

Observation

The physical examination starts with observation. Much of this can be done while taking the history. Note whether the patient appears to be in distress. Unlike acute pain, most patients with chronic pain do not look distressed on the outside. Do not let this allow you to minimize the patient's suffering. Observe the individual's posture and movement during the interview. People with chronic musculoskeletal pain will often move frequently during the interview to try to find a position of comfort.

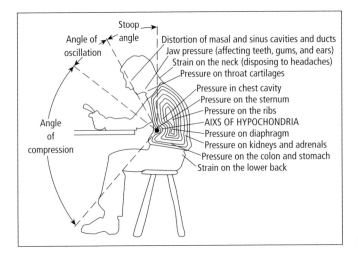

Figure 7.1 Posture theory diagram.

We always invite them to move as they need to at the beginning of the history and physical assessment. Posture should be noted in sitting and standing positions. For example, the protracted or rolled shoulder and protruded chin is common in individuals presenting with back, neck and shoulder pain (Figure 7.1). Observe the gait. A lurch or limp may indicate a musculoskeletal (MSK) or neurologic impairment that could be contributing to pain and may be corrected or improved with treatment such physical therapy or orthotics.

Musculoskeletal examination

The MSK examination should be detailed for regions identified as painful and should include inspection of the joint(s) and surrounding soft tissues, range of motion, palpation and special tests for that region. Limitations in range of motion or MSK abnormalities may be fixed and require accommodation or flexible in which case correction may be possible. For a more detailed presentation of the MSK examination the reader is referred to MaGee [8].

Inspection

Note muscle wasting and asymmetry, which may result from disuse or neurologic impairments. Observe for swelling and redness especially around joints that are symptomatic. Note any unusual

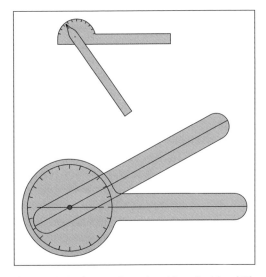

Figure 7.2 Goniometer. Reproduced from Braddom [10], with permission from Elsevier.

rashes or pigmentation. A quick screen of the asymptomatic joints is appropriate, followed by a more detailed review of symptomatic areas. If the patient is suspected to have sympathetically maintained pain, one should look for color, temperature and trophic changes as well as dystonia.

Range of motion

A goniometer is an inexpensive easy to use tool for assessing range of motion (ROM) (Figure 7.2).

Always start with active ROM as this is within the control of the individual and the safest way to proceed. If there is restriction of ROM you can then add a gentle passive assist to the joint to see if there is any further movement. If there is restricted ROM it is important to distinguish if it is due to pain, weakness or tightness. Figure 7.3 shows ROM testing for the apendicular joints. ROM of the lumbosacral spine is best measured using Schober's test which examines the movement of the lumbosacral spine during flexion (Figure 7.4). The normal excursion should be greater than 4.5 cm. There are a wide range of published values that are considered "normal" for cervical ROM. In general, for flexion the individual should be able to bring the chin to the chest or within two fingerbreadths of the chest (40–60°). For extension, they should be able to look up at the ceiling with their eyes in the straightforward position (55°). Lateral bending should be 45° to either side and lateral rotation 70–90° to the right and left (Figure 7.5).

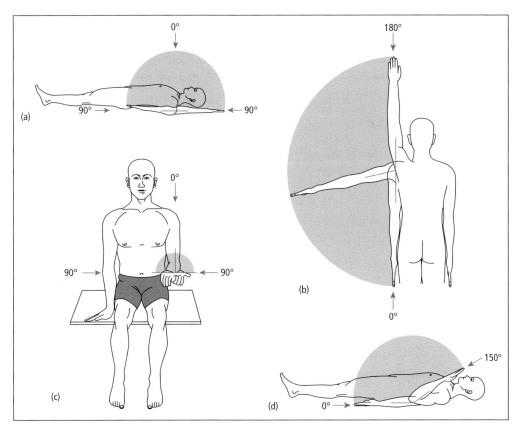

Figure 7.3 Range of motion testing for the apendicular joints. (a) Shoulder flexion; (b) shoulder abduction; (c) elbow supination; (d) elbow flexion and extension; (e) wrist adduction (30°) and abduction (20°); (f) wrist flexion and extension; (g) finger flexion; (h) metacarpophalangeal flexion; (i) knee flexion; (j) ankle dorsi (20°) and plantar (50°) flexion; (k) hip flexion; (l) hip external (45°) and internal (35°) rotation; (m) hip abduction; (n) hip adduction. Reproduced from Braddom [10], with permission from Elsevier.

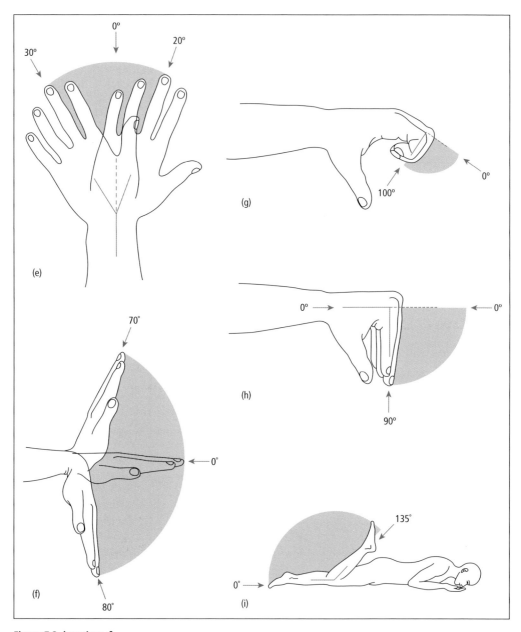

Figure 7.3 (*continued*)

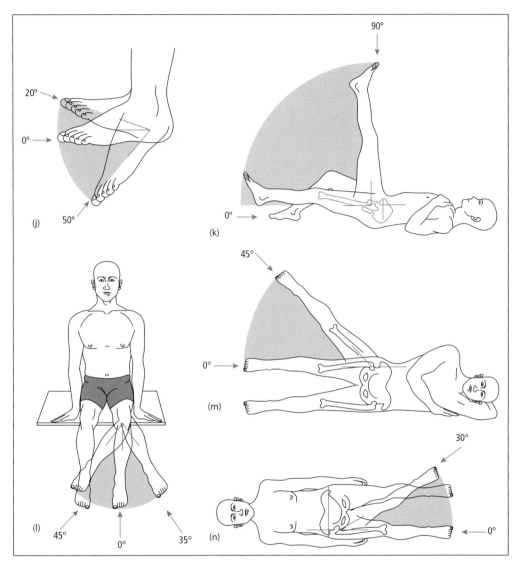

Figure 7.3 (*continued*)

Palpation

Palpate for swelling to define its character and note increased heat. Palpate joints and bony deformities for crepitus. Palpate soft tissues for tenderness and presence of myofascial trigger points [9] or fibromyalgia tender points. When palpating apply firm pressure (about 4 kg of pressure or enough pressure to blanch the nail on your palpating finger). There is a difference between tender points of fibromyalgia and trigger points of myofascial pain (Chapter 27).

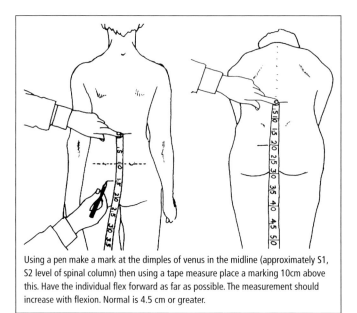

Using a pen make a mark at the dimples of venus in the midline (approximately S1, S2 level of spinal column) then using a tape measure place a marking 10cm above this. Have the individual flex forward as far as possible. The measurement should increase with flexion. Normal is 4.5 cm or greater.

Figure 7.4 Illustration of Schober's test for range of motion of the lumbosacral spine. Using a pen make a mark at the dimples of Venus in the midline (approximately S1,S2 level of spinal column) then, using a tape measure, place a marking 10cm above this. Have the individual flex forward as far as possible. The measurement should increase with flexion. Normal is 4.5cm or greater. *Source:* McRae R. (1997) *Clinical Orthopaedic Examination*, 4th edn. Churchill Livingstone, New York. p. 133, reproduced with permission from Elsevier.

Special tests

There are special tests for many MSK disorders and several tests for each joint which can be quite overwhelming to the assessor (for a full list and descriptions see MaGee [8]). In most cases if you remember your basic anatomy and biomechanics then you will be able to identify the pathology. For example, if you are considering a tendonopathy as a source of ongoing pain then:

1 Palpate the tendon for tenderness;
2 Stretch or stress the tendon, trying to reproduce the clinical symptom of pain.

Neurological examination

In most patients presenting with pain a good neurological examination is also essential. Again, a general screening examination is appropriate followed by a more detailed examination of symptomatic areas.

Cranial nerves

Most of the cranial nerve assessment can be observed during the history, with later examination of vision, visual fields and oral and pharyngeal function on the physical examination.

Motor examination

Observe muscle wasting and fasiculations; a regional or radicular pattern of wasting and weakness may suggest an underlying neurological disorder. Pain can cause disuse which can lead

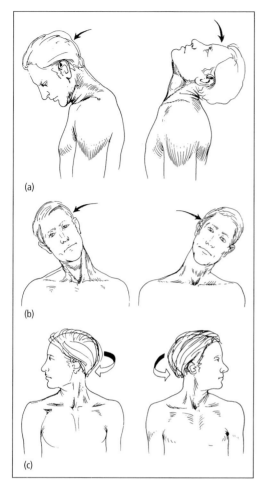

(a)

(b)

(c)

Figure 7.5 C-spine range of motion. (a) Flexion and extension; (b) lateral flexion; (c) lateral rotation. Reproduced from Hoppenfeld [12], with permission from Pearson Education.

to diminished strength and wasting. This is usually less profound than that seen with lower motor neuron damage and is not associated with fasiculations. Motor tone should be observed as normal, increased or decreased. If a region is painful it is often difficult for the individual to relax fully and this will make assessment of tone more difficult to interpret. As much as possible let the individual you are examining move within their range of comfort (for more detail see Braddom [10]).

Sensory examination

A good sensory examination includes an assessment of light touch and response to sharp stimulation. Regional areas of numbness are commonly associated with regional soft tissue pain especially in the presence of muscle tightness and spasm. These do not necessarily mean that there is neurological dysfunction related to the pain. Areas of sensory abnormality that follow a specific dermatome or peripheral nerve distribution suggest an underlying neurological injury or compressive neuropathy that may be potentially reversible (Figure 7.6). The presence of allodynia or hyperalgesia may suggest a component of neural sensitization and will assist in identifying whether there is a neuropathic component to the individual's pain. Further detail regarding the neurosensory examination is covered in Chapter 9.

Reflexes

The deep tendon reflexes should be described as normal, increased or decreased and assist in identifying a neurological problem involved in the pain process; note any asymmetry.

Cerebellar examination

The screening examination includes observation regarding balance, coordination, tremor and smoothness of motion during the other aspects of the physical examination.

Table 7.4 summarizes some pearls of the physical examination for chronic pain.

Conclusions

A complete biopsychosocial history followed by an appropriate physical examination will give you the diagnosis in over 90% of cases. Further investigations, where available, are used primarily to confirm your working diagnosis. Once this thorough assessment has been completed you now have the data to build a comprehensive treatment plan.

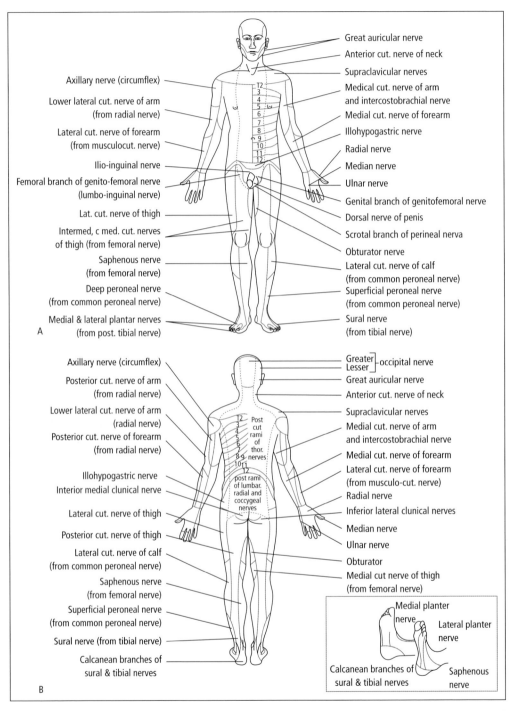

Figure 7.6 Areas of sensory abnormality that follow a specific dermatome or peripheral nerve distribution. Reproduced from Braddom [10], with permission from Elsevier.

Table 7.4 Physical examination pearls.

Presenting complaint	Examination pearl	Comments
Hip or back pain	Check for LLD, palpate GT area for signs of bursitis	LLD can change the biomechanics of the lower extremity and back and contribute to ongoing pain and dysfunction. With GT bursitis pain often radiates into the lateral upper leg
Back or lower extremity joint pain	Check the feet	Foot deformities like LLD put abnormal strain on the low back and lower extremity structures. This can lead to knee, hip and/or low back complaints
Neck pain	Posture! Posture! Posture!	Even subtle poor posture can greatly increase the strain on the neck and increase discomfort
Neck and back pain	Ask about the pillow and mattress	Proper support during sleep can alleviate a multitude of symptoms
Neck pain	Always do a neurological screen for myelopathy	The neurologic screen for myelopathy in neck pain should include upper extremity and lower extremity strength and sensation and reflex examination. The Babinski sign may be an important sign for myelopathy
Persistent shoulder pain	Do not forget to examine the long head of the biceps in the bicipital groove (see examining tendons above)	This is often missed when rotator cuff tendonopathy is diagnosed. Pain coming from the biceps tendon needs to be treated as well

GT, greater trochanteric; LLD, leg length discrepancy.

References

1 Carr DB, Loeser JD, Morris DB. (2005) *Narrative, Pain, and Suffering*. IASP Press, Seattle, WA.

2 Charon R. (2005) A narrative medicine for pain. In: Carr DB, Loeser JD, Morris DB, eds. *Narrative, Pain, and Suffering*. IASP Press, Seattle, WA. pp. 29–44.

3 Cleeland CS, Ryan KM. (1994) Pain assessment: global use of the Brief Pain Inventory. *Ann Acad Med Singapore* **23(2)**:129–38.

4 Melzack R. (1987) The short-form McGill Pain Questionnaire. *Pain* **30(2)**:191–7.

5 Ware JE Jr, Sherbourne CD. (1992) The MOS 36-item short-form health survey (SF-36). I. Conceptual framework and item selection. *Med Care* **30(6)**:473–83.

6 Melzak R, Katz J, (2005) Pain assessment in adult patients. In: McMahon SB, Koltzenburg M, eds. *Melzack & Wall's Textbook of Pain*, 5th edn. Churchill Livingstone. pp. 291–304.

7 Dworkin RH, Turk DC, Farrar JT *et al.* (2005) Core outcome measures for chronic pain clinical trials: IMMPACT recommendations. *Pain* **113(1–2)**:9–19.

8 MaGee DJ. (2008) *Orthopedic Physical Assessment*, 5th edn. Saunders, St. Louis, MO.

9 Travell JG, Simons DG. (1992) *The Lower Extremities*. Media: Williams and Wilkins.

10 Braddom RL. (2004) In: Peterson AT, Kornbluth I, Marcus DB *et al.* eds. *Handbook of Physical Medicine and Rehabilitation*, 2nd edn. Saunders, Philadelphia, PA.

11 American Psychiatric Association. (1994) *Diagnostic and Statistical Manual of Mental Disorders*. American Psychiatric Association, Washington, DC.

12 Hoppenfeld S. (1976) *Physical Examination of the Spine and Extremities*. Appleton Century Crofts, East Norwalk.

Chapter 8

Measurement and assessment of pain in pediatric patients

Jennifer N. Stinson[1,2,3] & Patrick J. McGrath[4,5]

[1] Child Health Evaluation Sciences, The Hospital for Sick Children, Toronto
[2] Department of Anesthesia and Pain Medicine, The Hospital for Sick Children, Toronto
[3] University of Toronto, Toronto, Ontario
[4] IWK Health Centre
[5] Dalhouse University, Halifax, Nova Scotia

Introduction

This chapter provides an overview of the assessment of pain in children from neonates to adolescents. The difference between pain assessment and pain monitoring is highlighted and the key steps in pain assessment identified. Self-report, behavioral and physiological indicators of pain in children are reviewed. Information about commonly used pain tools is provided and the factors that need to be considered when choosing a pain assessment tool are outlined. Finally, the need for clear documentation about pain assessment and how regularly pain assessment should be undertaken are also discussed.

Assessing pain in children

Pain in children occurs across a spectrum of conditions including everyday pains, acute injuries and medical events, recurrent or chronic pain, and pain related to chronic disease. Pain assessment is the first step in the management of pain. Accurate assessment of children's pain is needed to diagnose medical conditions and to guide pain management interventions [1,2]. To treat pain effectively,

Clinical Pain Management: A Practical Guide, 1st edition.
Edited by Mary E. Lynch, Kenneth D. Craig and
Philip W.H. Peng.
© 2011 Blackwell Publishing Ltd.

ongoing monitoring of the presence and severity of pain and the child's response to treatment is essential.

Pain assessment poses many challenges in infants and children because of: (a) the subjective and complex nature of pain; (b) developmental and language limitations that preclude comprehension and self-report; and (c) dependence on others to infer pain from behavioral and physiological indicators. The important steps in assessing pain in children include:

1 recording a comprehensive pain history;
2 assessing the child's pain using a developmentally appropriate pain assessment tool; and
3 selection of an appropriate intervention [3].

Assessment should be followed by ongoing monitoring of pain, having allowed time for pain-relieving interventions to work. Parents and significant family members know their child best and often can recognize subtle changes in manner or behavior. They have a particularly important role in pain assessment [1].

Pain measurement generally describes the quantification of pain intensity (e.g. "How much does it hurt?"). The emphasis is on the quantity, extent or degree of pain. Pain assessment is a broader concept than measurement and involves clinical judgment based on observation of the nature, significance and context of the child's pain experience [4]. Comprehensive pain assessment involves exploring the intensity of pain, location of pain, its duration, the sensory qualities (e.g. word descriptors), cognitive (e.g. perceived impact of pain on aspects of everyday life) and affective aspects of the pain experience (e.g. pain unpleasantness) [3]. Furthermore, contextual and situational factors that may influence children's perception of pain should also be explored. This helps healthcare professionals to make decisions regarding the most likely cause of the pain (nociceptive, neuropathic or mixed) and to choose the most appropriate intervention.

Obtaining a pain history

Conducting a thorough history of the child's prior pain experiences and current pain complaints is the first step in pain assessment. Standardized pain history forms have been developed for talking with children and parents about the pain [5]. To assess pain of relatively brief duration, instruments measuring pain intensity, location and affect are typically used. For a child with chronic pain, a more detailed pain history needs to be taken that measures the frequency, duration, time course and activity interference due to pain (Table 8.1) [2,3].

Approaches to measuring pain in children

The three approaches to measuring pain are self-report (what the child says), behavioral (how the child behaves) and physiological indicators (how the child's body reacts) [3]. These measures are used separately (unidimensional) or in combination (multidimensional or composite) in a range of pain assessment tools that are available to use in practice. The ideal would be a composite measure including self-report and one or more of these other approaches. However, this approach would not be applicable for preverbal children or non-verbal or cognitively impaired children for whom behavioral observation must be the source for pain measurement [6,7].

Children's self-report of their pain is the preferred approach and should be used with children who are old enough to understand and use self-report scales (e.g. 3 years of age and older) and not overtly distressed [8]. With infants, toddlers, preverbal, cognitively impaired and sedated children who are unable to self-report, an appropriate behavioral or composite pain assessment tool should be used. If the child is overtly distressed, no meaningful self-report can be obtained at that point in time. The child's pain can be estimated using a behavioral pain assessment tool until such time as the child is less distressed [6].

Tools for assessing pain in children

In adults, pain intensity is most often assessed by asking patients to rate their pain on a numerical rating scale, with 0 indicating no pain and 10 indicating the worst pain possible. Because of children's more limited understanding of number concepts, a variety of other rating scales have been developed.

Self-report tools

The types of self-report tools that have been designed for use with school-aged children and adolescent are outlined below. For a more in-depth review of self-report measures and their psychometric properties see the two reviews by Cohen *et al.* [2] and Stinson *et al.* [8].

Faces pain scales

Faces pain scales present the child with drawings or photographs of facial expressions representing increasing levels of pain intensity. The child is asked to select the picture of a face that best represents their pain intensity and their score is the number of the expression chosen. Faces scales have been well validated for use in children aged 5–12 years [8]. There are two types of faces scales: line drawings (e.g. Faces Pain Scale – Revised [9]) and photographs. Faces pain scales with a happy and smiling no pain face or faces with tears for most pain possible have been found to affect the pain scores recorded [8]. Therefore, faces pain scales with neutral expressions for no pain are generally recommended [8].

Table 8.1 Pain history questions for children with chronic pain and their parents/caregivers.

Description of pain	**Type of pain** *Is the pain acute (e.g. postoperative pain), recurrent (e.g. headaches) or chronic (e.g. arthritis)?* **Onset of pain** *When did the pain begin? What were you doing before the pain began? Was there any initiating injury, trauma or stressors?* **Duration** *How long has the pain been present* (e.g. hours/days/weeks/months)? **Frequency** *How often is pain present? Is the pain always there or is it intermittent? Does it come and go?* **Location** *Where is the pain located? Can you point to the part of the body that hurts?* (Body outlines can be used to help children indicate where they hurt). *Does the pain go anywhere else* (e.g. radiates up or down from the site that hurts)? Pain radiation can also be indicated on body diagrams. **Intensity** *What is your pain intensity at rest? What is your pain intensity with activity?* *Over the past week what is the least pain you have had? What is the worst pain you have had? What is your usual level of pain?* **Quality of pain** School-aged children can communicate about pain in more abstract terms. *Describe the quality of your pain* (e.g. word descriptors such as sharp, dull, stabbing, burning, throbbing). Word descriptors can provide information on whether the pain is nociceptive or neuropathic in nature or a combination of both.
Associated symptoms	*Are there any other symptoms that go along with or occur just before or immediately after the pain* (e.g. nausea, vomiting, tiredness or difficulty ambulating)? *Are there any changes in the color or temperature of the affected extremity or painful area?* (These changes most often occur in children with conditions such as complex regional pain syndromes).
Temporal or seasonal variations	*Is the pain affected by changes in seasons or weather?* *Does the pain occur at certain times of the day?*
Impact on daily living	*Has the pain led to changes in daily activities and/or behaviors* (e.g. sleep disturbances, change in appetite or mood, decreased physical activity, social interactions or school attendance)? *What level would the pain need to be so that you could do all your normal activities* (e.g. tolerability)? *What level would the pain need to be so that you won't be bothered by it?* (Rated on similar scale as pain intensity.) *What brings on the pain or makes the pain worse* (e.g. movement, stress, etc.)?
Pain relief measures	*What has helped to make the pain better?* *What medication have you taken to relieve your pain? If so what was the medication and did it help? Were there any side effects?* It is important to also ask about the use of physical, psychological and complementary and alternative treatments tried and how effective these methods were in relieving pain (Chapter 5). The degree of pain relief or intensity of pain after a pain-relieving treatment/intervention should be determined.

Source: Stinson J. (2009) [3]. Reproduced with permission.

Numerical pain scales

A numerical rating scale (NRS) consists of a range of numbers (e.g. 0–10 or 0–100) which can be represented in verbal or graphic format. Children are told that the lowest number represents no pain and the highest number represents the most pain possible. The child is instructed to circle, record or state the number that best represents their level of pain intensity. Verbal NRS tend to be the most frequently used pain intensity measure with children over 8 years of age in clinical practice. They have the advantage that they can be verbally administered without a print copy and are easy to score. They do require numeracy skills and therefore should only be used in older school-aged children and adolescents. While there is evidence of their reliability and validity in adults, verbal NRS have undergone very little testing in children [8]. Von Baeyer et al. [10] recently reported on datasets from three studies on acute pain in which the NRS was used together with another self-report scale and conclude that use of the NRS is tentatively supported for clinical practice with children of 8 years and older.

Graphic rating scales

The most commonly used graphic rating scale is the Pieces of Hurt Tool. This tool consists of four red poker chips, representing a little hurt to the most hurt you could ever have. The child is asked to select the chip that represents his/her pain intensity and the tool is scored from 0 to 4. The Pieces of Hurt Tool has been well validated for acute procedural and hospital-based pains and is recommended for use in young preschool children. The Pieces of Hurt Tool is easy to use and score and the instructions have been translated into several languages. Drawbacks to its use include cleaning the chips between patient use and the potential for losing chips [11].

Visual analog scales

Visual analog scales (VAS) require the child to select a point on a vertical or horizontal line where the ends of the line are defined as the extreme limits of pain intensity. The child is asked to make a mark along the line to indicate the intensity of their pain. There are many versions of VAS for use with children. In addition, creative strategies have been employed to improve the reliability and validity of VAS for use in children by using graphic (color analog scales) or other methods to enhance the child's understanding of the measure. VAS have been extensively researched and have been recommended for most children aged 8 years and older [8]. While VAS are easy to reproduce, photocopying may alter length of line and they require the extra step of measuring the line which increases the burden and likelihood for errors.

Verbal rating scales

Verbal rating scales (VRS) consist of a list of simple word descriptors or phases to denote varying degrees or intensities of pain. Each word or phrase has an associated number. Children are asked to select a single word or phrase that best represents their level of pain intensity and the score is the number associated with the chosen word. One example of a VRS is using word descriptors of not at all = 0, a little bit = 1, quite a lot = 2 and most hurt possible = 3 [3].

Multidimensional pain tools

Although pain intensity is the most commonly recorded measure of a painful episode, a more comprehensive pain assessment is often necessary for children with recurrent or chronic pain. In this situation it is necessary to assess factors such as pain triggers, types of sensations that are experienced and how the pain interferes with aspects of everyday life. More recently, the Bath pain questionnaire was developed to assess the impact of chronic pain on the range of pertinent psychosocial functions [12]. The self-report measure consists of 61 items that cover seven domains of functioning affected by pain: social functioning, physical functioning, depression, general anxiety, pain-specific anxiety, family functioning and development. There is beginning evidence of the reliability and validity of this measure and a parent version of this tool has been developed and tested.

Behavioral tools

The tools developed to assess pain in infants and young children generally use behavioral indicators of pain. A wide range of specific expressive behaviors have been identified in infants and young children that are indicative of pain: individual behaviors (e.g. crying and facial expression); large movements (e.g. withdrawal of the affected limb, touching the affected area, and tensing of limbs and torso); changes in social behavior or appetite; and changes in sleep–wake state or cognitive functions [6,7,13].

Observational tools are indicated for children who are too young to understand and use self-report scales (<4 years); too distressed to use self-report scales; impaired in their cognitive or communicative abilities; very restricted by bandages, surgical tape, mechanical ventilation or paralyzing drugs; whose self-report ratings are considered to be exaggerated, minimized or unrealistic due to cognitive, emotional or situational factors [6].

Physiological indicators

Neonates and children clearly display metabolic, hormonal and physiological responses to pain. These physiological reactions all indicate the activation of the sympathetic nervous system, which is part of the autonomic nervous system, and is responsible for the fight or flight response associated with stress. Physiological changes can include changes in heart rate, respiratory rate, blood pressure, oxygen saturation, sweating and dilated pupils. These indicators usually reflect stress reactions and are only loosely correlated with self-report of pain. They can occur in response to other states such as exertion, fever and anxiety or in response to medications. On their own, physiological indicators do not constitute a valid clinical pain measure for children [6]. A multidimensional or composite measure that incorporates physiological and behavioral indicators, as well as self-report is therefore preferred whenever possible [6,7,13].

Pain assessment tools for neonates

Several pain assessment tools combine behavioral and physiological indicators as well as contextual factors (e.g. gestational age, sleep–wake state) for assessing pain in neonates. The Premature Infant Pain Profile (PIPP) has been the most rigorously validated of these measures [14]. Facial activity has been the most comprehensively studied behavioral pain assessment measure in neonates. It is the most reliable and consistent indicator of pain across populations and types of pain. The facial actions associated with acute pain in neonates include bulging brow, eyes squeezed tightly shut, deepening of nasolabial furrow, open lips, mouth stretched vertically and horizontally and taut tongue [7]. For a more in-depth review of the assessment of pain in neonates and infants see Stevens *et al.* [7].

Pain assessment in cognitively delayed children

Infants and children with cognitive impairment or developmental delay who are unable to report pain may be at greater risk for under-treatment of pain. Pain experienced by these children is particularly difficult to assess accurately. While these children are generally unable to report pain, credible assessment can usually be obtained from the parent or another person who knows the child well [2,7]. Behavioral cues used to identify pain in neurologically impaired children include facial expression, vocalizations, changes in posture and movements, physiological changes, alterations in sleeping and eating, and change in mood and sociability. The most well-validated measure is the Non-Communicating Children's Pain Checklist – Revised [15]. For more detailed information about the assessment of pain in cognitively delayed children see Chapter 39 and Oberlander & Symons [16].

Other approaches for assessing pain in children

Pain diaries in which children track their pain can be either paper or electronic. While paper-based

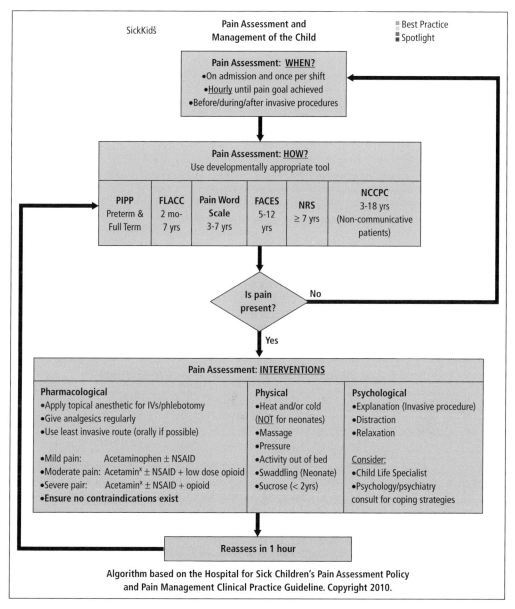

Figure 8.1 Example of an organization-specific pain assessment algorithm. Reproduced with permission.

diaries have been used in clinical and research practice for decades, they are prone to recall biases and poor compliance. More recently, real-time data collection methods using electronic handheld diaries have been developed which allow patients to report how they feel at that time, minimizing recall bias and improving compliance. Despite their appeal, few studies have examined their use in children with recurrent and chronic pain [17]. Electronic pain diaries need to be comprehensively studied in children, with particular attention given to how developmental issues (age and developmental stage) influence the usability, feasibility (acceptability and compliance) and validity of these measures [17].

Choosing the right pain assessment measure

There are many reliable, valid and clinically useful pain assessment tools for assessing pain in neonates, infants [7,13], children and adolescents [2,8]. However, no easily administered, widely accepted, uniform technique exists for assessing pain for all children [3]. Perhaps the most important consideration is to choose a single set of tools for a given institution and then to use these tools consistently. Organizations should develop clinical practice guidelines that clearly outline the tools that should be used for each age group (see Figure 8.1 for an example of the clinical practice guidelines for assessing pain in children developed by the Hospital for Sick Children [18]).

Frequency of pain assessment and documentation

Effective pain management depends on regular assessment of the presence and severity of pain and the patient's response to pain management interventions. Every patient should have their pain assessed: (a) on admission to hospital; (b) when they visit an emergency department; (c) at least once per shift (if they are an inpatient); (d) before, during and after an invasive procedure; and (e) at each office visit for ambulatory care. Pain should be assessed very regularly following surgery and/or if the patient has a known painful medical condition. Pain should be assessed hourly for the first 6 hours. After this, if the pain is well controlled it can be assessed less frequently (e.g. every 4 hours). If the pain is fluctuating, regular assessment should continue for 48–72 hours; after this the pain intensity will normally have peaked and be starting to subside [3,19].

Regular assessment and documentation facilitates effective treatment and communication among members of the healthcare team, patient and family. Pain is considered to be the fifth vital sign and therefore should be assessed and documented along with the other vital signs. Putting mechanisms in place that make documentation of pain easy for clinicians helps ensure consistent documentation. Standardized forms/tools for the documentation of pain allow for the initial assessment and ongoing reassessment. They can also be used for the documentation of the efficacy of pain-relieving interventions. Including pain intensity as part of the vital signs record allows for pain to be assessed, documented and taken as seriously as other vital signs [3,19].

Conclusions

Pain assessment is vital for effective pain management. The first step in assessing pain is recording a pain history. The second step in pain assessment is assessing the child's pain using a developmentally appropriate pain assessment tool. The third step is monitoring the effectiveness of the pain-relieving interventions used or implemented. Validated and reliable pain assessment tools are available for children of all ages. However, no individual tool can be broadly recommended for pain assessment in all children and across all contexts. The child's self-report of pain is considered the gold standard for those who are able self-report. Physiological, behavioral and self-report indicators can all be used to assess children's pain. Pain should be assessed regularly to detect the presence of pain and to evaluate the effectiveness of treatments. Finally, documentation of pain facilitates regular reassessment of pain and enhances communication about a patient's pain to all members of the multidisciplinary care team.

References

1 Moon E, McMurtry M, McGrath PJ. (2008) Assessment of pain in children. In: Hunsley J, Mash EJ, eds. *A Guide to Assessments That Work*. Oxford University Press, New York. pp. 51–575.

2 Cohen LL, Lemanek K, Blount RL *et al.* (2008) Evidence-based assessment of pediatric pain. *J Pediatr Psychol* **33**:939–55.

3 Stinson J. (2009) Pain assessment. In: Twycross A, Bruce L, Dowden S, eds. *Managing Pain in Children: A Clinical Guide*. Wiley-Blackwell, Oxford. pp. 85–108.

4 Johnston CC. (1998) Psychometric issues in the measurement of pain. In: Finley GA, McGrath PJ, eds. *Measurement of Pain in Infants and Children*. IASP Press, Seattle, WA. pp. 5–21.

5 Acute Pain Management Guideline Panel. (1992) *Acute Pain Management in Infants, Children, and Adolescents: Operative and Medical Procedures – Quick Reference Guide for Clinicians*. AHCPR No. 92-0020. Agency for Health Care Policy and Research, Public Health Service, US Department of Health and Human Services, Rockville, MD.

6 von Baeyer C, Spagrud LJ. (2007) Systematic review of observational (behavioral) measures of pain for children and adolescents aged 3 to 18 years. *Pain* **127**:140–50.

7 Stevens BJ, Pillai Riddell RR, Oberlander TE *et al.* (2007) Assessment of pain in neonates and infants. In: Anand KJS, Stevens BJ, McGrath PJ, eds. *Pain in Neonates and Infants*, 3rd edn. Elsevier, Edinburgh. pp. 67–90.

8 Stinson JN, Kavanagh T, Yamada J *et al.* (2006) Systematic review of the psychometric properties, interpretability and feasibility of self-report pain intensity measures for use in clinical trials in children and adolescents. *Pain* **125**:143–57.

9 Hicks CL, von Baeyer CL, Spafford PA *et al.* (2001) The Faces Pain Scale – Revised: toward a common metric in pediatric pain measurement. *Pain* **93**:173–83.

10 von Baeyer CL, Spagrud LJ, McCormick JC *et al.* (2009) Three new datasets supporting use of the Numerical Rating Scale (NRS-11) for children's self-reports of pain intensity. *Pain* **143**:223–7.

11 Hester N, Foster R, Kristensen K. (1990) Measurement of pain in children: generalizability and validity of the pain ladder and poker chip tool. *Adv Pain Res Ther* **15**:79–84.

12 Eccleston E, Jordan A, McCrackena LM *et al.* (2005) The Bath Adolescent Pain Questionnaire (BAPQ): development and preliminary psychometric evaluation of an instrument to assess the impact of chronic pain on adolescents. *Pain* **118**:263–70.

13 Duhn LJ, Medves JM. (2004) A systematic integrative review of infant pain assessment tools. *Adv Neonatal Care* **4**:126–40.

14 Stevens B, Johnston C, Petryshen P *et al.* (1996) Premature Infant Pain Profile: development and initial validation. *Clin J Pain* **12**:13–22.

15 Breau LM, McGrath PJ, Camfield C *et al.* (2002) Psychometric properties of the Non-communicating Children's Pain Checklist – Revised. *Pain* **99**:349–57.

16 Oberlander TF, Symons F. (2006) *Pain in Children and Adults with Developmental Disabilities*. Paul H. Brookes, Baltimore, MD.

17 Stinson JN. (2009) Improving the assessment of pediatric chronic pain: harnessing the potential of electronic dairies. *Pain Res Manag* **14**:59–64.

18 The Hospital for Sick Children. (2008) *Pain Assessment and Management of the Child: Pain Assessment Policy and Pain Management Clinical Practice Guidelines*. The Hospital for Sick Children, Toronto.

19 Clinical Practice Guidelines. (2009) *The Recognition and Assessment of Acute Pain in Children: Update of Full Guideline*. Royal College of Nursing, London.

Acknowledgments

Dr. Stinson's work is supported by an Ontario Ministry of Health and Long-term Career Scientist Award. Dr. McGrath's work is supported by a Canada Research Chair.

Chapter 9

Laboratory investigations, imaging and neurological assessment in pain management

Pam Squire[1], David Walk[2], Gordon Irving[3] & Misha Bačkonja[4]

[1] University of British Columbia, Vancouver, Canada
[2] Department of Neurology, University of Minnesota, Minneapolis, USA
[3] University of Washington Medical School, Seattle, USA
[4] Department of Neurology, University of Wisconsin, Madison, USA

General principles

No test shows pain. Currently, there are no clinically useful biomarkers for pain, nor can imaging or any other technique localize or characterize pain. Furthermore, chronic pain is usually a multifactorial problem. In a patient with chronic low back pain, for example, contributing factors may include degenerative joint disease, root entrapment, myofascial pain, muscle deconditioning, central sensitization, and the effects of mood and psychosocial circumstances. For this reason pain must be evaluated in a multidimensional context, including the medical diagnosis, or diagnoses, most directly responsible for the pain complaint, medical and psychological comorbidities, and the social and occupational context [1].

Many patients present with pain that is poorly correlated with clinical findings and clinical investigations that are negative or non-diagnostic. One of the essential roles of the pain practitioner is to

care for patients with either no identifiable source of pain or sustained pain despite treatment of an identified source of pain. Clinicians must recognize when the cost of further investigation exceeds diminishing returns.

Diagnostic studies provide supportive evidence for a clinical diagnosis but are not pathognomonic. Investigations must always be interpreted in the clinical context. This chapter reviews common laboratory, imaging and neurological investigations for assessment of patients with chronic pain disorders.

Common laboratory, imaging and neurological investigations for the patient with chronic pain

Laboratory investigations

Laboratory studies are conducted to identify disorders that could be primary or contributory causes of a chronic pain disorder. Relatively few laboratory studies contribute substantially to the diagnosis of painful conditions. Inflammatory markers may be among the most important.

Erythrocyte sedimentation rate (ESR) and C-reactive protein (CRP) are acute phase reactants

Clinical Pain Management: A Practical Guide, 1st edition.
Edited by Mary E. Lynch, Kenneth D. Craig and
Philip W.H. Peng.
© 2011 Blackwell Publishing Ltd.

that function as relatively non-specific indicators of a systemic inflammatory response. ESR is usually, but not universally, elevated in polymyalgia rheumatica, and CRP is often elevated in this condition as well [2]. Both ESR and CRP are commonly used as markers of active rheumatoid arthritis [3]. Active inflammatory processes that consume complement can be identified by a reduction in circulating complement (C3, C4) levels. Hepatitis C antibody testing is warranted in individuals with unexplained polyarticular pain and idiopathic neuropathy, particularly if clinical or laboratory evidence of hepatic disease is present [4].

Sjögren's syndrome is an inflammatory disorder that is probably under-recognized and is commonly associated with widespread pain as well as pain from associated sensory neuropathy [5]. Dry eyes and dry mouth (sicca symptoms) are the fundamental clinical feature. Diagnostic criteria include a combination of clinical, paraclinical and laboratory parameters including autoantibodies against Ro (SS-A) and/or La (SS-B) antigens [6]. Many patients who fulfill criteria are seronegative. Nonetheless, Sjögren's antibody testing should be obtained in patients with unexplained myofascial or neuropathic pain and sicca symptoms.

Vasculitides can present with unexplained pain, from diffuse aches and pains that are difficult to pinpoint to more specific pain from nerve infarction or gastrointestinal ischemia. Protoplasmic or classic staining antineutrophil cytoplasmic antibodies (p-ANCA and c-ANCA) are more specific markers of systemic vasculitides. c-ANCA is a highly sensitive marker for Wegener's granulomatosis, polyarteritis nodosa and Churg–Strauss vasculitis, while p-ANCA is a sensitive marker for vasculitis due to systemic lupus erythematosus, rheumatoid arthritis and Sjögren's syndrome. Vasculitis is a tissue diagnosis and must be confirmed pathologically; however, these serologic markers can be helpful in providing justification for tissue biopsy and, on occasion, therapeutic intervention pending a tissue diagnosis in the appropriate clinical setting.

There is a strong correlation between spondyloarthritis (a spectrum of conditions including ankylosing spondylitis and reactive arthritis) and HLA B27 positivity. HLA B27 testing can be very helpful in patients with an appropriate clinical syndrome, particularly if imaging studies are non-diagnostic (see below).

Many rheumatological conditions, such as rheumatoid arthritis, cause chronic multifocal or widespread pain on the basis of inflammatory joint and connective tissue disease. These are diagnosed principally on the basis of clinical criteria with laboratory support.

The following laboratory abnormalities are occasionally obtained, with little evidence of value, in chronic pain states:

• There is, to our knowledge, no compelling evidence that evaluating thyroid function, serum cortisol or growth hormone levels is of value in the investigation of fibromyalgia [7].

• It has been proposed that reduced levels of 1,25-OH vitamin D can be responsible for a reversible widespread pain syndrome, although the evidence supporting this assertion is modest [8].

• Creatine phosphokinase (CPK) is commonly elevated in inflammatory muscle disease, but these conditions are usually painless. CPK is normal in myofascial pain syndromes.

To date neither biomarkers for pain, such as substance P or other inflammatory cytokines, nor known genetic information (such as the role of the pain protecting haplotype for guanosine triphosphate [GTP] cyclohydrolase 1) [9], can be used as independent indicators of pain or the transition from acute to chronic pain [10].

Imaging studies

X-rays

X-rays are inexpensive, readily available in any medical facility and can provide information about the skeletal system but provide little information about soft tissues. They remain useful investigations to demonstrate degenerative changes in joints, pathologic fractures, diffuse idiopathic skeletal hyperostosis (DISH), scoliosis, tumors with osseous involvement, or calcified tendons or cystic and sclerotic changes where tendons insert into bone.

Computed tomography scan

Computed tomography (CT) scan is a two-dimensional gray-scale representation of the relative densities of tissues usually acquired axially. CT can provide information regarding both bony structures and soft tissues. Three-dimensional reconstructions are possible as are multiplanar images that reconstruct axial slices into three-dimensional images. The main limitation of CT scanning is that it may provide a significant dose of radiation and does not visualize soft tissues as well as magnetic resonance imaging (MRI). CT scanning, often with contrast, may be the investigation of choice when MRI scanning is contraindicated.

Magnetic resonance imaging

Magnetic resonance imaging (MRI) evaluates soft tissues such as discs, tendons, ligaments, cartilage and nerve roots and is sensitive for imaging tumors. A non-contrast MRI is sufficient in the majority of cases. The addition of intravenous gadolinium allows better imaging of infection, tumor or fibrosis. MRI scans are not good for showing bony cortex architecture because bone cortex has little water content and hence appears as black on MRI scans. MRI scans can show change in marrow signal and can demonstrate bone marrow edema, a non-specific finding associated with a variety of painful conditions including insufficiency or fatigue fractures, inflammatory or ischemic disorders, degenerative conditions such as osteoarthritis, cartilage defects, tendon abnormalities and complex regional pain syndrome but this is only a surrogate marker of bony cortex architecture. MRI cannot diagnose osteoporosis but quantitative CT (QCT) scanning can be used to evaluate bone density. MRI is more sensitive than bone scan for detection of vertebral compression fractures but CT scans are the investigations of choice for demonstrating abnormalities within bone, a radiodense material.

MRI has a few important limitations. First, the strong magnetic field precludes investigation of patients with metallic fragments in the eye, pacemakers, cochlear implants or some intracranial vascular clips. Most metal placed as part of orthopedic procedures, including spine procedures, is considered permissible. Administration of gadolinium-containing MRI contrast agents should be avoided in patients with moderately or severely impaired renal function (e.g. estimated glomerular filtration rate <15–30 mL/min).

Myelography and post-myelogram CT

Myelography and post-myelogram CT scanning allows visualization of bony structures and neural elements and are indicated when both are needed and MRI is contraindicated. Myelography and upright MRI scanning enable imaging of the thecal sac and emerging nerve roots while weight-bearing and/or while performing flexion–extension movements. If an infiltrative, malignant or infectious process is being considered, cerebrospinal fluid should be withdrawn for analysis during the procedure.

Nuclear imaging

Nuclear imaging involves detection of gamma radiation produced either as the direct result of radioactive decay (e.g. ^{99m}Tc) or positron-electron annihilation (e.g. ^{15}O).

Bone scanning

Bone scanning uses technetium agents that affix to the bone surface by attaching to the hydroxyapatite crystals in bone and calcium crystals in mitochondria. Tracer is increased locally where there is new bone formation because these regions are hyperemic, and increased blood flow exposes the bone to more tracer over a given period of time. Bone scanning can be very sensitive but not very specific, as fractures, degenerative disease and other benign findings may also produce a positive scan and up to 40% of positive findings occur at sites that are asymptomatic. Painful lesions identified by bone scanning include malignancies, prosthetic loosening in a cemented prosthesis (a normal bone scan essentially rules out prosthetic complications), pars defects and complex regional pain syndrome (CRPS), although the yield in early CRPS is limited.

Single photon emission computed tomography

Single photon emission computed tomography (SPECT) scanning allows three-dimensional views and may improve the localization and characterization of an image. SPECT of known facet joint disease may help to predict which patients are most likely to respond to facet joint injections [11].

Positron emission tomography

Positron emission tomography (PET) scanning is based on the principle that specific radio-labeled tracers can bind to specific receptors on various tissues, and depending on which tissue and its metabolic step is being studied highly specific tracers are produced. Synthesis of tracers is technologically very involved and available only at imaging centers that specialize in nuclear imaging. PET scanning is most useful in differentiation of malignant and non-malignant lesions but otherwise has limited use in pain management. False positive results are generally due to metabolically active infectious or inflammatory lesions such as granulomas (fungal or tuberculous) or rheumatoid nodules and are more common than false negative results [12]. PET scanning will have a lower specificity in areas where these types of infection are endemic.

Neurological investigations

Electromyography

Electromyography (EMG) is performed by recording spontaneous discharges of muscle cells, indicative of muscle disease or denervation, and the configuration and firing pattern of motor unit potentials, which represent the coordinated discharge of muscle cells all innervated by a common motor neuron. Nerve conduction studies (NCS) are performed by passing a depolarizing current through individual named nerves and recording the evoked nerve action potential, in the case of sensory conduction studies, or the compound muscle action potential (response from muscle) in the case of motor conduction studies. EMG/NCS is highly sensitive at addressing the following questions:

- Is nerve or muscle disease present?
- In the case of nerve disease, is the primary process a disorder of axons or myelin?
- Does the condition involve motor nerves, sensory nerves, or both?
- What is the localization and distribution of the process?

Examples of pain states that can be reliably identified by NCS/EMG include radiculopathy, plexopathy, multifocal polyneuropathy, distal symmetric polyneuropathy and sensory neuropathy.

EMG/NCS has the following limitations:

- EMG/NCS only evaluates large myelinated axons. Because neuropathic pain is often due to disease of small myelinated Aδ and C fibers, EMG/NCS can be normal in patients whose condition principally affects these "small fibers." Approximately 30% of diabetic neuropathies can be small fiber neuropathies and will have a normal EMG/NCS [13]. Small fiber neuropathy can be assessed functionally with quantitative sensory testing and confirmed pathologically with determination of epidermal nerve fiber density (see below). Until these modalities became available, there was little awareness of the concept of small fiber neuropathy (SFN).
- Not all nerves can be readily studied using this technique. Truncal or inguinal mononeuropathies, for example, are not readily evaluated with EMG/NCS.
- EMG/NCS can be painful, especially in patients who have cutaneous mechanical allodynia and hyperalgesia.
- EMG/NCS provides information about peripheral nerve physiology but not about pain. Many patients with substantial EMG/NCS evidence of neuropathy have no pain, and many patients with normal EMG/NCS studies, particularly those with SFN (see below) have neuropathic pain.

Quantitative sensory testing

Quantitative sensory testing (QST) refers to testing of sensory perception in response to standardized stimuli. The goal of testing is to quantitate both sensory loss (e.g. hypoalgesia or hypoesthesia) and sensory gain (e.g. hyperalgesia, allodynia and hyperpathia) within small and large fiber sensory modalities. Pain QST protocols utilize a broad range of cutaneous stimuli, including brush, punctate, pressure, vibration, warm, cool, painful hot and painful cold. Some stimuli, such as thermal, vibration and punctate stimuli, can be delivered in a graded fashion to allow determination of thresholds for perception of innocuous sensation or pain [14]. Stimulus intensity can also be fixed at a supra-threshold intensity, in which case the patient is asked to rate the perceived intensity of the modality in question [15]. When evaluated in conjunction with typical symptoms of neuropathic pain, demonstration of sensory loss or sensory gain is one defining feature of neuropathic pain. Some QST findings are felt to have specific mechanistic significance. For example, heat hyperalgesia is thought to reflect peripheral sensitization, while dynamic mechanical allodynia (report of pain from innocuous light brushing of the skin) is thought to reflect central sensitization. Abnormal thermal or punctate sensation can provide supportive evidence of SFN when nerve conduction studies, which evaluate large nerve fibers, are normal [16,17].

QST has several limitations at present. First, control values are limited to certain methods and body sites, and data on test–retest reproducibility are inadequate for interpretation of data across time and across centers. Second, the test is a psychophysical evaluation and therefore it is critically dependent on the instruction and training of the subject as well as the person performing QST testing. Patients who are unable (because of neurological conditions such as dementia or intoxication) or unwilling (because of psychological factors) to concentrate or for other reasons are not able to fully participate in testing will provide invalid results. For similar reasons, both patients and personnel performing the test must be adequately trained to perform the testing. The testing should be preceded by standardized instructions to subjects and performed in a designated quiet room without distractions.

Epidermal nerve fiber density

Epidermal nerve fiber density (ENFD) analysis is based on immunostaining a 3-mm punch biopsy of skin for PGP 9.5, a pan-neuronal marker, and quantifying the density of nerve fibers in the epidermis. Epidermal nerves are the terminals of C and Aδ fibers, most of which are nociceptors. ENFD determination provides pathological confirmation of epidermal nerve fiber loss, and is therefore often used to support the diagnosis of neuropathy, particularly when EMG/NCS is normal. Another strength of ENFD is that skin biopsy can be performed in sites where nerve conduction studies are not performed, such as the trunk, and results can be compared with established norms or, if none exist and the contralateral side is clinically unaffected, a control biopsy from the contralateral side of the same patient. Unfortunately, appropriate tissue processing is available in relatively few centers. See Table 9.1 for a list of some laboratories that perform this testing and accept samples from outside institutions.

ENFD determination has proven to be a valuable tool in the diagnosis of neuropathy due to diabetes, impaired glucose tolerance and the metabolic syndrome, HIV infection and Sjögren's syndrome, among others [17–19].

The development of ENFD determination and, to a lesser extent, QST, is largely responsible for a revolution in neuromuscular and pain medicine. Until a short time ago, EMG/NCS was viewed by clinicians as the sine qua non of peripheral nerve diagnosis, and it was commonly assumed that patients with normal EMG/NCS did not have neuropathy. This resulted in a diagnostic and management conundrum for patients with neuropathic pain and normal EMG/NCS studies. It is now well recognized that specific features of neuropathic pain (punctate and thermal sensory deficits in combination with hyperalgesia, allodynia and hyperpathia, as well as spontaneous paresthesias

Table 9.1 Laboratories that perform epidermal nerve fiber density processing.

North America	Josef-Schneider-Str. 11
William R. Kennedy, MD	D-97080 Würzburg
Professor, Department of Neurology	Germany
University of Minnesota	Tel. +49 931 201 23763
MMC 295	Fax +49 931 201 23697
420 Delaware St. S.E.	sommer@uni-wuerzburg.de
Minneapolis MN USA 55455	www.klinik.uni-wuerzburg.de/neurologie
612.624.5131	
kenne001@umn.edu	Dr. Giuseppe Lauria
	Dr. Raffaella Lombardi
Michael Polydefkis, MD MHS	IRCCS. Foundation "Carlo Besta" Neurological Institute
Associate Professor, Department of Neurology	Via Celoria 11
Johns Hopkins Medical Institutions	20133 Milan
Tel 410-502-2909;	Italy
Fax 410-502-5560	Tel +390223942254
mpolyde@jhmi.edu	Fax +390270633874
Contact: Jennie at jichnio1@jhmi.edu	glauria@istituto- besta.it
www.hopkinsmedicine.org/CutaneousNerveLab	Contact: lombardi.r@istituto-besta.it
Therapath	Maria Nolano, MD
545 W. 45th Street	Skin Biopsy Laboratory
New York New York 10036	Neurology Department
Tel 800 681 4338	"S. Maugeri" Foundation
Fax 917 441 9116	Via Bagni Vecchi, 1
LaboratoryServices@Therapath.com	82037 Telese Terme (BN)
	Italy
Europe	Tel. +39 (0)824 909 257
Professor Dr. Claudia Sommer	Fax. +39 (0)824 909 614
Neurologische Klinik	Email: maria.nolano@fsm.it
Universitätsklinikum Würzburg	Email: vincenzo.provitera@fsm.it

and pain) in the absence of other neurological symptoms or signs are a common presentation of what is now known as small fiber neuropathy (SFN), and that EMG/NCS are normal in pure SFN [20]. While there is no "gold standard" for the diagnosis of SFN, it has been proposed that the diagnosis be confirmed by the presence of two of the following three findings: deficits in punctate or thermal sensation on neurological examination, abnormal ENFD and thermal QST abnormalities (Figure 9.1) [21].

Somatosensory evoked potential studies

Somatosensory evoked potential studies (SEPs) are performed by passing a depolarizing current through a peripheral nerve and recording the evoked neural response. Unlike NCS, in which recording electrodes are placed over a peripheral nerve, in SEPs recordings are made over the spine and scalp in order to record traveling and stationary waves evoked by the peripheral stimulus and thereby assess conduction through the somatosensory pathways in the central nervous system. SEPs are delayed or absent in the presence of structural or metabolic pathology in the central nervous system pathways under study. SEPs are the only physiological test of conduction through sensory pathways of the central nervous system, and can be a useful procedure in selected patients with unexplained sensory symptoms and normal peripheral conduction and non-diagnostic imaging studies [22].

The principal limitation of SEPs in the context of pain evaluation is that clinically available SEPs

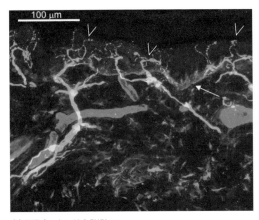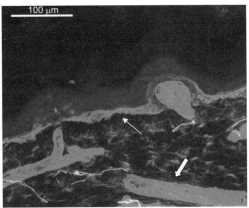

(a) ENF density: 40.3 ENF/mm

QST (°C):		
warm perception threshold	32.9	
cool perception threshold	31.8	
heat pain threshold	40.3	
cold pain threshold	24.9	

(b) ENF density: 0.0 ENF/mm

QST (°C):		Normal
warm perception threshold	48.3	(<40.2)
cool perception threshold	27.8	(>29.2)
heat pain threshold	50	
cold pain threshold	<0	

Figure 9.1 ENFD and QST for evaluation of neuropathic pain due to possible small fiber neuropathy. Both patients presented with spontaneous burning pain and allodynia. Nerve conduction studies and cutaneous perception of touch, vibration and position were normal in both patients. Patient A demonstrated normal threshold determination QST, normal foot ENF density, and both thermal allodynia and multimodality hyperalgesia on suprathreshold QST. She has no evidence of functional or structural neurological deficit. Her symptoms and signs suggest sensitization but the mechanism is unknown. Patient B demonstrated elevated thermal thresholds, reduced foot ENF density, and reduced mechanical and thermal perception in the foot. The diagnosis is small fiber neuropathy.

Dermal and epidermal nerves are stained in white, basement membrane and blood vessels (collagen IV) in gray. Epidermis is at the top of the images. In (a), epidermal nerves (arrowheads) are plentiful, and arise from robust subepidermal nerves. In (b), no epidermal nerves are seen and there is a paucity of dermal innervations as well. Thin arrows: epidermal basement membrane. Thick arrow: dermal arteriole. Normal ENF density is > 12.2 ENF/mm (5th percentile cutoff).

Reference for QST controls: Getz Kelly K, Cook T, Backonja MM. (2005) Pain ratings at the threshold are necessary for quantitative sensory testing. *Muscle Nerve* **32**:179–84.

Reference for skin biopsy technique: Kennedy WR, Wendelschafer-Crabb G, Johnson T. (1996) Quantitation of epidermal nerves in diabetic neuropathy. *Neurology* **47**:1042–8.

evaluate large myelinated fibers and the posterior column-lemniscal system, and therefore do not assess transmission in tracts critical to nociception. To overcome this limitation, several SEP techniques for assessment of the small-fiber-spinothalamic system have been developed in recent years. These include laser evoked potentials (LEPs), contact-heat evoked potentials (CHEPs) and pain-related evoked potentials (PREPs). Like SEPs, these all utilize scalp-recorded evoked potentials; the principal difference is in the nature of the stimulus. LEPs utilize a very brief laser radiant heat pulse to activate A-δ fibers. There is evidence that scalp-recorded LEP amplitudes reflect the integrity of pain processing pathways in the peripheral and central nervous system [23] and may prove useful as a surrogate marker for analgesia [24]. CHEPs use a short pulse of painful heat applied directly to the skin as the stimulus or painful stimulus. The amplitude of the CHEPs scalp-evoked response has been shown to correlate with perceived pain intensity in normal subjects [25]. A CHEPs device is commercially available (Medoc Ltd., Ramat Yishai, Israel). PREPs use a small electrical stimulus with high current density to depolarize cutaneous afferents, and has been used in studies of HIV neuropathy [26]. While these are all emerging techniques, their promise lies in their ability to assess both central and peripheral pain pathways and their putative correlation with perceived pain intensity. It is hoped that pain-evoked potentials, in combination with ENF density, QST and pain questionnaires, will contribute to a powerful comprehensive assessment of pain peripheral anatomy, psychophysics and neurophysiology.

Magnetic resonance neurography and peripheral nerve ultrasonography

Magnetic resonance neurography (MRN) and peripheral nerve ultrasonography are emerging techniques for imaging individual peripheral nerves for identification of localized structural abnormalities, such as edema, focal entrapment or hypertrophy due to infiltration or demyelination [27,28]. MRN in particular holds promise as a diagnostic adjunct in conditions affecting proximal nerve segments, where the value of EMG/NCS is limited in some cases.

Interventional diagnostic procedures

Diagnostic neural blockade

Diagnostic neural blockade are usually fluoroscopic, CT or ultrasound guided injections that are used to demonstrate the contribution of a particular anatomic structure (e.g. facet, nerve or disc) in the evaluation of pain. The role of diagnostic blockade in the investigation of chronic pain is discussed in detail in Chapter 19.

Conclusions

In summary, chronic pain is a biopsychosocial phenomenon and no test shows pain. Pain clinicians must be prepared to care for their patients with either no identifiable source of pain or sustained pain despite treatment for an identified source of pain.

Nonetheless, there are a number of imaging and neurological investigations as well as specific diagnostic procedures that may assist in the overall assessment of the patient presenting with chronic pain. Currently available tests have been presented along with developing technologies such as QST, ENFD and SEPs.

References

1 Backonja M, Argoff C. (2005) Neuropathic pain-definition and implications for research and therapy. *J Neuropathic Pain Symptom Palliation* **1(2)**:11–17. Available online at http://www.haworthpress.com/web/JNPSP

2 Cantini, F, Salvarani, C, Olivieri, I. (1998) Erythrocyte sedimentation rate and C-reactive protein in the diagnosis of polymyalgia rheumatica. *Ann Intern Med* **128**:873.

3 Donald F, Ward MM. (1998) Evaluative laboratory testing practices of United States rheumatologists. *Arthritis Rheum* **41**:725–9.

4 Sharara AI, Hunt CM, Hamilton JD. (1996) Hepatitis C. *Ann Intern Med* **125**:658–68.

5 Segal B, Carpenter A, Walk D. (2008) Involvement of nervous system pathways in primary Sjögren's syndrome. *Rheum Dis Clin North Am* **34(4)**:885–906.

6 Vitali C, Bombardieri S, Jonsson R *et al.* (2002) Classification criteria for Sjögren's syndrome: a revised version of the European criteria proposed by the American-European Consensus Group. *Ann Rheum Dis* **61**:554–8.

7 Geenen R, Jacobs JW, Bijlsma JW. (2002) Evaluation and management of endocrine dysfunction in fibromyalgia. *Rheum Dis Clin North Am* **8(2)**:389–404.

8 Straube S, Moore RA, Derry S. (2009) Vitamin D and chronic pain. *Pain* **141**:10–13.

9 Tegeder I, Costigan M, Griffin RS *et al.* (2006) GTP cyclohydrolase and tetrahydrobiopterin regulate pain sensitivity and persistence. *Nat Med* **12**:1269–77.

10 Mao J. (2009) Translational pain research: achievements and challenges. *J Pain* **10(10)**: 1001–11.

11 Pneumaticos SG, Chatziioannou SN, Hipp JA *et al.* (2006) Low back pain: prediction of short term outcome of facet joint injection with bone scintigraphy. *Radiology* **238**:693.

12 Casey KL, Bushnell MC. (2000) Pain Imaging. *IASP* Press, Seattle, WA.

13 England JD, Gronseth GS, Franklin G *et al.* (2009) Practice Parameter: evaluation of distal symmetric polyneuropathy. Role of autonomic testing, nerve biopsy, and skin biopsy (an evidence-based review). Report of the American Academy of Neurology, American Association of Neuromuscular and Electrodiagnostic Medicine, and American Academy of Physical Medicine and Rehabilitation. *Neurology* **72(2)**: 177–84.

14 Rolke R, Magerl W, Andrews CK *et al.* (2006) Quantitative sensory testing: a comprehensive protocol for clinical trials. *Eur J Pain* **10**:77–88.

15 Walk D, Sehgal N, Moeller-Bertram T *et al.* (2009) Quantitative sensory testing and mapping: a review of nonautomated quantitative methods for examination of the patient with neuropathic pain. *Clin J Pain* **25(7)**:632–40.

16 Hansson P, Backonja M, Bouhassira D. (2007) Usefulness and limitations of quantitative sensory testing: clinical and research application in neuropathic pain states. *Pain* **129**: 256–9.

17 Dyck PJ, Dyck PJ, Larson TS *et al.* (2000) Patterns of quantitative sensation testing of hypoesthesia and hyperalgesia are predictive of diabetic polyneuropathy: a study of three cohorts. Nerve Growth Factor Study Group. *Diabetes Care* **23**:510–7.

18 Smith AG, Rose K, Singleton JR: (2008) Idiopathic neuropathy patients are at high risk for metabolic syndrome. *J Neurol Sci* **273**:25–8.

19 Zhou L, Kitch DW, Evans SR *et al.* (2007) Correlates of epidermal nerve fiber densities in HIV-associated distal sensory polyneuropathy. *Neurology* **68**:2113–9.

20 Vlčková-Moravcová E, Bednařík J, Ladislav D *et al.* (2008) Diagnostic validity of epidermal nerve fiber densities in painful sensory neuropathies. *Muscle Nerve* **37**:50–60.

21 Devigili G, Tugnoli V, Penza P *et al.* (2008) The diagnostic criteria for small fibre neuropathy: from symptoms to neuropathology. *Brain* **131**:1912–25.

22 Walk D, Zaretskaya M, Parry GJ. (2003) Symptom duration and clinical features in painful sensory neuropathy with and without nerve conduction abnormalities. *J Neurol Sci* **214**:3–6.

23 Treede RD, Lorenz J, Baumgärtner U. (2003) Clinical usefulness of laser-evoked potentials. *Neurophysiol Clin* **33(6)**:303–14.

24 Truini A, Panuccio G, Galeotti F *et al.* (2010) Laser-evoked potentials as a tool for assessing the efficacy of antinociceptive drugs. *Eur J Pain* **14(2)**:222–5.

25 Granovsky Y, Granot M, Nir RR *et al.* (2008) Objective correlate of subjective pain perception by contact heat-evoked potentials. *J Pain* **9**:53–63.

26 Katsarava Z, Yaldizli O, Voulkoudis C *et al.* (2006) Pain related potentials by electrical stimulation of skin for detection of small-fiber neuropathy in HIV. *J Neurol* **253**:1581–4.

27 Filler A. (2009) Magnetic resonance neurography and diffusion tensor imaging: origins, history, and clinical impact of the first 50,000 cases with an assessment of efficacy and utility in a prospective 5000-patient study group. *Neurosurgery* **65**:29–43.

28 Koenig RW, Pedro MT, Heinen CPG *et al.* (2009) High-resolution ultrasonography in evaluating peripheral nerve entrapment and trauma. *Neurosurg Focus* **26(2)**:E13.

Acknowledgments

The authors thank Dr. Owen Williamson and Dr. Rob DeCosta for their extremely valuable comments.

Chapter 10

Psychological assessment of persons with chronic pain

Robert N. Jamison[1] & Kenneth D. Craig[2]

[1] Departments of Anesthesia and Psychiatry, Brigham and Women's Hospital, Harvard Medical School, Chestnut Hill, USA
[2] Department of Psychology, University of British Columbia, Vancouver, Canada

Introduction

A number of psychological and social risk factors have been identified that correlate with greater risk for pain severity and longevity as well as poorer outcomes from treatment of pain: pain chronicity, psychological distress, a history of abuse or trauma, poor social support and significant cognitive dysfunction and deficits [1]. In particular, psychopathology and/or extreme emotionality have been recognized as contraindications for certain therapies [2]. Outcome studies highlight poor response to treatment among patients with psychiatric comorbidity, with this prevalent among persons with chronic pain. For example, spinal pain patients with both anxiety and depression have a 62% worse return-to-work rate than those with no psychopathology. Similarly, cognitive processes such as maladaptive beliefs and pessimistic expectations are associated with poorer functional outcomes among patients with chronic low back pain [3].

Psychological assessment is designed to identify problematic emotional reactions, maladaptive thinking and behavior, and social problems that contribute to pain and disability. When psychosocial issues are identified, treatment can be tailored to addressing these challenges in the patient's life, thereby improving the likelihood and speed of recovery and prevention of ongoing or more severe problems.

There are many theoretical and empirically based arguments for early assessment of psychosocial well-being. Success of biomedical interventions is often determined by the psychological status of the patients. Psychosocial issues typically become more important the longer pain remains a problem in the patient's life. Early psychological assessment typically provides a statement of treatment objectives and allows ongoing assessment so as to establish treatment effectiveness.

Components of a psychological assessment

A number of themes should be addressed during thorough psychological assessment of a person with pain. Semistructured clinical interviews (Table 10.1) and self-report instruments allow for assessment of the different domains of the pain experience:

1 *Somatosensory qualities* of the experience, with this usually best understood through description of the severity, location and temporal characteristics of painful experiences. Individuals who use many pain descriptors and are highly pain-sensitive are at

Clinical Pain Management: A Practical Guide, 1st edition.
Edited by Mary E. Lynch, Kenneth D. Craig and Philip W.H. Peng.
© 2011 Blackwell Publishing Ltd.

Table 10.1 Categories to be addressed during an interview.

1 Pain description
2 Aggravating and minimizing factors
3 Past and current treatments, including medication use
4 Daily activities: content and level
5 Relevant medical history
6 Development, education and employment history
7 Compensation status, engagement in litigation
8 History of drug or alcohol abuse
9 History of psychiatric disturbance
10 Current emotional status
11 Financial and social support
12 Perceived directions for treatment

greater risk for poor long-term pain outcomes. Quantitative sensory testing (QST) also can be useful in assessing an individual's response to light touch, pressure, heat and cold threshold and tolerance.

2 *Affective qualities* of the experience. Distressing emotional qualities of a painful experience as well as pre-existing emotional dispositions such as a mood disorder with associated anxiety, fear and depression contribute to heightened response to pain.

3 *Cognitive features*, with patterns of thinking able to exacerbate and maintain dysfunctional pain, or, on the contrary, able to facilitate coping. Catastrophizing is a set of cognitive and emotional processes encompassing magnification of pain-related stimuli, feelings of helplessness and a generally pessimistic orientation to pain outcomes. Higher catastrophizing predicts greater pain-related disability and healthcare utilization.

4 *Pain behavior.* There is substantial variability in the extent to which chronic pain interferes with activities of daily living or contributes to functional impairment. Astute clinicians have long relied upon a careful appraisal of pain behavior through observation of patients both during and outside the examining situation, for example, when engaged in spontaneous activity in everyday situations.

5 *Personal history.* Ethnic and cultural background, family socialization and important life experiences

influence the capacity to cope with pain. A history of trauma or physical or sexual abuse can have an adverse effect on coping with pain. For example, when significant others in a person's family have had a history of chronic or particularly severe pain, there may be a predisposition to similar patterns in the patient.

6 *Psychosocial stressors* tend to negatively impact coping and result in increased healthcare utilization. Similarly, the current social contexts in which patients may be experiencing social distress (e.g. with employers or family members) either directly affected by painful episodes (e.g. unemployment, social isolation) or indirectly related to painful episodes (e.g. dysfunctional relationships).

7 *Social context of the assessment* can be very important. While clinicians must be aware of the objectives of referral sources, patients similarly are typically aware of the expectations and goals of referral agencies and those engaged in the assessment. Patients frustrated with lack of success from treatment and hampered by financial concerns and negative experiences may react differently in assessment situations than those without such experiences or concerns.

Assessment measures

Selected assessment categories and frequently used reliable and valid psychometric measures to assess the domains mentioned above are listed in Table 10.2.

Pain intensity

There are a number of ways to measure pain intensity, including numerical pain ratings, visual analog scales (VAS), verbal rating scales, pain drawings and a combination of standardized questionnaires, with self-monitored pain intensity ratings often demonstrably reliable and valid [4]. Daily monitoring of multiple measures of pain intensity over a 1- to 2-week period prior to therapy has a number of benefits: averaging multiple measures of pain intensity over time increases the reliability and validity of the assessment, they serve as a baseline to establish whether continued treatment is

Table 10.2 Selected assessment categories and frequently used psychometric measures.

---

1 *Psychosocial history*
Comprehensive pain questionnaire
Structured clinical interview
2 *Pain intensity*
Numerical rating scales (NRS)
Visual analog scales (VAS)
Verbal rating scales (VRS)
Pain drawings (PD)
3 *Mood and personality*
Minnesota Multiphasic Personality Inventory (MMPI)*
Symptom Checklist 90 (SCL-90)
Millon Behavior Health Inventory (MBHI)
Beck Depression Inventory (BDI)
Center for Epidemiologic Studies Depression Scale (CES-D)
Hospital Anxiety and Depression Scale (HADS)
4 *Functional capacity*
Short-Form Health Survey (SF-36)
Multidimensional Pain Inventory (WHYMPI)
Pain Disability Index (PDI)
5 *Pain beliefs and coping*
Coping Strategies Questionnaire (CSQ)
Pain Management Inventory (PMI)
Pain Self-Efficacy Questionnaire (PSEQ)
Survey of Pain Attitudes (SOPA)

---

* See text for potential disadvantages in interpreting results in patients with chronic pain.

needed after an appropriate trial period and they allow assessing the overall impact of treatment for pain.

Numerical pain ratings provide the patient's pain rating on a 0–10 or 0–100 scale. External validity is improved by descriptive anchors that establish the meaning of numerical values. Another popular means of measuring pain intensity is the VAS, which uses a straight line (often 10 cm long) with extreme limits of pain at either end [5]. The patient marks the point on the line that best indicates present pain severity. Scores are obtained by measuring the distance from the end labeled "no pain" to the mark provided by the patient. Although evidence exists for the validity of the VAS it can be difficult to use with older people [4]. Concerns have been addressed by the

use of electronic VAS diaries, which have been shown to be as reliable as paper measures [6].

There are a number of verbal rating scales that consist of phrases (as few as 4 or as many as 15, often ranked in order of severity from "no pain" to "excruciating pain") chosen by the patients to describe the intensity of their pain [4]. Other verbal scales can be used to describe the quality of pain (e.g. piercing, stabbing, shooting, burning, throbbing) [7]. Among the self-report measures, numerical rating scales are most popular among professionals. However, there is no evidence to suggest that VAS or verbal rating scales are any less sensitive to treatment effects.

Mood and personality

Patients with chronic pain often report depression, anxiety, irritability, a history of physical or sexual abuse or a past history of a mood disorder. Up to half of patients with chronic pain have a comorbid psychiatric condition, and 35% of patients with chronic back and neck pain have a comorbid depression or anxiety disorder. In surveys of chronic pain clinic populations, 50–80% of patients with chronic pain had signs of psychopathology, making this the most prevalent comorbidity in these patients [8].

Psychopathology and/or extreme emotionality have been seen as contraindications for certain therapies [9]. Mental health professionals continue to debate the best way to measure psychopathology and/or emotional distress in patients with chronic pain. Although most measures are helpful in ruling out severe psychiatric disturbance, unfortunately no measure can boast validity in predicting treatment outcome. The measures most commonly used to evaluate personality and emotional distress include the Minnesota Multiphasic Personality Inventory (MMPI-2) [10], the Symptom Checklist 90 (SCL-90-R) [11], the Millon Behavior Health Inventory (MBHI) [12], the Beck Depression Inventory (BDI) [13] and the Hospital Anxiety and Depression Scale (HADS) [14].

The MMPI is an instrument traditionally used in assessing psychopathology [10]. This 567 true–false item measure yields a distinct profile for each patient that can predict return-to-work in males as well as response to surgical treatment. Although this test has been widely used to measure psychopathology, the profiles obtained in people living with pain can be misinterpreted because of the physical symptoms reported by these patients. This is because the test is standardized on the basis that no physical illness is present and so when a person with pain or other physical illness endorses questions that confirm back pain or pain in other joints this increases scores on hypochondriasis and hysteria scales that may be incorrectly interpreted as evidence of psychological illness [15]. Patients may also dislike the test's emphasis on psychopathology.

The SCL-90 is a 90-item checklist general assessment of emotional distress that provides a global index score as well as nine subscale scores. It is a relatively brief measure including individual items that may pertain specifically to persons with chronic pain. Its disadvantages include the high correlation between subscales and the absence of validity scales to detect subtle inconsistencies in responses.

The MBHI, another popular measure for assessing mood and personality among patients with pain, includes 150 true–false items and offers 20 subscales that measure: (a) styles of relating to providers; (b) psychosocial stressors; and (c) response to illness. The scales are not subject to misinterpretation due to physical symptoms. Unlike other measures, the MBHI emphasizes medical rather than emotional concerns.

The BDI assesses depressive symptoms in patients with chronic pain. This 21-item self-report questionnaire measures the severity of depression and is commonly used to evaluate the outcome of treatment. It is easy to administer and score, although one limitation is the potential for misinterpretation of an elevated depression score as a result of the frequent endorsement of somatic items (e.g. fatigue, sleep disturbances and loss of sexual interest) by patients with chronic pain. The Center for Epidemiologic Studies Depression Scale (CES-D) is an additional tool for assessment of depressive symptoms in patients with pain [16].

The HADS is a 14-item scale designed to assess the presence and severity of anxious and depres-sive symptoms. Seven items assess anxiety and seven items measure depression, each coded 0–3. The HADS has been used extensively in clinics and has adequate reliability and validity.

Functional capacity and activity interference

Some clinicians consider pain reduction meaningless unless accompanied by a noticeable change in function. Thus, some reliable measurement of functional capacity should be used before the onset of therapy. Physical impairment itself is not very predictive of disability, with beliefs about injury predicting physical performance better than pain ratings [17]. Measures that assess activity level and function include the Short-Form Health Survey (SF-36) [18], the West Haven-Yale Multidimensional Pain Inventory (WHYMPI) [19] and the Pain Disability Index (PDI) [20].

The SF-36, which was initially developed to survey health status, includes eight scales that measure:

1 Limitations in physical activities due to health problems;

2 Limitations in social activities due to physical and emotional problems;

3 Limitations in usual role activities due to physical health problems;

4 Bodily pain;

5 General mental health;

6 Limitations in usual role activities due to emotional problems;

7 Vitality (energy and fatigue); and

8 General health perceptions.

The SF-36 is a short test with excellent reliability and validity; however, pain patients tend to score very low (severe limitations) such that modest improvements can go undetected. An expanded measure known as the Treatment Outcomes of Pain System (TOPS) [21], which incorporates the SF-36, has been modified specifically for patients with pain to improve sensitivity and reliability of measurement of treatment outcome.

The WHYMPI, a 56-item measure, provides subscales assessing activity interference, perceived support, pain severity, negative mood and perceived control. This self-report instrument was created specifically for patients with chronic pain and can be useful in classifying those patients into three categories: dysfunctional, interpersonally distressed and adaptive copers. Strong evidence supports the presence of these three groups in the assessment of patients with chronic pain. Other functional measures include the Oswestry Disability Questionnaire [22], Chronic Illness Problem Inventory [23], the Waddell Disability Instrument [24], the Functional Rating Scale [25] and the Back Pain Function Scale [26].

Pain beliefs and coping

Pain perception, beliefs about pain and coping mechanisms are important in predicting the outcome of treatment. Unrealistic or negative thoughts may contribute to increased pain and emotional distress, decreased functioning and greater reliance on medication. Certain patients presenting with chronic pain are prone to maladaptive beliefs about their condition incompatible with the physical nature of their pain [27]. Patients with adequate psychological functioning exhibit a greater tendency to ignore their pain, use coping self-statements and remain active in order to divert their attention from their pain [27].

Because efficacy expectations have been shown to influence the efforts patients will make to manage their pain, measures of self-efficacy or perceived control are useful in assessing a patient's attitude. A number of self-report measures assess coping and pain attitudes. The most popular tests used to measure maladaptive beliefs include the Coping Strategies Questionnaire (CSQ) [28], the Pain Management Inventory (PMI) [29], the Pain Self-Efficacy Questionnaire (PSEQ) [30], the Survey of Pain Attitudes (SOPA) [5] and the Inventory of Negative Thoughts in Response to Pain (INTRP) [31]. Patients who have a high score on the Catastrophizing Scale of the CSQ, who endorse passive coping on the PMI, who demonstrate low self-efficacy regarding their ability to manage their pain on the PSEQ, who describe themselves as disabled by their pain on the SOPA and who report frequent negative thoughts about their pain on the

INTRP are at greatest risk for poor treatment outcome.

Substance abuse assessment

A variety of traditional assessment measures are used to identify patients with pain who are addicted, although most were developed for other purposes. The Minnesota Multiphasic Personality Inventory and related scales (e.g. MacAndrew Alcoholism Scale) have been used to detect medication abuse in patients with pain, but the results have been equivocal. Structured interview measures have been published for assessment of alcoholism and drug abuse based on DSM-IV criteria [32], but they have not been validated in persons with chronic pain. Although traditional substance abuse assessment tools may be useful for persons with a severe substance abuse disorder (e.g. the CAGE Questionnaire or Michigan Alchoholism Screening Test), they are not the best for persons with chronic pain because they may be insensitive to medication abuse or indicate abuse when none exists.

Other measures were developed to screen patients with pain for addiction risk or potential. The 5-item Opioid Risk Tool, a checklist completed by the clinician, is a validated questionnaire that predicts which patients will display aberrant drug-related behaviors [33]. The Pain Assessment and Documentation Tool, a scale also completed by the clinician, provides a detailed means of documenting patient progress that helps record a patient's care objectively [34].

The Screener and Opioid Assessment for Patients with Pain (SOAPP-R), a 24-item self-administered screening tool developed and validated for patients with chronic pain being considered for long-term opioid therapy predicts aberrant medication-related behaviors [35]. The Current Opioid Misuse Measure (COMM) is a 17-item questionnaire that recently was developed and validated for patients with chronic pain already receiving long-term opioid therapy [36]. Reasonably good sensitivity and specificity have established the COMM as a brief but useful self-report measure of current aberrant drug-related behavior.

Electronic diaries and web-based assessment

Electronic diaries have much promise for future psychological assessment of pain patients. They allow for improved communication between patients and providers and may be an efficient means of evaluating and tracking important clinical information. With the advent of personalized digital assistants (PDAs) and the ability to capture time-stamped data and store it for uploading to the web or to a larger computer, more clinicians are exploring options of capturing data throughout the day. Studies have shown that "natural" data are less prone to fabrication and may be a truer indicator of patient responses in the environment. Patients have been shown to demonstrate remarkably high compliance with electronic diary monitoring [37]. Ever-evolving technological methods of tracking in real time can address the need for improved evaluation and treatment of persons with chronic pain. Portable monitors such as cell phones using customized software have made the collection and storage of serial data about health behaviors both convenient and affordable. Electronic diaries allow two-way communication between patients and providers and are an efficient means of evaluating and tracking medication use and associated symptoms [37].

There are currently a number of reliable web-based pain assessment and information programs (e.g. WebMD.com; PainAction.com; ReliefInsite. com; Theacpa.org). A recent review of 240 websites related to pain found the overall quality to be poor [38], suggesting that some caution is needed. Certain sites are designed for all pain conditions and others are targeted for individuals with specific pain conditions (e.g. migraine). Unfortunately, not all give the date of the last update and although most of the websites have company sponsors, rarely do the websites present easily assessable information about the sponsors and conflicts of interest. Thus, the reliability of these programs is variable and the information and education associated with these programs can be dated without any outside rigorous evaluation [38].

Future directions

Rapid changes in the way healthcare services are offered have led to a need for brief, reliable and valid measures that establish need for service and monitor efficacy of treatment. A focus on accountability and efficacy has encouraged implementation of ongoing assessment, with preference given to treatments tailored to the individual with evidence of improvement.

In light of these changes, the economic efficiency of treatment for chronic non-cancer pain will be under increased scrutiny. While evidence exists for the cost-effectiveness of therapy for chronic pain, such treatment may not meet the criterion of increased benefit with limited cost. Early and ongoing psychological assessment may help in identifying those individuals who will and do benefit most from certain pain therapies. Documentation of increased function and decreased healthcare utilization among certain patients as a result of pain therapy would support the continuation of pain management programs. The role of electronic and web-based assessment may play an important part in addressing these needs in the future.

References

1 Mannion AF, Elfering A. (2006) Predictors of surgical outcome and their assessment. *Eur Spine J* **15**:S93–108.
2 Main CJ, Spanswick CC. (2000) *Pain Management: An Interdisciplinary Approach.* Churchill Livingstone, New York.
3 Iles RA, Davidson M, Taylor NF. (2008) Psychosocial predictors of failure to return to work in non-chronic non-specific low back pain: a systematic review. *Occup Environ Med* **8**:507–17.
4 Jensen MP, Karoly P. (2001) Self-report scales and procedures for assessing pain in adults. In: Turk DC, Melzack R, eds. *Handbook of Pain Assessment.* 2nd edn. Guilford Press, New York. pp. 15–34.
5 Karoly P, Jensen MP. (1987) *Multimethod Assessment of Chronic Pain.* Pergamon Press; New York.

6 Jamison RN, Gracely RH, Raymond SA *et al.* (2002) Comparative study of electronic vs. paper VAS ratings: a randomized, crossover trial using healthy volunteers. *Pain* **99(1–2)**:341–7.

7 Jamison RN, Vasterling JJ, Parris WC. (1987) Use of sensory descriptors in assessing chronic pain patients. *J Psychosom Res* **31(5)**:647–52.

8 Kalso E, Edwards JE, Moore RA *et al.* (2004) Opioids in chronic non-cancer pain: systematic review of efficacy and safety. *Pain* **112(3)**: 372–80.

9 Celestin J, Edwards RR, Jamison RN. (2009) Pretreatment psychosocial variables as predictors of outcomes following lumbar surgery and spinal cord stimulation: a systematic review and literature synthesis. *Pain Med* **10(4)**: 639–53.

10 Hathaway SR, McKinley JC, Butcher JN *et al.* (1989) *Minnesota Multiphasic Personality Inventory-2:ManualforAdministration.*University of Minnesota Press, Minneapolis, MN.

11 Derogatis LR, Melisaratos N. (1983) The Brief Symptom Inventory: an introductory report *Psychol Med* **13**:595–605.

12 Millon T, Green CJ, Meagher RBJ. (1979) The MBHI: a new inventory for the psychodiagnostician in medical settings. *Prof Psychol* **10**: 529–39.

13 Beck AT, Ward CH, Mendelson M *et al.* (1961) An inventory for measuring depression. *Arch Gen Psychiatry* **4**:561–71.

14 Zigmond AS, Snaith RP. (1983) The Hospital Anxiety and Depression Scale. *Acta Psychiatr Scand* **37**:361–70.

15 Merskey H. (1987) Pain, personality and psychosomatic complaints. In: Burrows GD, Elton D, Stanley GV, eds. *Handbook of Chronic Pain Management.* Elsevier Science Publishers, Amsterdam. pp. 137–46.

16 Radloff LS. (1977) The CES-D scale: a self-report depression scale for research in the general population. *Appl Psychol Meas* **1**:385–401.

17 Turk DC, Okifuji A, Sinclair JD *et al.* (1998) Differential responses by psychosocial subgroups of fibromyalgia syndrome patients to an interdisciplinary treatment. *Arthritis Care* **11**:397–404.

18 Ware JE, Sherbourne CD. (1992) The MOS 36-item short-form health survey (SF-36). I. Conceptual framework and item selection *Med Care* **20**:473–83.

19 Kerns RD, Turk DC, Rudy TE. (1985) The West Haven-Yale Multidimensional Pain Inventory (WHYMPI). *Pain* **23**:345–56.

20 Pollard CA. (1984) Preliminary validity study of the pain disability index. *Percept Mot Skills* **59**:974.

21 Ho MJ, LaFleur J. (2004) The treatment outcomes of pain survey (TOPS): a clinical monitoring and outcomes instrument for chronic pain practice and research. *J Pain Palliat Care Pharmocother* **18**:49–59.

22 Leclaire R, Blier F, Fortin L *et al.* (1997) A cross-sectional study comparing the Oswestry and Roland-Morris Functional Disability scales in two populations of patients with low back pain of different levels of severity. *Spine* **22**:68–71.

23 Kames LD, Naliboff BD, Heinrich RL *et al.* (1984) The chronic illness problem inventory: problem-oriented psychosocial assessment of patients with chronic illness. *Int J Psychiatry Med* **14**:65–75.

24 Waddell G, Main CJ. (1984) Assessment of severity in low-back disorders. *Spine* **9**:204–8.

25 Evans JH, Kagan A 2nd. (1986) The development of a functional rating scale to measure the treatment outcome of chronic spinal patients. *Spine* **11**:277–81.

26 Stratford PW, Binkley JM. (2000) A comparison study of the Back Pain Function Scale and the Roland Morris Questionnaire. *J Rheumatol* **27**:1924–36.

27 Waddell G. (1998) *The Back Pain Revolution.* Churchill Livingstone, Edinburgh.

28 Rosenstiel AK, Keefe FJ. (1983) The use of coping strategies in chronic low back pain patients: relationship to patient characteristics and current adjustment. *Pain* **17**:33–44.

29 Brown GK, Nicassion PM, Wallston KA. (1989) Pain coping strategies and depression in rheumatoid arthritis. *J Consult Clin Psychol* **57**: 652–7.

30 Lorig K, Chastain RL, Ung E *et al.* (1989) Development and evaluation of a scale to

measure perceived self-efficacy in people with arthritis. *Arthritis Rheum* **32**:37–44.

31 Gil K, Williams DA, Keefe FJ *et al.* (1990) The relationship of negative thoughts to pain and psychological distress. *Behav Ther* **21**:349–62.

32 Helzer JE, Robins LN. (1988) The Diagnostic Inteview Schedule: its development, evaluations, and use. *Soc Psychiatry Psychiatr Epidemiol* **23**:6–16.

33 Webster LR, Webster RM. (2005) Predicting aberrant behaviors in opioid-treated patients: preliminary validation of the Opioid Risk Tool. *Pain Med* **6(6)**:432–42.

34 Passik SD, Kirsch KL, Whitcomb RK *et al.* (2004) A new tool to assess and document pain outcomes in chronic pain patients receiving opioid therapy. *Clin Ther* **26(4)**:552–61.

35 Butler SF, Budman SH, Fernandez KC *et al.* (2009) Cross-validation of a screener to predict opioid misuse in chronic pain patients. *J Addict Med* **3**:66–73.

36 Butler SF, Budman SH, Fernandez KC *et al.* (2007) Development and validation of the Current Opioid Misuse Measure. *Pain* **130 (1–2)**:144–56.

37 Jamison RN, Raymond SA, Levine JG *et al.* (2001) Electronic diaries for monitoring chronic pain: 1-year validation study *Pain* **91(3)**:277–85.

38 Washington TA, Fanciullo GJ, Sorensen JA *et al.* (2008) Quality of chronic pain websites *Pain Med* **9(8)**:994–1000.

Further reading

Turk DC, Melzack R. (2001) *Handbook of Pain Assessment*, 2nd edn. Guilford Press, New York.

Jamison RN. (2003) Psychological evaluation and treatment of chronic pain. In: Samuels MA, Feske S, eds. *Office Practice of Neurology*, 2nd edn. Churchill Livingston, New York. pp. 1448–53.

Part 3

Management

Chapter 11

Introduction to management

Mary Lynch

*Dalhousie University, Halifax, Nova Scotia, Canada; Pain Management Unit,
Queen Elizabeth II Health Sciences Center, Halifax, Nova Scotia, Canada*

Overview

All pain management should take place within the context of a biopsychosocial approach where the role of the clinician is to assist the patient in becoming an active participant in their own healthcare. The following chapters address in detail pain management from different biological, psychological and social perspectives, with the interest in this chapter focusing on integration of the approaches so as to assure all facets of care are addressed. The principles of healthful living and therapeutic exercise should be a part of every patient's care. In addition, most people living with pain will benefit from strategies for relaxation along with cognitive approaches to deal with the pain day to day. Details of treatment approaches are presented in the following chapters. This chapter provides an overview of the four steps needed in the management of pain (Table 11.1).

Start with the basics

Step 1: Listen

Pain management begins the minute you start to listen

The importance of facilitating the patient's narrative was reviewed in Chapter 7. This is a therapeu-

Clinical Pain Management: A Practical Guide, 1st edition.
Edited by Mary E. Lynch, Kenneth D. Craig and
Philip W.H. Peng.
© 2011 Blackwell Publishing Ltd.

tic way to collect information as there "is the need of ill people to tell their stories, in order to construct new maps and new perceptions of their relationship to the world" [1]. The Stone Center Study Group on Women with Chronic Illness and Disability state that "Giving voice to one's experience with illness is courageous" and note that courage can inspire growth [2]. In this way the "therapy" starts the minute you start to listen.

Step 2: Communicate the diagnosis clearly

Establish and communicate the diagnosis

In determining treatment one must first establish the diagnosis as far as possible. As presented in more detail in previous chapters, chronic pain may or may not have a definitive explanation in tissue pathology. In the former case, the pain and related disability may result from a sustained sensory abnormality occurring as a result of ongoing peripheral pathology, such as chronic inflammation. It may also be autonomous and independent of the trigger that initiated it as in post-traumatic or postsurgical neuropathic pain. Thus, patients may present with nociceptive pain (pain due to tissue damage), neuropathic pain (pain due to pathology in neural systems) or a combination of both. When there is no identifiable medical or biological explanation, the biopsychosocial model encourages a stronger emphasis on psychophysiological and social explanations of functional symptoms [3]. In addressing management it is important

Table 11.1 The four steps of good pain management.

Step 1: Listen
Narrative or telling one's story of pain is therapeutic so the treatment starts the minute you start to listen
 	
Step 2: Communicate the diagnosis clearly
In order to come to terms with a chronic pain diagnosis, understanding regarding the cause along with an active plan for management are essential
 	
Step 3: Review healthful living
Proper nutrition
Quit smoking
Balance of activities and rest
Good sleep hygiene
Exercise program within pain tolerance
 	
Step 4: Consider pain reduction treatment options in biological, psychological and social domains
Medical
  Pharmacotherapy
  Neuromodulation
  Surgery
Psychological: assure psychosocial issues are identified and addressed in management
Physical and rehabilitation

to consider both disease-based (e.g. diabetic neuropathy, lumbar radiculopathy, cervical sprain) and mechanistic (e.g. nociceptive, inflammatory, neuropathic) aspects of the pain. It is also important to reassure the patient as to the reality of their experience even when there is not an identifiable etiology. One must also consider comorbidities (e.g. medical, psychiatric or substance abuse conditions), as well as additional aspects relating to the consequences of pain and disability and the state of the patient's overall health (e.g. psychosocial issues, metabolic and circadian factors, deconditioning) all of which can influence the experience of pain. For this reason all management should take place within a holistic active participatory context.

You must communicate the diagnosis to the patient in clear unambiguous terms. In most cases the pain will have come on in the context of illness or injury and will have persisted beyond the time where healing should have taken place. The presence of allodynia or hyperalgesia may support a

diagnosis of a neuropathic component to the pain. In this case it is appropriate to explain that the nerves that convey pain-related information are alive and can be changed after injury such that they become sensitized or "stuck in the on" position like a light switch that cannot be turned off. The patient may have been previously diagnosed with Crohn's disease or recurrent renal stones and suffering from pain in the absence of a documented Crohn's exacerbation or presenting with pain that persists between renal stones. In this case it is important to explain to the patient that they are probably suffering from visceral hyperalgesia [4] or neuropathic pain in the gut. When one is unable to make a specific diagnosis it is important to explain that cancer and other structural pathologies have been ruled out, that you believe the patient is in pain and support them in developing a plan for management. There are many excellent self-help books about pain as well as resources online. Encourage your patient to read about the pain and self-management strategies, but do so actively with the patient as there also is considerable misinformation online.

As you discuss the diagnosis, be as precise as possible. Avoid the term chronic pain syndrome. As described by Merskey over a decade ago, this term "encourages the practitioner to neglect the responsibility for establishing the precise contribution of physical and psychological problems to the overall state of the patient. It is much better to make two diagnoses and estimate their importance" [5]. In this case, one might make a diagnosis of lumbar spinal or radicular pain after failed spinal surgery complicated by depression, anxiety or grief. There may also be a component of grief related to job loss complicated by significant financial stress. Explain all of this to the patient along with the importance of addressing all in treatment.

It is unusual for there to be no explanation for the pain. In most patients there will be an identifiable precipitating event or series of events that will assist with the diagnosis, along with physical findings such as postural or muscular asymmetries, sensory abnormalities or abnormalities on palpation. However, in some cases it may be difficult to establish a diagnosis. In these cases it is important to remember that medically unexplained pain is not caused by psychopathology [6–8]. The biopsychosocial explanations needed are developed elsewhere in this volume. The therapeutic process in patients with medically unexplained symptoms depends on a process of negotiation which requires dialog [9]. As with all patients, the therapeutic process thrives within an atmosphere of trust between healthcare professional and patient. Clear direct communication is critical. It is best to acknowledge that we as health professionals cannot explain everything, that we have ruled out serious illness such as cancer, inflammatory arthritis, etc., and that we are going to assist the patient with management of their pain to the best of our ability. The multidisciplinary approach to pain management supported in this volume encourages utilizing the resources of other healthcare professionals when appropriate. Patients report a high level of satisfaction with pain care even when the pain remains and research has suggested this is related to the patient–provider relationship and their appreciation for the providers mere voicing of interest in adequate pain treatment [10,11].

Step 3: Review healthful living

Pain management is a joint effort

Emphasize that pain management must involve a joint effort where the patient will have to do their part in managing their own pain. As healthcare professionals we will do everything we can do to reduce the pain where possible but there are key steps the patient must take to reduce pain and improve health.

There is growing support that self-management approaches are efficacious and cost effective in chronic diseases including pain. Self-management is reviewed in more detail in Chapter 22. Here I emphasize that all clinicians, regardless of background or setting, should review the basics of healthful living. People living with pain are as heterogeneous as the general population so for some there will already be an understanding of the need to live a healthy lifestyle. For others it will take some time for them to "get it." In this case the

Table 11.2 Basic principles of sleep hygiene.

Regular sleep–wake pattern
Arise same time every day
Avoid long naps (keep to <30 minutes/day)
Regular meals and avoid large meals before bed
Limit bedroom activities to sleep and sex
Establish relaxing bedtime ritual
Environmental factors
Adequate light in morning
Hot bath1.5–2 hours before bed (to raise core temperature)
Keep clock face turned away
Keep environment dark and cool
Use white noise machine to ↓ background noise
Regular exercise
Drugs
Avoid nicotine several hours before bed
Limit alcohol as it fragments sleep as metabolized
No caffeine for 8 hours before bed
Avoid over-the-counter sleep medications
Assure no stimulants before bed

Source: Summarized from Smith & Haythornthwaite [22].

patient must understand that before chronic pain they may have been able to get away with abusing their body. Now that they have pain it is important to "live right." This includes proper nutrition, quitting tobacco smoking, pacing activities, adequate sleep or down time and a basic exercise program. Nutrition and exercise are reviewed in Chapters 13 and 24, respectively. The majority of people living with chronic pain report problems with sleep. Recent research and management are reviewed in the excellent IASP Press book, *Sleep and Pain* [12]. At the primary care level all practitioners should review the basics of sleep hygiene with the patient and these are summarized in Table 11.2. The importance of quitting smoking is obvious with regards to general health but what many patients may not know is that chronic exposure to nicotine increases the chances of neural sensitization and they may be making their pain worse. In addition, it is well established that chronic smoking exacerbates autoimmune disease including rheumatioid arthritis [13], Crohn's disease [14] and multiple sclerosis [15] which often present with severe pain.

Step 4: Consider pain reduction treatment options in biological, psychological and social domains

Medical: pharmacological, interventional and surgical

In many cases patients may benefit from medical approaches including medications, interventional therapies such as injection, or surgical approaches.

Pharmacotherapy

Recent reviews have identified several key groups of medication for which there is high quality evidence supporting efficacy in the management of chronic pain [16]. This evidence has been used to develop recommendations and treatment algorithms for pharmacological management of chronic neuropathic pain [17,18] and chronic pain in general [16,19].

The agents for which there is well-established evidence of analgesic efficacy include the nonsteroidal anti-inflammatory drugs (NSAIDs), the tricyclic antidepressants, specific anticonvulsants and the opioids. The cannabinoids have good support to justify their use as a second or third line treatment and there is growing evidence that specific topically delivered agents are effective as sole agents in mild to moderate pain with potential to be used in combination with systemic therapy in moderate to severe pain.

Once the physician has established the working diagnosis and has identified that analgesic medication is necessary, the usual approach is to start with a non-opioid analgesic such as a NSAID or acetaminophen for mild to moderate pain. If this is inadequate, and if there is an element of sleep loss, the next step is to add an antidepressant with analgesic qualities. If there is a component of neuropathic pain, then a trial of one of the anticonvulsant analgesic agents is appropriate. If these steps are inadequate, then an opioid analgesic may be added. Cannabinoids and topical agents may also be appropriate as single agents or in combination [16]. In an individual patient, one or several mechanisms may be at play in the etiology of the pain and more than one agent may be necessary for pain control. There is also significant individual variation in response to medications. For this reason it is important to take an individual approach to each patient and adjust dosage according to treatment response while minimizing side effects. It is also appropriate to use a combination of agents with different mechanisms of action in an effort to obtain adequate pain control. This combination approach has been supported by randomized double blind placebo controlled trials which found that gabapentin and morphine combined achieved better analgesia at lower doses than when the agents were used alone [20] and a combination of nortriptyline and gabapentin was superior to the single agent [21]. Details regarding these agents and other emerging medications are presented in the following chapters.

Interventional and surgical therapies

In properly selected patients, diagnostic or therapeutic blocks, neuromodulation or surgical approaches may be appropriate. The details regarding these approaches and appropriate indications are presented in Chapters 19–21.

Exercise management and physical strengthening

Pain will often lead to decreased movement, postural asymmetry, loss of strength and eventually deconditioning. This will lead to additional problems complicating the patient's original pain condition and must be addressed. Approaches offered through physiotherapy and rehabilitation programs are reviewed in Chapter 21.

Psychological therapies

The assessment and management of psychosocial aspects of pain are critical in assisting the patient presenting with pain (Chapters 10 and 23). Chapter 24 reviews the fact that psychosocial variables such as catastrophic thinking and fear of movement are significant determinants of persistent pain and disability and response to all forms of treatment. Psychological and self-management interventions have demonstrable effectiveness in painful distress and pain-related disability.

Complementary therapies and integrative healthcare

Many patients seek relief through complementary therapies such as acupuncture, Qigong, massage, osteopathy and other complementary therapeutic approaches. The field of "integrative medicine," using a combination of conventional medical approaches along with the complementary therapies, has application in pain management. The growing research regarding an integrative approach has been reviewed in Chapter 25.

Conclusions

The steps to good pain management include listening, communicating the diagnosis of the pain clearly and, where the diagnosis is unclear after appropriate investigation, assuring the patient there is no serious medical pathology with support for broader lifestyle management and engagement in self-management care. Reassure the patient you believe they are in pain and use a biopsychosocial approach where the role of the clinician is to assist the patient in becoming an active participant in their own healthcare using treatments presented in the following chapters.

References

1 Frank A. (1995) *The Wounded Storyteller*. University of Chicago Press, Chicago.

2 Reid-Cunningham M, Snyder-Grant D, Stein K et al. (1999) *Women with Chronic Illness: Overcoming Disconnection*. Stone Center Work in Progress Paper 80:1–8.

3 Williams SE, Smith CA, Bruehl SB et al. (2009) Medical evaluation of children with chronic abdominal pain: impact of diagnosis, physician practice orientation, and maternal trait anxiety and mother's response to evaluation. *Pain* **146**:283–92.

4 Gebhart GF. (1995) *Visceral Pain*. IASP Press, Seattle, WA.

5 Merskey H. (1989) Psychiatry and chronic pain. *Can J Psychiatry* **34**:329–35.

6 Crombez G, Beirens K, Van Damme S et al. (2009) The unbearable lightness of somatization: a systematic review of the concept of somatisation in empirical studies of pain. *Pain* **145**:31–5.

7 Gagliese L, Katz J. (2000) Medically unexplained pain is not caused by psychopathology. *Pain Res Manag* **5**:251–7.

8 Merskey H. (2009) Somatization: or another God that failed. *Pain* **145**:4–5.

9 Kirmayer LJ, Groleau D, Looper KJ et al. (2004) Explaining medically unexplained symptoms. *Can J Psychiatry* **49**:663–72.

10 Dawson R, Spross JA, Jablonski ES et al. (2002) Probing the paradox of patients' satisfaction with inadequate pain management. *J Pain Symptom Manag* **23**:211–20.

11 Carr DB. (2009) What does pain hurt? *IASP Pain Clinical Updates* **XVII(3)**:1–6.

12 Lavigne G, Sessle B, Choiniere M et al. (2007) *Sleep and Pain*. IASP Press, Seattle, WA.

13 Baka Z, Buzás E, Nagy G. (2009) Rheumatoid arthritis and smoking: putting the pieces together. *Arthritis Res Ther* **11(4)**:238.

14 Cosnes J, Carbonnel F, Carrat F et al. (1999) Effects of current and former cigarette smoking on clinical course of Crohn's disease. *Aliment Pharmacol Ther* **13(11)**:1403–11.

15 Healy BC, En A, Guttman CR et al. (2009) Smoking and disease progression in multiple sclerosis. *Arch Neurol* **66**:858–64.

16 Lynch ME, Watson CP. (2006) The pharmacotherapy of chronic pain: a review. *Pain Res Manag* **11**:11–38.

17 Finnerup NB, Otto M, McQuay HJ et al. (2005) Algorithm for neuropathic pain treatment: an evidence based proposal. *Pain* **118**:289–305.

18 Moulin DE, Clark AJ, Gilron I et al. (2007) Pharmacologic management of chronic neuropathic pain concensus statement and guidelines from the Canadian Pain Society. *Pain Res Manag* **12**:13–21.

19 Griffin RS, Woolf CJ. (2005) *Pharmacology of Analgesia. Principles of Pharmacology: The Pathophysiologic Basis of Drug Therapy*. Lippincott,

Williams and Wilkins, Philadelphia, PA. pp. 229–43.

20 Gilron I, Bailey JM, Dongsheng T *et al.* (2005) Morphine, gabapentin, or their combination for neuropathic pain. *N Engl J Med* **352**: 1324–34.

21 Gilron I, Bailey JM, Tu D *et al.* (2009) Nortriptyline and gabapentin, alone and in combination for neuropathic pain: a double-blind, randomised controlled crossover trial. *Lancet* **374**:1252–61.

22 Smith MT, Haythornthwaite JA. (2007) Cognitive behavioral treatment for insomnia and pain. In: Lavigne G, Sessle B, Choiniere M *et al.* eds. *Sleep and Pain.* IASP Press, Seattle, WA.

Chapter 12

Managing chronic pain in primary care

Blair H. Smith[1], Alexander J. Clark[2] & Beverly Collett[3]

[1] *University of Aberdeen, Scotland, UK*
[2] *Dalhousie University, Halifax, Nova Scotia, Canada*
[3] *University Hospitals of Leicester, Leicester, UK*

Introduction

The impact of chronic pain on the individual, the family, society and health services is impressive and frightening. In an ideal world, every individual with chronic pain would have the opportunity for assessment and treatment at a specialist pain clinic, where the management strategies described in this book can be utilized effectively. This is neither practical nor affordable.

Twenty percent of the population experiences chronic pain [1], and a more conservative 7% has "significant" chronic pain (needing frequent treatment and healthcare advice) [2]. In reality, only a small proportion of those with chronic pain are seen in a pain clinic [1]. For example, in the UK, a clinic serving a population of some 500,000 might expect to see 500 new referrals each year (0.1% of the population) and Peng *et al.* [3] noted 49,000 consultations per year to multidisciplinary Pain Treatment Centres in Canada (also 0.15% of the population).

Between 0.5% and 2% of those with chronic pain are seen each year in a pain clinic [1]. The great majority of the remainder are treated in

primary care, if at all [4]. Many attend complementary or other community-based therapists, and others attend other specialist clinics for specific diagnoses. Nonetheless, the majority are in some form of communication with their primary care physician, on a regular or ad hoc basis [5], and even those attending other clinics are generally referred from, and return to, primary care. Given the high prevalence and impact of chronic pain in their practice population (Chapter 2) and the fact that individuals with chronic pain consult their primary care physician up to five times more frequently than those without [6], it is important that every general practitioner (GP, or family doctor) has some knowledge of chronic pain and the ability to manage it in a holistic context. This knowledge and skill should be shared by the wider primary care or community-based team, including nurse practitioners and other health professionals.

The aim of this chapter is to address this management in primary care, and takes as its starting point the assumption that the pain in question has been brought to the GP and that all reasonable attempts have been made to investigate and treat its cause, where appropriate.

A specific diagnosis or cause of chronic pain will often not be possible or feasible to confer in primary care. For example, there are over 100 diagnostic pathophysiological subclassifications of chronic back pain [7], one of the most prevalent of which is "idiopathic." For most primary care

Clinical Pain Management: A Practical Guide, 1st edition.
Edited by Mary E. Lynch, Kenneth D. Craig and
Philip W.H. Peng.
© 2011 Blackwell Publishing Ltd.

physicians, investigation of these is neither possible nor fruitful, nor does it contribute importantly to decisions about primary care management. GPs should prepare patients at the outset for the possibility that no cause may be found for their chronic pain. In other words, "chronic pain" itself should be considered high on the list of differential diagnoses, but with sufficient weight and clinical relevance attached to that diagnosis.

Basic mechanisms and the scientific basis for understanding the subject

Management of chronic pain in primary care follows that of other chronic illness models. For this to be most effective, three things should ideally be in place:

1 An appreciation of the importance of chronic pain and comorbidities, its impact on function and quality of life, and its multidimensional assessment and management.

2 Access to an evidence-based range of effective management strategies in primary care.

3 Practical evidence-based consensus on referral guidelines from primary care to specialist clinics, and on follow-up after clinic attendance.

Unfortunately, none of these three requirements can be demonstrated. Education about chronic pain is poorly represented in undergraduate and postgraduate training in primary care medicine, and application of the principles of its assessment and management from tertiary care settings to GPs is often unsatisfactory [1]. There is also less opportunity for full assessment in primary care. For example, while a pain management program based on cognitive behavioral therapy can be shown to be effective in chronic pain [8], patients taking this program are first fully assessed for their suitability, and filtered accordingly, before they receive multidisciplinary care.

There is good evidence for the limited benefit of pharmaceutical interventions in many chronic pain conditions, with studies generally showing around 35% improvement in pain, and 40–50% of patients obtaining some benefit. Prescribing is one of the main responsibilities of the primary care physician, and therefore an opportunity for

effective management. However, the danger is that this becomes the focus of management in primary care, at the expense of a more holistic approach including other treatment modalities. Both physician and patient may collude in routine administration of repeat prescriptions without proper review, despite evidence that most chronic pain patients are dissatisfied with the benefit they are experiencing from medications [1].

The absence of widely agreed, evidence-based referral guidelines tends to promote the low profile of chronic pain in primary care, hamper its effective treatment, lead to inappropriate or insufficient referral and misses a major opportunity for educational intervention within primary care. There are several examples of evidence-based consensus statements that apply to aspects of primary care pain management, such as the use of opioids [9] and guidelines for the management of certain conditions such as back pain [10] or neuropathic pain [11]. Dissemination will be as important as their further development as new evidence becomes available to guide content.

Impact on clinical practice

Many of the principles outlined throughout this book represent the core of primary care medicine, including the biopsychosocial approach to whole-person care, and timely collaboration between the healthcare disciplines practicing in primary care. Assuming that the GP recognizes a diagnosis of "chronic pain," and has excluded and/or addressed underlying medical causes and "Red Flag" conditions (such as serious trauma, evidence of cancer or infection), he or she can quickly and expertly move to a rehabilitative model of management (Table 12.1). These management principles neither cease nor change after a referral has been made. The GP's involvement in the case must continue during specialist care and, ideally, the pain specialist and the GP should collaborate in the care of the patient.

Importantly, the GP is well placed to identify some of the psychosocial factors that tend to lead to chronicity, impairment in function and reduction in quality of life, and to address those that

Table 12.1 Components of a rehabilitative approach to chronic pain management [12]. In chronic pain, rehabilitation is often the aim of management, rather than cure. The overall aim is to maximize future quality of life.

Assessment
Education
Improving physical condition
Recovery or maintenance of activities
Relaxation and sleep management
Medication reduction
Improving mood and confidence
Improving social functioning
Improving socioeconomic circumstances
Managing relapse

Table 12.2 Psychosocial barriers to recovery.

Myth that pain and activity are harmful
"Sickness behaviors" (e.g. extended rest)
Low or negative mood, social withdrawal
Treatment expectations that do not fit best practice
Problems with claim and compensation
History of back pain, time off, other claims
Problems at work, poor job satisfaction
Heavy work, unsociable hours (shift work)
Overprotective family or lack of support

can be addressed. In back pain, psychosocial "Yellow Flags", psychosocial barriers to recovery, have been introduced [13]. Many of these are amenable to detection and modification in primary care (Table 12.2). Addressing "Yellow Flags" more widely may help prevent chronic pain and/or minimize disability.

Features of best clinical practice for managing chronic pain in primary care

General considerations

After excluding treatable causes of chronic pain, the starting point for its management in primary care is therefore the same as in secondary care: to manage the individual rather than the pain. Although time constraint is an important barrier to

a full physical, psychological and social assessment, an advantage in primary care is that the physician usually has known the patient and his or her family and circumstances for several years. Comorbidities including sleep disturbance, depression, anxiety or other psychiatric symptoms need to be assessed and treated.

The next important step is to determine, where possible, the type of pain: nociceptive, neuropathic or mixed. A full neurological examination is not required in primary care, but a basic clinical assessment can determine the extent of neuropathic involvement [14] and this will be an important guide to the most effective treatment to alleviate pain.

Pharmacological treatment

Although pharmacological treatment is likely an important component, it is important to recognize that it is only one component of the overall management. There is now good evidence and consensus available to support effective prescribing in musculoskeletal pain [15], neuropathic pain [11] and for the use of opiates for chronic pain in primary care [9]. GPs should be familiar with the use of analgesics, and the World Health Organization pain ladder (and particular care with the use of strong opioids) [16].

The most important part of prescribing for chronic pain is regular review of the patient, adjusting medicines and dosage according to apparent effectiveness (based not only on assessment of pain levels, but also on improvement in function), adverse reactions and interactions, and misuse/abuse behaviors. Regular review should be ongoing, must include repeated brief assessment of general health and contributes to the holistic approach while avoiding one of the frequent criticisms leveled at GPs in chronic pain – an apparent lack of concern or failure to address patients' full spectrum of needs [1]. Medication review must consist of more than simply initiating treatment then signing repeat prescriptions.

Opioids can be both under- and over-utilized in primary care. Moderate or strong opioids, if used appropriately, represent a safe and effective form of pain treatment in some patients [17]. With careful prescribing, regular review, titration and flexibility of dosage and attention to regulatory procedures, they can be prescribed by GPs, and can lead to improved outcomes in the long term [18]. Stigma, and concerns about addiction and side effects [11], often limit their use and should be addressed. However, opioids are frequently not effective, and side effects, dependence, tolerance, hyperalgesia and abuse/misuse do occur. Caution should be deployed in their initiation by GPs, with clear goals of care and adequate pre-emptive management of side effects, including constipation, being established. When there is a history of misuse or abuse of prescription or non-prescription drugs it is often best reserved for the specialist pain clinic to initiate these medications. In most situations the GP should be confident in continuing their prescription, under monitored conditions.

Specialist pain physicians should recognize that primary care physicians often feel uncomfortable prescribing opioid and other medications used in the management of chronic pain. Clear suggestions and/or instructions about how to prescribe these medications are needed in consultation reports and follow-up letters. Direct communication, for example by telephone, between physicians often leads to enhancement and clarity of care. Physicians in both settings need to "make the time" available to ensure this happens.

Irrespective of the drug(s) prescribed, it is important at the outset of treatment to discuss likely side effects (to prepare the patient and guard against treatment withdrawal) and agree on goals of treatment. These goals should be realistic – the patient should not normally expect complete resolution of pain, but can reasonably expect an improvement (30% reduction of a pain intensity score). The goals should form the basis of review, and if they are not being met, a re-evaluation or change of therapy is indicated. This strategy should also apply to the use of other non-drug treatments.

Non-pharmacological treatment

Other reasonable approaches to management are based on consensus, experience and extrapolation

Table 12.3 Primary care–community interventions.

Effective interventions in primary care or the community	*Ineffective*, or marginally effective, interventions in primary care
Pharmacological interventions in early back pain [20]	Training in lifting (systematic review) [26]
Pain management program for chronic back pain [21]	Physiotherapy in whiplash injury [27]
Back schools [22]	Manipulation +/– exercise in back pain [28]
Public information [23]	GP-based psychological intervention in back pain [29]
Alexander technique in chronic back pain [24]	
"Collaborative care"[25]	

of evidence from other conditions and settings. They include management of comorbidity, and referral within the multidisciplinary establishment that is primary care, for primary care is a team activity. The team includes, but is not restricted to, members of the following disciplines: GP, nurses (e.g. practice nurse, district nurse, health visitor), practice staff, physiotherapist, occupational therapist, pharmacist, counselor or behavioral therapist, social worker and complementary therapists.

It is most important to emphasize the need for individual tailoring of management, and its ongoing nature, before and after referral. Good personal knowledge of the patient, good communication skills (especially listening) and frequent review are essential.

Specific interventions have been found to be effective in primary care or the community. In contrast, many interventions have been found to be ineffective, or only marginally effective in primary care (Table 12.3). It is important to recognize that absence of evidence for effectiveness of these interventions is not the same as evidence of absence of effectiveness.

Primary care management must therefore be based on guidance [19], evidence, including non-randomized trials, expert consensus and individual experience. Examples of innovative primary care approaches that have not (yet) been subjected to

Table 12.4 Innovative primary care approaches.

Interdisciplinary primary care-based pain clinics
Nurse-led pain clinics
Pharmacist-led interventions ("Medicines Use Review" in a community pharmacy or a practice-based pharmacist)
"Fast track" back pain services
Training of non-psychologist professionals (e.g. physiotherapists) in cognitive behavioral training
Formal/informal education of health professionals, including "GPs with a specialist interest" in pain
Community pain management programs
Telemedicine and teleconsult programs between GPs and specialists
Mentorship programs between GPs and specialists
GP liaison with occupational health services to maximize function, work capacity and minimize disability

Table 12.5 Broad reasons for referral.

Inadequate pain control achieved despite treatment according to the above principles
Consideration of specialist interventions (spinal cord stimulation, nerve block or strong opioids)
Access to a specialist interdisciplinary team and/or pain management program
Specific patient request (for reassurance or "second opinion")
Confirmation that all reasonable approaches have already been explored

full randomized controlled trials are shown in Table 12.4. Other coordinated primary–secondary care collaborations can be explored, such as Managed Clinical Networks, an 18-week Commissioning Pathway for Chronic Pain and multidisciplinary review during incidental hospitalization, with a view specifically to subsequent liaison with primary care teams.

This list is not exhaustive, but portrays some of the imaginative approaches that can be applied collaboratively in primary care, based on reasonable expectation of effectiveness.

Referral to specialist pain clinic

Referral to a pain specialist clinic should be considered in some cases. Broad reasons for referral are shown in Table 12.5.

Many patients attend secondary and/or tertiary pain management services with high expectations that their pain will be cured. This is often not realized, and realistic goal-setting is important at the time of referral. On discharge, the patient should have a greater understanding of why they have pain, the external influences that aggravate their symptoms and both a self-management and a crisis plan. Many patients with continuing symptoms find difficulty in accepting that nothing further

can be offered. Some pain services have strategies for patients to be reviewed in person, in a group setting or by phone to reinforce coping strategies. Resources need to be given to community practitioners to support these strategies to avoid repeated fruitless referrals.

Usually, the patient will continue to attend primary care throughout his or her period of attendance at the specialist clinic. During this stage, management of chronic pain should be regarded as a collaboration between GP and specialist.

How else can specialists support primary care?

The most important functions of a specialist pain clinic or physician are to be accessible to and to collaborate with the primary care physician. Often, specialist pain clinics have long waiting lists, are overburdened and unable to respond to requests for assistance. New approaches to dealing with these requests are needed. Many can be addressed by a short telephone call between physicians or between a primary care physician and another care provider (e.g. psychologist, nurse) in a specialist pain clinic. Telephone consultation programs that can be easily accessed on short notice would allow care options to be discussed and then initiated by the primary care physician. Mentoring programs, whereby one specialist can mentor a number of primary care physicians, have been shown to be beneficial in mental health care and are now being introduced into chronic pain care.

Another approach is to provide fax or email advice to the referring primary care physician, based on the information provided in the referral which can then be initiated while the patient waits for assessment. Good documentation needs to be provided in the referral. Triaging at the specialist clinic by a nurse or physician can enhance this process. Specialist pain clinics can develop collaborative approaches to care with groups of primary care physicians to enhance clinical skills and resources at the primary care level.

Chronic conditions and chronic disease management are priorities in many healthcare systems. Chronic pain is a chronic disease. By providing multidisciplinary expertise and leadership, specialist pain clinics need to help develop programs in the community that allow patients to gain a better understanding of what pain is, comorbidities of pain, pain impact on the individual and families and to provide self-management skills to manage and cope with pain.

Conclusions

In conclusion, limited scientific evidence is available to support the management of chronic pain in primary care, the high prevalence and impact within the primary care population means priority must be attached to the relief of suffering. The application of core primary care skills and experience, combined with evidence and consensus that is available, provide a reasonable approach for the primary care physician. Communication within the primary care team, and between physicians in primary and secondary/tertiary care, can maximize the effectiveness of available care. New innovative management approaches continue to be developed, and scientific evaluation in a community-based or primary care context is important to enable improved management of this important public health condition.

References

1 Breivik H, Collett B, Ventafridda V *et al.* (2006) Survey of chronic pain in Europe: prevalence, impact on daily life, and treatment. *Eur J Pain* **10**:287–333.
2 Smith BH, Elliott AM, Chambers WA *et al.* (2001) The impact of chronic pain in the community. *Fam Pract* **18**: 292–299.
3 Peng P, Choiniere M, Dion D *et al.*; STOPPAIN Investigators Group. (2007) Challenges in accessing multidisciplinary pain treatment in Canada. *Can J Anaesth* **54**:977–84.
4 Green LA, Fryer GE, Yawn BP *et al.* (2001) The ecology of medical care revisited. *N Engl J Med* **344**:2021–5.
5 Haetzman M, Elliott AM, Smith BH *et al.* (2003) Chronic pain and the use of conventional and alternative therapy. *Fam Pract* **20**:147–54.
6 Von Korff M, Dworkin SF, Le Resche L. (1990) Graded chronic pain status: an epidemiologic evaluation. *Pain* **40**:279–91.
7 Merskey H, Bogduk N, eds. (1994) IASP Task Force on Taxonomy. *Classification of Chronic Pain*, 2nd edn. IASP Press, Seattle, WA.
8 Morley S, Williams Ade C, Hussain S. (0000) Estimating the clinical effectiveness of cognitive behavioural therapy in the clinic: evaluation of a CBT informed pain management programme. *Pain* **137**:670–80.
9 The Pain Society, the Royal College of Anaesthetists, the Royal College of General Practitioners and the Royal College of Psychiatrists. (2004) *Recommendations for the appropriate use of opioids for persistent non-cancer pain.*
10 http://www.topalbertadoctors.org/cpgs/back_pain.html Accessed September 18, 2009.
11 Dworkin RH, O'Connor AB, Backonja M *et al.* (2007) Pharmacological management of neuropathic pain: evidence-based recommendations. *Pain* **132**:237–51.
12 Sullivan MD, Turner JA, Romano J. (1991) Chronic pain in primary care: identification and management of psychosocial factors. *J Fam Pract* **32**:193–9.
13 Kendall NAS, Linton SJ, Main CJ. (1997) *Guide to Assessing Psychological Yellow Flags in Acute Low Back Pain, Risk Factors for Long Term Disability and Work Loss.* Accident Compensation Corporation and the New Zealand Guidelines

Group, Wellington, New Zealand. http://www.chiro.org/LINKS/GUIDELINES/FULL/NEW_ZEALAND/Guide_to_Assessing/full_text.html Accessed September 19, 2009.

14 Haanpää M, Backonja MM, Bennett M *et al.* (2009) Assessment of neuropathic pain in primary care. *Am J Med* **122(10 Suppl)**:S13–21.

15 http://clinicalevidence.bmj.com/ceweb/conditions/msd/msd.jsp Accessed September 19, 2009.

16 World Health Organization (WHO). (1984) *WHO Draft Interim Guidelines. Handbook on Relief of Cancer Pain.* WHO Technical Document CAN/84.2. WHO, Geneva.

17 Kalso E, Edwards JE, Moore RA *et al.* (2004) Opioids in chronic non-cancer pain: systematic review of efficacy and safety. *Pain* **112**:372–80.

18 Kalso E, Allan L, Dobrogowski J *et al.* (2005) Do strong opioids have a role in the early management of back pain? Recommendations from a European expert panel. *Curr Med Res Opin* **21**:1819–28.

19 British Pain Society and Royal College of General Practitioners. (2004) A practical guide to the provision of Chronic Pain Services for adults in Primary Care. BPS, RCGP http://www.britishpainsociety.org/NAPP_RESOURCEPACK.pdf Accessed September 29, 2009.

20 National Institute for Health and Clinical Excellence (UK). (2009) *Low Back Pain. Early Management of Persistent Non-specific Low Back Pain.* NICE Clinical Guideline 88. http://www.nice.org.uk/nicemedia/pdf/CG88NICEGuideline.pdf Accessed September 20, 2009.

21 Von Korff M, Balderson B, Saunders K *et al.* (0000) A trial of an activating intervention for chronic back pain in primary care and physical therapy settings. *Pain* **113**:323–30.

22 Heymans M, van Tulder MW, Esmail R *et al.* (2004) Back schools for non-specific low-back pain. *Cochrane Database Syst Rev* **4**:CD000261.

23 Buchbinder R, Jolley D. (2004) Population-based intervention to change back pain beliefs: three year follow up population survey. *Br Med J* **328**:321.

24 Little P, Lewith G, Webley F *et al.* (2008) Randomised controlled trial of Alexander technique lessons, exercise, and massage (ATEAM) for chronic and recurrent back pain. *Br Med J* **337**:a884.

25 Dobscha SK, Corson K, Perrin NA *et al.* (2009) Collaborative care for chronic pain in primary care: a cluster randomized trial. *JAMA* **301**:1242–52.

26 Martimo KP, Verbeek J, Karppinen J *et al.* (2008) Effect of training and lifting equipment for preventing back pain in lifting and handling: systematic review. *Br Med J* **336**:429–31.

27 Scholten-Peeters GG, Meeleman-van der Steen CW, van der Windt DA *et al.* (2006) Education by general practitioners or education and exercises by physiotherapists for patients with whiplash-associated disorders? A randomized clinical trial. *Spine* **31**:723–31.

28 United Kingdom Back Pain Exercise and Manipulation (UK BEAM) Trial Team. (2004) UK BEAM randomised trial: effectiveness of physical treatments for back pain in primary care. *Br Med J* **329**:1377–81.

29 Jellema P, van der Windt DA, van der Horst HE *et al.* (2005) Why is a treatment aimed at psychosocial factors not effective in patients with (sub)acute low back pain? *Pain* **118**:350–9.

Part 4

Pharmacotherapy

Chapter 13

Nutrition and pain management: dietary soy as an analgesic modality

Alexis Codrington[1], Stéphanie Chevalier[2] & Yoram Shir[1]

[1] *Alan Edwards Pain Management Unit, McGill University Health Centre, Montreal, Canada*
[2] *McGill Nutrition & Food Science Centre, McGill University Health Centre, Montreal, Canada*

Your medicine shall be your food and your food shall be your medicine (Hippocrates)

Diet as an analgesic modality

Dietary habits have a crucial role in the prevention or aggravation of multifactorial illnesses such as cancer, and coronary heart and rheumatic diseases. For example, the consumption of a Mediterranean diet, characteristically low in saturated fatty acids and high in unsaturated fatty acids, is associated with a lower incidence of coronary heart disease [1]. Less explored, but no less plausible, is the idea that diet could also have a significant role in the prevention of other multifactorial diseases such as chronic pain. Indeed, there are preliminary animal and human data associating diet with analgesia. Although a comprehensive review of these data is beyond the scope of this chapter, a few examples are worth mentioning.

Animal studies

In rodents, changes in basic dietary ingredients have been shown to modify pain perception:

sweetened liquid attenuated the responses of intact rats to experimental noxious heat stimuli [2]; rats fed with soybean oil developed increased tolerance to noxious heat [3]; tryptophan and taurine-rich diets decreased visceral and chronic neuropathic-like pain [4]; dietary supplements such as ginseng root [5] and tart cherry anthocyanins [6] decreased nociception in multiple acute and persistent pain models; and vitamin B complex reduced neuropathic-like pain in nerve-injured rats [7].

Human studies

Although most reports in humans are anecdotal, there are some solid scientific data supporting the use of diet as an analgesic modality: sucrose supplementation decreased acute pain behavior in newborn infants undergoing painful procedures [8]; daily supplementation of fish oil was as effective as ibuprofen for relieving neck and back pain, and was beneficial in reducing inflammatory joint pain [9]; and daily supplementation of vitamin C decreased the risk of developing complex regional pain syndrome (CRPS) Type I in patients with wrist fractures [10].

Unfortunately, the limited amount of substantiated data related to dietary analgesia is in stark contrast to public interest in this topic. The lack of interest among the scientific community is surprising considering the prevalence of chronic pain, its

Clinical Pain Management: A Practical Guide, 1st edition.
Edited by Mary E. Lynch, Kenneth D. Craig and Philip W.H. Peng.

devastating physical, emotional and social consequences, and modern medicine's limited ability to alleviate it. In this chapter we focus on the analgesic properties of a single food, soy, and its derived products. The research program described later in the chapter, from initial experiments in laboratory animals to clinical studies in chronic pain patients, could serve as a model for future studies testing potential analgesic properties of other dietary candidates.

Soybeans: their significance and destiny in the human diet

The spread of soybean cultivation, its multiplicity of uses, and its global economic, political and medical significance set it apart from all other major food plants. The American Soybean Association reported that in the USA alone, 80.5 million metric tons of soy were harvested in 2008. Soybeans are still perceived by many in the Western world as primarily an industrial crop or animal feed rather than as human food. However, they are in reality an extraordinarily versatile and rich food source, gradually attaining growing importance in the world's food future. Widely available choices in today's market, including shelves of soy dietary supplements and nutraceuticals containing soy isoflavones, are sufficient proof of the increasing role of soybeans in our diet.

One of the advantages of soybeans over other plant foods is that they contain 30–40% protein, including all the amino acids essential for human nutrition. Soy products are almost equivalent to animal sources in protein quality but contain less saturated fat and no cholesterol. Traditional soy foods include tofu, miso and tempeh while "second generation" soy products, produced following chemical extractions and other forms of processing, include soy protein isolate and soy flour. There are numerous foods incorporating these products as primary ingredients such as meatless burgers, dietary protein supplements and infant formula. Soy protein, soy oil and soy lecithin have also become an often-unnoticed presence in countless food items as additives or food extenders.

An increased interest in soy has stemmed from evidence of its many health benefits. The observation that Asian populations have lower rates of breast and prostate cancer as well as cardiovascular disease drew great attention to traditional Asian diets and soy consumption. Asians consume significant amounts of soy protein, up to 80 g per day. While 25% of Americans consume soy foods or beverages at least once per week, per-capita soy protein consumption is less than 1 g per day. Although controversial, epidemiological and experimental data were strong enough to support a recommendation by the US Food and Drug Administration to increase daily dietary amounts of soy protein to at least 25 g for positive health benefits.

Hyponociceptive effect of soy: preclinical evidence

An inadvertent finding in the laboratory more than a decade ago ignited interest in the effect of diet, especially soy, on nociception. At the time, the authors' research group had established a neuropathic-like pain model in rats by partial sciatic nerve ligation (PSL), mimicking CRPS Type II in humans [11]. It was found that certain rat chows possessed a selected capability to decrease chronic neuropathic-like nociception in these rats. Unexpectedly, the common denominator of the analgesic diets was the amount of soy protein that the rat chow contained. The relationship between dietary soy and analgesia was thus extensively studied in two chronic pain models.

Neuropathic pain model

Both soy protein and soy fat possess antinociceptive properties in the PSL model of neuropathic pain. The perioperative consumption of diets consisting of 20% soy protein, rather than milk casein protein (used as a comparative control), suppressed the development of chronic neuropathic-like pain behavior and strikingly reduced levels of allodynia and hyperalgesia in PSL-injured rats [12]. Dietary soy protein may be a unique preemptive modality to prevent the development of

PSL hypernociception; the pain-suppressive properties of soy protein were predominantly the result of preoperative rather than postsurgical soy consumption [13].

Soy fat also possesses hyponociceptive properties. Both soy protein and soy fat interact synergistically to decrease neuropathic-like hypernociception following nerve injury [14]. The consumption of diets rich in soy fat brings about significant changes in the fatty acid composition of the injured sciatic nerve. These changes are significantly associated with hypoesthesia following PSL nerve injury in rats, with an inverse correlation between neural levels of omega-3 polyunsaturated fatty acids and levels of nociception [15]. It is therefore possible that dietary analgesia is partially mediated through specific changes in the fatty acid content of the injured nerve.

Bone cancer pain model

The analgesic properties of soy have also been examined using a murine model of bone cancer pain, created by injecting sarcoma cells into the medullary cavity of the femur [16]. Soy protein-enriched diets were able to decrease nociception and reduce secondary hyperalgesia in this model. As in humans, bone cancer pain in rats can be of a mixed nociceptive–neuropathic type, where neurochemical changes in the bone lead to central sensitization and secondary hyperalgesia. It is possible that the same analgesic mechanisms of soy in the PSL model of neuropathic-like pain are also involved in the hypoalgesic effect in this model.

Hyponociceptive mechanisms of soy

The identification of specific antinociceptive soybean components is quite difficult given that soy protein alone contains numerous bioactive components, many of which could possess analgesic properties. While few pharmacological data exist for intact soy protein, details on certain components found in commercial protein preparations are available.

Phytoestrogens (isoflavones and lignans)

Soy is a unique source of an abundance of phytoestrogens, mainly isoflavones. Out of all the components of soy, the health benefits of phytoestrogens, especially genistein and daidzein isoflavones, have received the most attention from health experts and much public interest. Phytoestrogens inhibit various types of protein-kinase enzymes [17], have antioxidative properties [18] and possess immunomodulatory as well as anti-inflammatory qualities [19]. Indeed, genistein, a natural isoflavone from soy, reversed pain hypersensitivity in an animal model of human sciatic neuritis [19]. In the PSL model, mid-range isoflavone plasma levels were associated with decreased nociception [20]. Interestingly, the consumption of a traditional soy diet based on tofu, natto and miso results in median plasma levels of the isoflavones genestein and daidzein (approximately 280 nmol/L) [21] that are within the range of effective isoflavone plasma levels measured in rats [20].

Phenolic acids

Soy products contain numerous phenolic acids, mainly salicylic, chlorogenic, caffeic and ferulic acids. These compounds might have antinociceptive effects due to their anti-inflammatory and antioxidant properties [22].

Phytates

Commercial soy preparations contain substantial amounts of phytates, accounting for 60–90% of the seed phosphorus content. Phytates also possess antioxidative properties [23].

Saponins

These complex polysaccharides, bound to compounds like steroids, have direct antinociceptive effects in addition to possessing anti-inflammatory and immunostimulatory properties [24].

Soy fat

Fat-mediated analgesia could be related to the fact that the composition of fatty acids in the diet in general has a critical role in determining tissue fatty acid composition [25]. Tissue fats, specifically polyunsaturated fatty acids, have two main biological roles:

1 They are crucial components of cell membranes, where they are incorporated into phospholipids, playing an important part in maintaining structural integrity and function. Since the physical state of the neuronal membrane is pivotal for information transmission, dietary fatty acids may induce changes in neurophysiological, cognitive and behavioral variables, all of which can be implicated in nociceptive response.

2 They serve as substrates for bioactive molecules such as prostaglandins, thromboxanes and leukotrienes, thus affecting immune and inflammatory responses [26].

Analgesic effect of soy protein: clinical evidence

The applicability of preclinical findings to humans remains to be firmly established. To the best of our knowledge, no population studies have been conducted comparing the prevalence of neuropathic pain in populations consuming soy-rich and soy-deficient diets. Only a few studies have examined the possible association between soy protein and analgesia.

Diets enriched with soymilk, taken orally each day for 3 months (34 g soy protein/day), had a mild analgesic effect on cyclical menstruation-associated breast pain; 56% of healthy women reported favorable results [27]. Daily consumption of 40 g soy protein for 3 months was found to be safe and effective in partially relieving pain and discomfort associated with osteoarthritis [28]. However, daily consumption of beverages containing 20 g soy protein and 160 mg isoflavones for 6 weeks did not improve fibromyalgia symptoms [29].

The analgesic effect of soy-enriched diets in patients with chronic postsurgical or post-traumatic neuropathic pain has been investigated in a multi-ple-case pilot study. The main inclusion criterion was the existence of tactile allodynia, regardless of its location or exact etiology [30]. For 6 weeks, half of the patients' daily protein consumption was exchanged with isolated soy protein powder (30–55 g proportional to body weight), dissolved into their usual foods and drinks. In addition, patients' added fat was replaced with soy sources such as soy oil and margarine. To maintain the diet isoenergetic and isonitrogenous, portion sizes of meat, fish, poultry and eggs were reduced by half and dairy products were omitted. At the end of the 6-week dietary manipulation period, patients were followed for an additional 6 weeks, during which time they resumed their regular diet. Fifteen out of 20 patients recruited to the study were able to adhere to the study protocol despite the major dietary change and no serious adverse events were recorded.

A decrease in pain levels, although not significant, was recorded for the whole group (baseline visual analog scale [VAS]: $71.8 \pm 4.8/100$ vs. post-soy VAS: $66.8 \pm 5.0/100$). However, there was a significant positive correlation between the total amount of soy protein consumed and change in pain intensity ($r = 0.525$; $p = 0.045$). As well, disability levels (Pain Disability Index) decreased significantly after 6 weeks of soy-rich diet ($p < 0.001$) and correlated to the amount of consumed soy protein ($r = 0.631$; $p = 0.012$). Unexpectedly, the average size of the dynamic tactile allodynia area decreased from $178 \pm 40 \, cm^2$ to $99 \pm 25 \, cm^2$ but this decrease did not reach statistical significance ($p = 0.09$). Mood changes (Profile of Mood States Questionnaire) and static tactile allodynia had not changed significantly at the end of the 6-week soy consumption period. These results do not negate the fact that upon individual assessment certain patients did find relief from this therapeutic approach; in five out of the 15 patients the area of tactile allodynia decreased by more than 30% and in one patient it completely disappeared at the end of the soy period.

Case illustration

A 64-year-old woman sustaining a bimalleolar ankle fracture of the left foot underwent open reduction and internal fixation. Following the surgery she developed constant, sharp and burning pain at the medial aspect of the left leg, radiating down to the 2nd, 3rd and 4th toes over the dorsum of the foot. Spontaneous pain levels were reported to be 80/100 (VAS) with tactile allodynia, atrophic skin changes and edema. The patient was diagnosed as CRPS Type II due to a saphenous nerve injury. Physical examination prior to joining the study revealed a cold and mildly edematous left foot with tactile allodynia in the dorsum of the foot, extending proximally to the medial aspect of the leg, 20 cm above the malleolus. Past therapeutic trials with physiotherapy, local lidocaine and Depo-Medrol® injections, saphenous nerve blocks, a variety of non-opioid and opioid analgesics, and adjuvant medications did not bring significant pain relief. At the end of the 6-week soy period the following changes were documented: the ongoing pain proximal to the ankle had completely disappeared; pain intensity levels in the foot and ankle decreased by 44% from baseline (8.1–4.5/10; VAS); McGill Pain Questionnaire scores decreased from 48 to 8 (number of words chosen) and the area of dynamic tactile allodynia decreased from 346 to 56 cm^2. Two weeks after stopping soy consumption and having resumed her regular diet, the patient reported increased pain extending proximally from the ankle to the leg. Upon recommencing the soy-rich diet the new pain symptoms subsided. Three years after adopting an out of study soy-rich diet routine, the patient still reported acceptable pain levels.

Clinical considerations in using soy protein

Drug interactions

Some concern exists relating to isoflavones and their effect on the antitumor properties of selective estrogen receptor modulators, such as tamoxifen. Soy protein may also interact with warfarin (Coumadin®) and simultaneous consumption with levothyroxine (Synthroid®) may reduce hormone absorption. To be safe, soy protein should not be consumed within 1 hour of taking the thyroid medication.

Adverse reactions

Adverse events related to soy consumption are generally minor and rare. Mild gastrointestinal side effects have been reported in adults including bloating, nausea, constipation and flatulence. This effect is due to an inability to digest the natural carbohydrates found in the whole soybean; however, more than 99% of the soy carbohydrates are removed in isolated soy protein products. Concerns have been expressed about the reduced bioavailability of minerals such as zinc, iron and calcium in diets rich in soy products. However, soy products incorporated into a diverse and balanced diet should have little effect on mineral status.

Bioavailability of isoflavones

Glycoside isoflavones, genestin and daidzin, cannot be absorbed unless hydrolyzed and converted to the bioactive aglycone forms, genistein and daidzein, by intestinal microflora or *in vitro* fermentation. Because antibiotics alter the gut flora metabolism of isoflavones, it is advisable not to undertake soy protein supplementation following recent antibiotic use.

Current and future research endeavors

The minimal amount of clinical data supporting the use of soy as an analgesic modality necessitates additional controlled studies to determine: (a) its efficacy; (b) the optimal amount of soy required to reduce pain; and (c) the minimum time-window of exposure required to obtain an analgesic effect both before and after the pain condition has developed. Two clinical studies are currently underway at Johns Hopkins University and the research unit at McGill University to assess the effect of pre-emptive soy supplementation on the development of chronic postoperative pain. An additional study to test the analgesic effect of soy supplementation in patients with established neuropathic facial pain is set to commence shortly. Finally, comparative population studies comparing the prevalence of neuropathic pain in societies customarily consuming soy-rich and soy-deficient diets would be of great value in contributing to the notion of soy as a novel therapeutic approach for pain management.

References

1 Roehm E. (2009) The evidence-based Mediterranean diet reduces coronary heart disease risk, and plant-derived monounsaturated fats may reduce coronary heart disease risk. *Am J Clin Nutr* **90**:697–8.

2 Ren K, Blass EM, Zhou Q *et al*. (1997) Suckling and sucrose ingestion suppress persistent hyperalgesia and spinal Fos expression after forepaw inflammation in infant rats. *Proc Natl Acad Sci U S A* **94**:1471–5.

3 Yehuda S, Carasso RL. (1987) Effects of dietary fats on learning, pain threshold, thermoregulation and motor activity in rats: interaction with the length of feeding period. *Int J Neurosci* **32**:919–25.

4 Belfer I, Davidson E, Ratner A *et al*. (1998) Dietary supplementation with the inhibitory amino acid taurine suppresses autotomy in HA rats. *Neuroreport* **9**:3103–7.

5 Mogil JS, Shin YH, McCleskey EW *et al*. (1998) Ginsenoside Rf, a trace component of ginseng root, produces antinociception in mice. *Brain Res* **792**:218–28.

6 Tall JM, Seeram NP, Zhao C *et al*. (2004) Tart cherry anthocyanins suppress inflammation-induced pain behavior in rat. *Behav Brain Res* **153**:181–8.

7 Wang ZB, Gan Q, Rupert RL *et al*. (2005) Thiamine, pyridoxine, cyanocobalamin and their combination inhibit thermal, but not mechanical hyperalgesia in rats with primary sensory neuron injury. *Pain* **114**:266–77.

8 Stevens B, Yamada J, Ohlsson A. (2004) Sucrose for analgesia in newborn infants undergoing painful procedures. *Cochrane Database System Rev* CD001069.

9 Maroon JC, Bost JW. (2006) Omega-3 fatty acids (fish oil) as an anti-inflammatory: an alternative to nonsteroidal anti-inflammatory drugs for discogenic pain. *Surg Neurol* **65**: 326–31.

10 Zollinger PE, Tuinebreijer WE, Breederveld RS *et al*. (2007) Can vitamin C prevent complex regional pain syndrome in patients with wrist fractures? A randomized, controlled, multi-center dose–response study. *J Bone Joint Surg* **89**:1424–31.

11 Seltzer Z, Dubner R, Shir Y. (1990) A novel behavioral model of neuropathic pain disorders produced in rats by partial sciatic nerve injury. *Pain* **43**:205–18.

12 Shir Y, Ratner A, Raja SN *et al*. (1998) Neuropathic pain following partial nerve injury in rats is suppressed by dietary soy. *Neurosci Letts* **240**:73–6.

13 Shir Y, Raja SN, Weissman CS *et al*. (2001) Consumption of soy diet before nerve injury preempts the development of neuropathic pain in rats. *Anesthesiology* **95**:1238–44.

14 Perez J, Ware MA, Chevalier S *et al*. (2004) Dietary fat and protein interact in suppressing neuropathic pain-related disorders following a partial sciatic ligation injury in rats. *Pain* **111**: 297–305.

15 Soleimannejad E, Tremblay-Mercier J, Cunane SC *et al*. (2008) Dietary analgesia in nerve-injured rats is associated with fatty acid changes in the peripheral nerve. *Pain Res Manag* **13**:148.

16 Zhao C, Wacnik PW, Tall JM *et al*. (2004) Analgesic effects of a soy-containing diet in three murine bone cancer pain models. *J Pain* **5**:104–10.

17 Huang J, Nasr M, Kim Y *et al*. (1992) Genistein inhibits protein histidine kinase. *J Biol Chem* **267**:15511–5.

18 Djuric Z, Chen G, Doerge DR *et al*. (2001) Effect of soy isoflavone supplementation on markers of oxidative stress in men and women. *Cancer Letts* **172**:1–6.

19 Valsecchi AE, Franchi S, Panerai AE *et al*. (2008) Genistein, a natural phytoestrogen from soy, relieves neuropathic pain following chronic

constriction sciatic nerve injury in mice: anti-inflammatory and antioxidant activity. *J Neurochem* **107**:230–40.

20 Shir Y, Campbell JN, Raja SN *et al.* (2002) The correlation between dietary soy phytoestrogens and neuropathic pain behavior in rats after partial denervation. *Anaesth Anal* **94**:421–6, table.

21 Arai Y, Uehara M, Sato Y *et al.* (2000) Comparison of isoflavones among dietary intake, plasma concentration and urinary excretion for accurate estimation of phytoestrogen intake. *J Epidemiol* **10**:127–35.

22 Han X, Shen T, Lou H. (2007) Dietary polyphenols and their biological significance. *Int J Molec Sci* **8**:950–88.

23 Graf E, Eaton JW. (1990) Antioxidant functions of phytic acid. *Free Radic Biol Med* **8**:61–9.

24 Moharram FA, El Shenawy SM. (2007) Antinociceptive and anti-inflammatory steroidal saponins from Dracaena ombet. *Planta Med* **73**:1101–6.

25 Kelly GS. (2001) Conjugated linoleic acid: a review. *Altern Med Rev* **6**:367–82.

26 Calder PC. (2006) Polyunsaturated fatty acids and inflammation. *Prostaglandins Leukot Essent Fatty Acids* **75**:197–202.

27 McFadyen IJ, Chetty U, Setchell KD *et al.* (2000) A randomized double blind-cross over trial of soya protein for the treatment of cyclical breast pain. *Breast* **9**:271–6.

28 Arjmandi BH, Khalil DA, Lucas EA *et al.* (2004) Soy protein may alleviate osteoarthritis symptoms. *Phytomedicine* **11**:567–75.

29 Wahner-Roedler DL, Thompson JM, Luedtke CA *et al.* (2008) Dietary soy supplement on fibromyalgia symptoms: a randomized, double-blind, placebo-controlled, early phase trial. *Evid Based Complement Alternat Med* Nov **6**:1–6.

30 Shir Y, Perez J. (2005) The effect of soy-enriched diets on neuropathic pain in humans: preliminary results. *Pain Res Manag* **10**:95.

Acknowledgments

The multiple-case soy pilot study was supported by the Montreal General Hospital Research Institute and the Louise and Alan Edwards Foundation.

Chapter 14

Antidepressant analgesics in the management of chronic pain

C. Peter N. Watson

Department of Medicine, University of Toronto, Toronto, Canada

Introduction

More than a quarter century of investigation has identified that antidepressants are effective for chronic non-cancer pain (CNCP). This chapter is a based on systematic reviews of quality randomized controlled trials (RCTs) in these conditions [1–5].

Historically, these RCTs first examined tricyclic antidepressants (TCAs) such as amitriptyline based on published observational data and because of their putative action on potentiating pain-inhibitory mechanisms involving serotonin and noradrenaline. Because of limitations in efficacy and concern about adverse effects, attention turned to the more selective serotonin reuptake inhibitors (SSRIs) such as fluoxetine and others and the more noradrenergic agents such as maprotiline, desipramine and nortriptyline. More recently, because of disappointing results regarding the superiority of most of these more specific antidepressants (except the more noradrenergic TCA nortriptyline), research has explored new drugs such as the serotonin noradrenaline reuptake inhibitors (SNRIs) venlafaxine, duloxetine and milnacipran (not yet approved in Canada) which,

Clinical Pain Management: A Practical Guide, 1st edition.
Edited by Mary E. Lynch, Kenneth D. Craig and Philip W.H. Peng.
© 2011 Blackwell Publishing Ltd.

like amitriptyline, have an effect on both serotonin and noradrenaline with the hope of fewer adverse effects and better analgesia.

This chapter addresses the scientific basis for the treatment of CNCP with antidepressants based on RCTs in CNCP such as neuropathic pain, fibromyalgia, arthritis, low back pain and headache.

Basic mechanisms

RCTs in neuropathic pain have repeatedly and clearly demonstrated the separation of the analgesic and antidepressant effects. The earliest concept of the mechanism of antidepressant analgesia was that this occurred via pain-inhibiting systems that descend from the brainstem onto the dorsal horn of the spinal cord. This earliest model involved an endorphin link from the periaqueductal gray area of the midbrain to the raphe nucleus lower in the brainstem and then a serotonergic connection from the raphe to the dorsal horn of the spinal cord. However, another inhibitory system extends from the locus ceruleus in the lateral pons to the dorsal horn which involves noradrenaline. The older antidepressants are relatively "dirty drugs" and act on multiple receptors and have multiple effects. Among several other actions reasonable mechanisms are the N-methyl-D-aspartate (NMDA) and sodium channel blocking effects of these drugs.

Basic understanding of mechanisms and their impact on clinical practice

A concept of the putative mechanism(s) of action of antidepressants is important clinically because these drugs have a moderate effect at best and are often accompanied by adverse effects limiting therapy. Combinations of drugs with differing actions such as gabapentinoids (act on the $\alpha_2\delta$ subunit of the calcium channel) and/or opioids (opioid receptors) and/or cannabinoids (cannabinoid receptors) are often required with the hope of an additive or even synergistic action.

Best clinical practice for antidepressants in some CNCP conditions

Neuropathic pain

Neuropathic pain can be defined as pain initiated or caused by a primary lesion or dysfunction in the nervous system. There are many examples of these disorders. Most antidepressant research has been carried out in neuropathic pain and 80% of neuropathic pain RCTs have been carried out in painful diabetic neuropathy (PDN) and post-herpetic neuralgia (PHN). Sixty-one RCTs of 20 antidepressants in neuropathic pain were identified [1]. Seventeen were conducted in PDN, 11 in PHN and 33 in other neuropathic pain pain conditions which included facial pain, neuropathic pain with cancer, central post-stroke pain, HIV neuropathy, spinal cord injury, cisplatinum neuropathy, painful polyneuropathy, phantom limb pain and chronic lumbar root pain. Of the trials of oral drugs, 13 antidepressants in 36 RCTs showed a significant effect. With TCAs, six drugs tested favorably, including amitriptyline, imipramine, nortriptyline, desipramine and nortriptyline. Of SNRIs, venlafaxine and duloxetine were superior to placebo [6]. SSRIs yielded favorable results over placebo with paroxetine, citaloprim and escitalopram. The tetracyclic, noradrenergic maprotiline (three RCTs) and the noradrenergic/dopaminergic bupropion (one RCT) also have shown a significant effect

versus placebo. These RCTs have repeatedly shown an analgesic effect independent of an effect on depression and the relief of the different pain qualities seen in neuropathic pain including steady pain, jabbing pain and skin pain (allodynia or pain on touch). RCT results in PDN and PHN are reasonably similar but negative trials in such neuropathic pain disorders as lumbar root pain, HIV and cisplatinum neuropathies and spinal cord injury may reflect the greater intractability of these neuropathic pain problems.

A significant difficulty for the clinician lies in interpreting the results of these many RCTs for translation to clinical practice in deciding which drug to use. One problem is the lack of clinical meaningful data in most studies such as the number of subjects with satisfactory relief. Another issue is the paucity of comparative data (most RCTs are a comparison with placebo). To deal with these deficiencies, number-needed-to-treat (NNT) figures for 50% or more relief and number-needed-to-harm figures for withdrawal for neuropathic pain RCTs have been calculated for both antidepressants and other analgesic classes (Table 14.1) [7]. In neuropathic pain these data indicate that balanced noradrenergic/serotonergic TCAs are superior to noradrenergic TCAs and SNRIs which in turn are superior to SSRIs. Also TCA NNTs are about equal to the opioids morphine and oxycodone and superior to gabapentinoids (gabapentin, pregabalin), the opioid-like drug tramadol and cannabinoids. These data are helpful in placing the different drugs in a treatment algorithm for neuropathic pain (Figure 14.1) [8] which places TCAs as a first choice along with gabapentinoids and SNRIs as a second choice.

Fibromyalgia

A systematic review of the effectiveness of antidepressants in fibromyalgia in 2008 [9] was based on 26 RCTs. The authors concluded that amitriptyline (10–50 mg/day) reduced pain, fatigue and depression in fibromyalgia and improved sleep and quality of life. They also found that some SSRIs and the SNRIs duloxetine and milnacipran were effective but that long-term data were lacking.

Table 14.1 Average numbers needed to treat among placebo controlled trials examining tricyclic antidepressants, and serotonin and noradrenaline reuptake inhibitor antidepressants for neuropathic pain for benefit (50% or more reduction of pain), and minor and major harm. After Lynch & Watson [4].

Agent[*]	NNT "benefit"	NNT "minor harm"	NNT "major harm"[†]	Number of studies[‡]
Amitriptyline	2.4	20.4	30.5	6
Imipramine	2.1	1.4	13.7	4
Desipramine	2.4	12.4	15.2	3
Nortriptyline	2.6	1.4	–	3
Clomipramine	2.1	No dichotomous data available	8.7	1
Average TCAs	2.3	8.9	17	
Venlafaxine	4.0			2
SSRIs	6.7			3

NNT, number-needed-to-treat; SSRI, selective serotonin reuptake inhibitor; TCA, tricyclic antidepressant.
* References for several sources of NNT figures are found in Lynch & Watson [4].
† Major harm consists of withdrawal from the study due to adverse effects.
‡ This column refers to the number of studies for which there was adequate information with which to calculate an average NNT. Please note that these figures derive from studies using different methodologies, different data analyses, with different numbers of patients. There are few comparative trials and the external validity may be poor because of selection that goes into trials. Thus, the NNT data is a rough guide only.

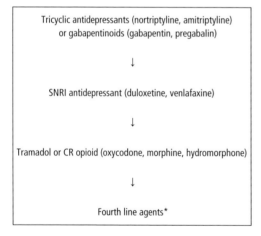

Figure 14.1 Stepwise pharmacological management of neuropathic pain [8]. *Cannabinoids, methadone, lamotrigine, topiramate, valproic acid.

A meta-analysis published in January 2009 [10] of 18 RCTs of antidepressants concluded that antidepressants were associated with improvements in pain, depression, fatigue, sleep and health-related quality of life in patients with fibromyalgia. Further, they noted large effect sizes for TCAs (mostly amitriptyline), a medium effect size for monoamine oxidase inhibitors (MAOs) (moclobemide, pirlindole) and a small effect size for SSRIs (fluoxetine, citalopram, paroxetine) and SNRIs (duloxetine, milnacipran).

The literature review for this chapter (July 2009) found further favorable results for three trials of the SNRIs duloxetine (20–120 mg/day) and four RCTs of milnacipran. As a class of drugs, dual uptake inhibitors improved pain, depression, sleep and quality of life in several of these studies. Duloxetine was approved for treatment of fibromyalgia by the US Food and Drug Administration (FDA) and Health Canada in 2008 and milnacipran for fibromyalgia by the FDA in January 2009.

Headache

Four antidepressants were favorable in 16 RCTs in tension-type headache, migraine, medication-induced and chronic daily headache. Of the commercially available drugs those with a mixed effect on serotonin and noradrenaline (e.g. amitriptyline, venlafaxine and mirtazapine) were superior in both migraine and tension headache. Amitriptyline was efficacious in one RCT in drug withdrawal headache. The SSRIs were found no more effective than placebo in migraine and less effective than TCAs in chronic tension-type headaches [3]. Thus, the TCA amitriptyline, the tetracyclic mirtazapine and the SNRI venlafaxine all seem useful for headache prevention of both migraine and tension-type headache. Most RCTs report a reduction in duration and frequency of headache and less commonly severity.

Low back pain

Three antidepressants were favorable for low back pain (amitriptyline, nortriptyline and doxepin) [2].

Arthritis

Amitriptyline, imipramine and trimipramine were found to be favorable for differing arthritis conditions (osteoarthritis, rheumatoid arthritis, ankylosing spondylitis) [5].

Adverse events

Table 14.2 summarizes monoamine profiles and common side effects for antidepressants used for pain; more details are available elsewhere [4,5,11]. Sedation is common with most TCAs but can be used therapeutically for those with comorbid insomnia when taken at bedtime. The presence of a seizure disorder precludes the use of bupropion. Allergic reactions are generally uncommon. Mild withdrawal reactions may occur and gradual withdrawal is prudent. Number-needed-to-harm (NNH) figures for TCAs do not indicate a worse side effect profile in RCTs than other drug choices for CNCP such as gabapentinoids [7].

SNRIs may aggravate hypertension, exacerbate seizures and trigger mania. More common are nausea, anorexia, weakness, drowsiness, nervousness, dizziness and dry mouth. SSRIs are less likely to cause anticholinergic, adrenergic and antihistaminic side effects, severe sedation, hypotension and weight gain. They may cause gastrointestinal upset (most common), insomnia, dry mouth, drowsiness, sweating, anxiety, agitation, headache, sexual dysfunction and tremor. A central serotonergic syndrome and an increased risk of gastrointestinal bleeding have been reported.

Drug interactions are a consideration with all antidepressants and the safety of most antidepressants in pregnancy and lactation has not been established.

Choice of agent

The few head-to-head RCTs indicate the superiority of non-selective TCA antidepressants over SNRIs and SSRIs. In order to further judge the relative efficacy and safety of these drugs in comparison with each other and with other analgesics, NNTs for 50% or more relief and NNHs for RCT withdrawal have been calculated in neuropathic pain where there are substantial numbers of RCTs (Table 14.1) [7]. NNT values from neuropathic pain trials have identified balanced serotonergic/noradrenergic TCAs as the strongest analgesics followed by noradrenergic antidepressants, then SNRIs and lastly SSRIs. For comparison with other analgesics, NNT values for gabapentinoids are 5.1 for gabapentin, 4.2 for pregabalin, 2.5 for opioids (morphine, oxycodone) and 4 for the dual mechanism agent tramadol. NNH figures for withdrawal from RCTs for TCAs are 14.7 for gabapentin 26.2 and 11.7 for pregabalin. An algorithm has been suggested for neuropathic pain (Figure 14.1) [8] recommending a TCA (e.g. amitriptyline or nortriptyline) or a gabapentinoid (e.g. gabapentin, pregabalin) as first choice, depending on age, concomitant disorders and side effects; an SNRI (venlafaxine, duloxetine) second; and an opioid (morphine, oxycodone, tramadol) next with other drugs as trial and error final options. In fibromyalgia, effect size data suggest that TCAs (amitriptyline) are superior to the other antidepressant groups studied [10]. Of commercially available drugs for migraine and tension headache, balanced drugs such as the TCA amitriptyline, the SNRI venlafaxine and the tetracyclic mirtazapine may be useful prophylactically. For chronic low back pain, arthritis and the miscellaneous CNCP group, general guidelines as for neuropathic pain appear reasonable as there are few studies.

Table 14.2 Analgesic antidepressants. Source: Lynch & Watson [4], reproduced with permission. This information was originally published in *Pain Research & Management* 2006; **11(1)**:11–38.

Drug	Common trade name	Therapeutic range for pain (mg/24h)	Half-life (h)	Neurotransmitter profile		Sedation	Most common side effects (%)				
				NA	5-HT		Orthostatic hypotension	Weight gain	Dry mouth	Consti-pation	GI distress nausea, diarrhea
Tricyclics											
Amitriptyline	Elavil†	10–150*	10–46	+++	+++	>30	>10	>30	>30	>10	>2
Doxepin	Sinequan‡	10–150*	8–36	+++	++	>30	>10	>10	>30	>10	<2
Trimipramine	Surmontil§	10–150*	7–30	++	+	>30	>10	>10	>10	>10	<2
Imipramine	Tofranil¶	10–150*	4–34	+++	+++	>10	>30	>10	>30	>10	>10
Clomipramine	Anafranil**	10–150*	17–37	+++	++++	>2	>10	>10	>30	>10	>10
Desipramine	Norpramin§	10–150*	12–76	+++++	++	>2	>2	>2	>10	>2	>2
Nortriptyline	Aventyl††	10–100*	13–88	++++	++	>2	>2	>2	>10	>10	<2
Serotonin/noradrenaline reuptake inhibitors											
Venlafaxine	Effexor‡‡	37.5–225	3–7 (parent) 9–13 (metabolite)	++	++++	>10	>10	<2	>10	>10	>30
Duloxetine	Cymbalta§§	60–120	10	++++	+++++	>10	<10	<2	>10	>10	>10

5-HT, 5-hydroxytryptamine; GI, gastrointestinal; NA, noradrenaline.
* The therapeutic range for depression is up to 200 mg/24 h for nortriptyline and to 300 mg/24 h for the remaining tricyclic antidepressants; generally, these doses are not required for an analgesic effect and the usual dose will consist of 75 mg/24 h or less.
† 1560678 Ontario Inc, Canada
‡ ERFA Inc, Canada.
§ Aventis Pharma Inc, Canada.
¶ Novartis Pharmaceuticals, Canada.
** Oryx Pharmaceuticals Inc, Canada.
†† Pharmel Inc, Canada.
‡‡ Wyeth Canada.
§§ Lily, USA.
Source: After Virani A, Bezchlibnyk-Butler KZ, Jeffries JJ. (2009) *Clinical Handbook of Psychotropic Drugs*, 18th edn. Hogrefe & Huber, Toronto.

The results of all analgesics in RCTs in CNCP indicate a moderate effect at best in the selected subjects chosen. Currently, for antidepressants it appears that either we have not struck the right balance of serotonin and noradrenaline or that descending monoamine systems are only one component of pain inhibition. Combinations of drugs may be necessary (tricyclics, gabapentinoids, opioids, cannabinoids) unless a "magic bullet" is found but this appears not to be imminent.

Approach to therapy

It is important in selecting an antidepressant such as a TCA for CNCP to individualize therapy and to obtain a complete assessment with attention to issues that may preclude these drugs such as advanced age, heart disease (recent myocardial infarction, conduction defects), urinary retention, glaucoma, other medications and alcohol intake. In deciding on antidepressant therapy a history of failed antidepressant usage should not dissuade one from a careful trial as many failures result from high initial dosing, non-compliance or an inadequate trial (too low a dose or too brief a trial). It is important to explain carefully the goals of treatment and adverse effects to patients. They need information that complete relief is possible but unlikely and that the aim is to take the pain from severe or moderate to mild (occurs in 50–60% in RCTs). Patients also need to know that the starting dose will be low and slowly increased (every week or so) until satisfactory relief occurs or an intolerable adverse effect is experienced. It is important to inform them that the effect of a dosage increase may not be fully experienced for a week or more, that side effects are probable and that, if stopped, drug withdrawal should be gradual. A sedating TCA (amitriptyline) may be useful with the total dose at bedtime if insomnia is a problem or to avoid daytime drug-induced drowsiness. Weight gain may occur with some agents in which case diet and appropriate weight monitoring are important, particularly in the already overweight population. Sexual dysfunction may be more important in the younger age

groups. Less common adverse effects are allergic reactions such as rash, tachycardia (usually supraventricular) and paradoxical insomnia. It is prudent to eliminate, if possible, all other ineffective analgesics and sedating drugs so that drug interactions such as sedation and constipation are minimized. Antidepressants may interact with other drugs such as those that either prolong the QT interval (e.g. methadone) or interfere with hepatic metabolism (via cytochrome P450), possibly causing ventricular tachycardia (antiarrythmics, antiretrovirals, antifungals, calcium channel blockers, macrolide and quinolone antibiotics, SSRIs, antipsychotics, tamoxifen and cisapride).

Useful baseline tests are blood pressure measurement supine and standing, hematology, liver and kidney function, electrolytes and an electrocardiogram (ECG). A good general principle is to "start low and go slow," keeping in mind that with TCAs the analgesic effect occurs at lower doses than the antidepressant effect (mean 50–75 mg). It is reasonable if starting with a TCA such as nortriptyline (less significant adverse events) or amitriptyline to start with 10 mg in those over 65 years and 25 mg in those under 65, and to slowly increase the dose every week or two by similar amounts until an endpoint of satisfactory pain relief or a significant adverse event. It may be helpful to try different antidepressants, moving from TCAs (nortriptyline, amitriptyline, desipramine, imipramine) to the SNRIs (venlafaxine and duloxetine) as individual differences in pain inhibitory mechanisms may mean that one drug is more efficacious for an individual patient. Close follow-up (every 2 weeks initially) is important to supervise compliance, dose increments and to deal with adverse effects. Pre-emptive prescription of a stool softener and an artificial saliva mouth spray are useful routine measures. There is no therapeutic range of blood levels for the analgesic effects of antidepressants but they can be useful to check compliance and as a guide to dose increments in some patients who require higher dosage. Good relief and blood levels may in some be achieved with low doses of 10–20 mg. This response may not always be age-related. A 3-month treatment trial is reasonable. Combination therapy is reasonable and necessary in refractory cases (gabapentinoids, opioids, cannabinoids, topical agents).

In summary, certain antidepressants are analgesic in CNCP. In head-to-head RCTs, NNT figures and effect size data indicate the superiority of the TCAs (amitriptyline, nortriptyline, imipramine, desipramine) and a lesser effect of the SNRIs (venlafaxine, duloxetine, milnacipran) and the SSRIs.

References

1 Saarto T, Wiffen PJ. (2009) Antidepressants for neuropathic pain. *Cochrane Database Syst Rev* **4**:CD005454. http://www.thecochranelibrary.com.

2 Urquhart DM, Hoving JL, Assendelft WJJ *et al.* (2008) Antidepressants for non-specific low back pain (Review). *Cochrane Database Syst Rev* **1**:CD001703. http://www.thecochranelibrary.com.

3 Moja L, Cusi C, Sterzi R *et al.* (2010) Selective serotonin re-uptake inhibitors for preventing migraine and tension headaches (Review). *Cochrane Database Syst Rev* **3**:CD002919. http://www.thecochranelibrary.com.

4 Lynch ME, Watson CPN. (2006) The pharmacotherapy of chronic pain: a review. *Pain Res Manag* **11(1)**:11–38.

5 Watson CPN, Chipman ML, Monks RC. (2006) Antidepressant analgesics: a systematic review and comparative study. In: McMahon JR, Koltzenberg M, eds. *Wall and Melzack's Textbook of Pain*, 5th edn. Elsevier Churchill Livingston. pp. 481–98.

6 Kajdasz DK, Iyengar S, Desaiah D *et al.* (2007) Duloxetine for the management of diabetic peripheral neuropathic pain: evidence-based findings from the post-hoc analysis of three multi-center, randomized, double blind, placebo-controlled, parallel-group studies. *Clin Ther* **29**:2536–46.

7 Finnerup NB, Otto M, McQuay HJ *et al.* (2005) Algorithm for neuropathic pain treatment: an evidence based proposal. *Pain* **118**:289–305.

8 Moulin D, Clark AJ, Gilron I *et al.* (2007) Pharmacological management of chronic neuropathic pain- consensus statement and guidelines from the Canadian Pain Society. *Pain Res Manag* **12(1)**:13–21.

9 Uceyler N, Hauser W, Sommer C. (2008) A systematic review of the effectiveness of treatment with antidepressants in fibromyalgia syndrome. *Arthritis Rheum* **59**:1279–98.

10 Hauser W, Bernardy K, Uceyler N *et al.* (2009) Treatment of fibromyalgia syndrome with antidepressants: a meta-analysis. *JAMA* **301**: 198–209.

11 Hardman JG, Limbird LE, eds. (2001) *Goodman and Gilman's Pharmacological Basis of Therapeutics*, 10th edn. Chapter 17. McGraw Hill, New York.

Chapter 15

Anticonvulsants in the management of chronic pain

Nanna Brix Finnerup[1], Cathrine Baastrup[1] & Troels Staehelin Jensen[1,2]

[1] *Danish Pain Research Center, Aarhus University Hospital, Aarhus, Denmark*
[2] *Department of Neurology, Aarhus University Hospital, Aarhus, Denmark*

Introduction

Anticonvulsant drugs were primarily introduced for the treatment of epilepsy. Many anticonvulsants have pharmacological actions that can interfere with the processes involved in neuronal hyperexcitability either by decreasing excitatory or increasing inhibitory transmission, thereby exerting a neuronal depressant effect. This may explain why some anticonvulsants are effective in bipolar mood disorders and chronic pain conditions, which may share complex pathophysiological mechanisms manifest in different areas of the nervous system.

Chronic pain can be divided according to etiology. Nociceptive pain, including inflammatory pain, is pain arising from activation of nociceptors [1], while neuropathic pain can be defined as pain arising as a direct consequence of a lesion or disease affecting the somatosensory system [2]. A group of pain conditions, which include fibromyalgia, temporomandibular disorders and irritable bowel syndrome, do not fall into these two categories of pain. The underlying mechanisms in these pain syndromes are unknown, but it has been suggested that they may be a result of an abnormal amplification of nociceptive signals or a more generalized hypervigilance in the central nervous system.

As reviewed in previous chapters, all pharmacotherapy for chronic pain should take place within the context of a multidisciplinary approach that addresses biopsychosocial aspects and begins with a review of active healthful strategies and treatments with the least potential for harm.

Anticonvulsants in chronic pain: mechanisms of action

The exact mechanisms by which anticonvulsant drugs relieve chronic pain are not known. Several mechanisms of action may be involved in altering neurotransmission by exerting a neuronal depressant effect in pain pathways [3]. This way, anticonvulsants may attenuate the neuronal hyperexcitability, peripheral and central sensitization and ectopic activity, which are likely the responsible mechanisms underlying chronic pain conditions. These mechanisms of action include modulation of ion channels (sodium, calcium and potassium channels), augmentation of inhibitory effects (particularly by potentiating the inhibitory neurotransmitter gamma-aminobutyric acid [GABA]) and suppression of abnormal neuronal excitability such as inhibition of glutamate receptors or suppression of neurotransmitter release (Table 15.1).

Clinical Pain Management: A Practical Guide, 1st edition.
Edited by Mary E. Lynch, Kenneth D. Craig and
Philip W.H. Peng.
© 2011 Blackwell Publishing Ltd.

Table 15.1 Main mechanism of action of commonly used anticonvulsants for chronic pain.

Drug	Main mechanism of action	Side effects
Carbamazepine	Sodium channel blockade	Somnolence, nausea, dizziness, ataxia, rash, hyponatremia Potential aplastic anemia, hepatitis, serious dermatologic reaction
Oxcarbazepine	Sodium channel blockade	Dizziness, somnolence, diplopia, ataxia, vomiting Potential hyponatremia, anaphylactic reactions
Lamotrigine	Sodium channel blockade	Headache, dizziness, rash, diplopia, ataxia Potential serious dermatologic reaction
Lacosamide	Sodium channel blockade	Dizziness, ataxia, fatigue, headache, diplopia, nausea
Pregabalin	Calcium channel blockade	Dizziness, somnolence, ataxia, weight gain
Gabapentin	Calcium channel blockade	Sedation, ataxia, dizziness, somnolence
Valproate	Increased GABA inhibition, decreased glutamate excitation, sodium channel blockade	Gastrointestinal side effects, headache, allergic skin reactions Potential hepatotoxicity
Topiramate	Sodium and calcium channel blockade, increased GABA inhibition, decreased glutamate excitation	Paresthesia, headache, dizziness, anorexia, weight loss, somnolence, difficulty with memory
Levetiracetam	Binds to a synaptic vesicle protein SV2A	Somnolence, asthenia

GABA, γ-aminobutyric acid.

The anticonvulsant drugs carbamazepine, oxcarbazepine and lamotrigine primarily act by blocking sodium channels. Slowing of the recovery rate of voltage-gated sodium channels and inhibition of sustained high-frequency repetitive firing will stabilize membranes and reduce neuronal excitability in the peripheral and central nervous systems [3]. A newer drug, lacosamide, enhances the slow inactivation of voltage-gated sodium channels and inhibits the collapsing response mediator protein 2 (CRMP-2).

Valproate is a first-generation anticonvulsant with a wide range of actions including potentiation of GABAergic functions [3], reduction in excitatory amino acids, sodium channel and glutamate receptor functions, modulation of potassium and calcium homeostasis, and enhancement of serotonergic neurotransmission.

Gabapentin and pregabalin are members of a new generation of anticonvulsants and are structural derivatives of the inhibitory neurotransmitter GABA, but do not appear to act through the GABAergic neurotransmitter system. The predominant mechanism of action is thought to be through its presynaptic binding to the $\alpha_2\delta$ subunit of voltage-gated calcium channels, which in turn leads to reduced release of neurotransmitters such as glutamate, substance P and calcitonin gene-related peptide [3]. Such a decrease in neurotransmitter release from synapses in several neuronal tissues in the spinal cord and brain is likely to attenuate the neuronal hyperexcitability and abnormal synchronization, which may explain the anticonvulsant, analgesic and anxiolytic activity.

Topiramate is another new-generation anticonvulsant, which modulates sodium channels but also enhances GABAergic transmission and inhibits glutamate receptors. Levetiracetam binds to the synaptic vesicle protein SV2A and interferes with vesicle exocytosis, thus impeding nerve conduction across synapses.

Both the first-generation anticonvulsants phenytoin, valproate and carbamazepine and the newer anticonvulsants lamotrigine, pregabalin, gabapen-

Table 15.2   Anticonvulsant drugs with documented efficacy (consistent outcome in Class I randomized double-blind controlled trials), possible efficacy (owing to inadequate or conflicting data) and evidence for no efficacy in neuropathic pain (other than trigeminal neuralgia), trigeminal neuralgia, migraine prophylaxis and fibromyalgia.

Pain condition	Documented efficacy	Possible efficacy	Probably no efficacy
Neuropathic pain	Gabapentin Pregabalin	Topiramate Carbamazepine Oxcarbazepine Lacosamide Lamotrigine	Levetiracetam
Trigeminal neuralgia	Carbamazepine Oxcarbazepine	Lamotrigine	
Migraine prophylaxis	Valproate Topiramate	Gabapentin Carbamazepine	Lamotrigine Tiagabine Oxcarbazepine
Fibromyalgia	Pregabalin Gabapentin		

tin, lacosamide, topiramate and levetiracetam have a range of mechanisms which may interfere with mechanisms involved in chronic pain. Yet not all anticonvulsant drugs seem to be effective in relieving chronic pain. The three main pain conditions where anticonvulsant drugs have a role in treatment or prevention are neuropathic pain, migraine and fibromyalgia (Table 15.2).

Anticonvulsants in neuropathic pain

Neuropathic pain is a heterogeneous group of chronic pain conditions arising from lesions of the peripheral or central nervous systems. Common neuropathic pain conditions include painful diabetic polyneuropathy, post-herpetic neuralgia, trigeminal neuralgia, phantom pain, pain following peripheral nerve injury and central pain following stroke, spinal cord injury and multiple sclerosis. The various symptoms of neuropathic pain do not seem to be strongly correlated to the underlying etiology. The pain may be spontaneous and/or evoked with allodynia to cold, warmth or touch. Pain descriptors include burning, pins and needles, squeezing, shooting and freezing pain.

Gabapentin and pregabalin have demonstrated well-documented efficacy in various neuropathic pain conditions, including painful polyneuropathy, post-herpetic neuralgia and central pain [4], and are considered first-line drug choices together with tricyclic antidepressants and serotonin noradrenaline reuptake inhibitors [4,5]. Pregabalin and gabapentin may especially have a primary role in patients with anxiety and sleep disturbances and in patients who are taking multiple drugs. The number-needed-to-treat (NNT) for 50% pain relief ranges from 3.3–7 in various neuropathic pain conditions [4], with a pooled NNT of 4.7 (4.2–5.4).

Lamotrigine had initially demonstrated efficacy in small trials in trigeminal neuralgia, HIV neuropathy, painful diabetic neuropathy and central post-stroke pain, but recent large parallel group trials have failed to find a pain-relieving effect of lamotrigine in mixed neuropathic pain and painful polyneuropathy [6]. Therefore, at present, lamotrigine seems not to have a primary role in the treatment of neuropathic pain.

There are also mixed reports for valproate in three studies. One group reported high efficacy while others failed to find an effect, therefore the question remains open as to whether valproate is effective in neuropathic pain [6].

Topiramate failed to relieve pain in three large trials involving 1259 patients with painful diabetic neuropathy [4]. Although these trials had a high placebo response, topiramate does not have a role at present in the treatment of neuropathic pain.

The most recently studied anticonvulsant, lacosamide, may have some effect in painful diabetic neuropathy, but the results from randomized controlled trials are conflicting [6].

Levetiracetam, despite some promising results from experimental animal and open-label trials, failed to find an effect in two recent trials of postmastectomy neuropathic pain and spinal cord injury pain [6], and there is no evidence to suggest the use of levetiracetam for neuropathic pain.

Carbamazepine is the mainstay of treatment for trigeminal neuralgia, but the evidence is sparse and based on old, poorly conducted trials [4,7]. Randomized controlled trials have documented comparable analgesic effects between oxcarbazepine and carbamazepine in trigeminal neuralgia, and a change to oxcarbazepine may be beneficial if carbamazepine is poorly tolerated. Furthermore, there is some evidence to suggest a combination of carbamazepine with lamotrigine or baclofen if monotherapy fails [7], although pharmacodynamic interactions of the drugs may increase the risk of severe side effects [8]. The role of carbamazepine and oxcarbazepine in other neuropathic pain conditions is still unclear because of conflicting results from a limited number of randomized controlled trials.

Anticonvulsants in migraine

Migraine is a common disorder characterized by episodic attacks of headache presenting with or without aura. In patients with migraine who experience a low frequency of attacks, avoidance of factors that trigger the migraine and acute treatment with analgesics or specific migraine medications such as triptans may be adequate [9]. In a subgroup of patients, however, preventive therapy is needed. This includes patients with severe and frequent attacks, overuse of acute therapies and certain migraine conditions such as hemiplegic migraine and migraine with prolonged aura [9].

Together with antidepressants, beta-blockers, calcium channel blockers and non-steroidal anti-inflammatory drugs (NSAIDs), anticonvulsants are recommended as preventive therapy for migraine because of the evidence of good efficacy and tolerability [9,10]. Introducing a prophylactic treatment for migraine has to be individualized and discussed carefully with the patient. The European Federation of Neurological Societies (EFNS) Task Force has recently recommended that drugs of first choice for migraine prophylaxis include beta-blockers, calcium channel blockers, valproate and topiramate [10]. These drugs have the best documented efficacy from randomized controlled trials, which have shown a significant reduction in the number and duration of migraine attacks and pain intensity.

Gabapentin is classified as probably effective and a third-line drug of choice based on one placebo-controlled trial. Lamotrigine did not reduce the frequency of migraine attacks but may be effective in reducing the frequency of migraine auras [10]. Carbamazepine is classified as possibly effective [9], while tiagabine, clonazepam and oxcarbazepine cannot be recommended for migraine prophylaxis [9].

Anticonvulsants in fibromyalgia

Fibromyalgia is a chronic pain condition in which the key symptoms are widespread pain, fatigue and sleep disturbances in association with muscle tender points [11]. Non-pharmacological treatments such as cognitive behavioral therapy and certain exercises as well as amitriptyline treatment have been recommended for the treatment of fibromyalgia.

A recent meta-analysis, which included four randomized placebo-controlled trials with pregabalin and one trial with gabapentin, concluded that there was a strong evidence supporting the efficacy of gabapentin and pregabalin in reducing pain and sleep disturbances, albeit small effect sizes and a pooled NNT for 30% pain reduction of 8 [11]. However, there was no effect of the gabapentinoids on depressed mood, anxiety and fatigue [11], and therefore the key symptoms in fibromyalgia were only partially relieved. There were also a large number of withdrawals because of side effects, which included neurocognitive side effects such as confusion, disturbed attention and anxiety, which may be of particular concern in patients with fibromyalgia because many already develop additional psychological symptoms [11]. The conclusion of this extensive review was that gabapentin and pregabalin can be considered for the treatment of pain and sleep disturbances, but clinicians should consider comorbidities, and the treatment should be multidisciplinary. While pregabalin has been approved for the treatment of fibromyalgia by the US Food and Drug Administration (FDA), the European Medicines Agency (EMEA) denied approval in 2009.

Other anticonvulsants currently not used for chronic pain treatment

The role of phenytoin as a therapeutic option is limited because other anticonvulsants are now available with better side effect profiles. Benzodiazepines have no established role in the treatment of chronic pain. Zonisamide acts on sodium and calcium channels and has only been evaluated in uncontrolled studies and in one small randomized trial in painful polyneuropathy where it was no more effective than placebo [4]. The treatment carries a risk of serious dermatological and hematological reactions. Other second-generation anticonvulsants still await clinical trials to clarify their role in the treatment of neuropathic pain conditions. These include tiagabine, vigabatrin (has a risk of retinal toxicity) and felbamate (risk of aplastic anemia and hepatic failure).

Safety and dosing

Gabapentin and pregabalin have no pharmacokinetic drug–drug interactions, low incidence of life-threatening side effects and no contraindications except for known hypersensitivity. The most common side effects are dose-related dizziness and somnolence, which may resolve in some. Other side effects include dry mouth, asthenia, blurred vision, ataxia, peripheral edema and weight gain not limited to patients with edema. Adverse events have usually been mild or moderate. There is an unsettled association of pregabalin with rhab-

domyolysis and creatine kinase elevations, and patients are advised to report unexplained muscle pain, particularly if accompanied with malaise and fever. Gabapentin should be initiated at a dosage of 300 mg/day and then increased slowly up to 1800–3600 mg/day according to patient response and side effects. Pregabalin is usually started at 75 mg once or twice daily and may be increased up to a final dosage of 600 mg/day in two or three divided doses. For the treatment of fibromyalgia, there was no superiority of 600 mg compared with 300 mg as seen in the treatment of neuropathic pain [11].

Older generation anticonvulsants, such as carbamazepine and valproate, have a narrow therapeutic index and serious side effects, while many newer anticonvulsants have better tolerability profiles and fewer drug interactions. The most common side effects of carbamazepine are sedation, dizziness, ataxia, blurred vision, hyponatremia, confusion in elderly patients and, in rare cases, blood dyscrasia. The starting dosage is usually 300 mg/day, and the dosage is increased by 100 mg every other day to 1500–2000 mg/day.

Oxcarbazepine is reported to have a better side effect profile than carbamazepine but is associated with dizziness, somnolence, ataxia, blurred vision and hyponatremia. From a starting dosage of 600 mg/day, oxcarbazepine may be increased by 150–300 mg every other day to 1500–3000 mg/day.

Side effects to valproate treatment include weight gain, nausea, tremor, hair loss and rare idiosyncratic reactions. Valproate for prophylactic treatment of migraine can be started at 250–500 mg/day and increased up to 500–1800 mg/day.

Side effects associated with the use of lamotrigine include dizziness, ataxia, diplopia, somnolence and nausea. The most concerning side effects are rash and other potentially life-threatening hypersensitivity reactions, and slow dose escalation is recommended to minimize the risk of serious hypersensitivity reactions. The final dosage in the treatment of neuropathic pain is 200–400 mg/day in two divided doses.

Side effects to topiramate treatment include sedation, weight loss, renal calculi, dizziness, ataxia, psychomotor slowing and cognitive difficulties. The recommended daily dosage of topiramate for prophylactic treatment of migraine is 25–100 mg/day given in two divided doses with a starting dose of 15–25 mg at bedtime.

Lacosamide is associated with dizziness, somnolence, nausea, tremor and headache. Caution is advised in patients with cardiac conduction disorders or severe cardiac diseases. A final dosage of 400 mg/day seems to be the optimal balance between side effects and pain relief in neuropathic pain.

Finding the drug that will produce the best possible pain relief for the individual patient may require administration of several of the mentioned drugs as monotherapy over many periods. Steady-state concentration of the anticonvulsant is obtained within days after reaching target dosage (e.g. 4–8 days for topiramate), although the maximal effect may not yet be achieved.

The FDA issued a warning in 2008 on the increased risk of suicidality in patients taking anticonvulsants [12]. Based on the analysis of 199 randomized controlled trials and 43,000 patients, anticonvulsants were associated with twofold increase in suicidal ideation and behavior. This risk was across all anticonvulsants and started as soon as after 1 week of therapy.

In some cases polytherapy may be favorable, especially with a combination of drugs with different modes of action. Special attention to dosage is required when polytherapy is initiated because several of the anticonvulsants increase the clearance of each other (e.g. carbamazepine, phenytoin, lamotrigine, tiagabine and topiramate) with a marked reduction of plasma concentration as a result. Thus, a dose increase of each administered drug may be necessary. In contrast, concomitant administration of lamotrigine and valproic acid results in decreased elimination, and the half-life of lamotrigine may be more than doubled [8].

Discontinuation of a drug, especially in polytherapy, must be done gradually through a dosage decrease regimen.

Conclusions

Anticonvulsant drugs are increasingly used in the treatment of neuropathic pain, fibromyalgia and migraine prophylaxis. As we have few treatments that influence the underlying disease processes in these pain conditions, drugs such as anticonvulsants and antidepressants which may suppress the neuronal hyperexcitability and symptomatic treatment are often used.

Currently, we know little about which patients will benefit from treatment with an anticonvulsant. While some patients will show a moderate to good effect, others will show no effect. Large trials are needed to further understand and evaluate a possible relationship between the symptomatology and presumed underlying mechanisms and efficacy from different drugs with different mechanisms. Also, we need more studies to evaluate the long-term efficacy and safety of anticonvulsants in various chronic pain conditions.

The exact pain-generating mechanisms underlying neuropathic pain, fibromyalgia and migraine are not known. However, these conditions seem to share to some extent the presence of allodynia in skin or deep tissue either within the painful affected dermatome or outside this and it has been suggested that a general neuronal hyperexcitability in the nervous system either peripherally or more centrally might be responsible for this shared allodynia. The fact that several anticonvulsants are effective in these three conditions lend support to the notion that a neuronal hyperexcitability does have a role in generating and maintaining pain in these conditions.

References

1 Loeser JD, Treede RD. (2008) The Kyoto protocol of IASP basic pain terminology. *Pain* **137**: 473–7.

2 Treede RD, Jensen TS, Campbell JN *et al.* (2008) Neuropathic pain: redefinition and a grading system for clinical and research purposes. *Neurology* **70**:1630–5.

3 Dickenson AH, Matthews EA, Suzuki R. (2002) Neurobiology of neuropathic pain: mode of action of anticonvulsants. *Eur J Pain* **6(Suppl A)**:51–60.

4 Finnerup NB, Otto M, McQuay HJ *et al.* (2005) Algorithm for neuropathic pain treatment: an evidence based proposal. *Pain* **118**:289–305.

5 Dworkin RH, O'connor AB, Backonja M *et al.* (2007) Pharmacologic management of neuropathic pain: evidence-based recommendations. *Pain* **132**:237–51.

6 Jensen TS, Madsen CS, Finnerup NB. (2009) Pharmacology and treatment of neuropathic pains. *Curr Opin Neurol* **22**:467–74.

7 Jorns TP and Zakrzewska JM. (2007) Evidence-based approach to the medical management of trigeminal neuralgia. *Br J Neurosurg* **21**:253–61.

8 Perucca E (2006) Clinically relevant drug interactions with antiepileptic drugs. *Br J Clin Pharmacol* **61**:246–55.

9 Silberstein SD. (2008) Treatment recommendations for migraine. *Nat Clin Pract Neurol* **4**:482–9.

10 Evers S, Afra J, Frese A *et al.* (2009) EFNS guideline on the drug treatment of migraine: revised report of and EFNS task force. *Eur J Neurol* **16**:968–81.

11 Häuser W, Bernardy K, Üceyler N, Sommer C. (2009) Treatment of fibromyalgia syndrome with gabapentin and pregabalin: a meta-analysis of randomized controlled trials. *Pain* **145**:69–81.

12 FDA. US Food and Drug Administration. http://www.fda.gov/Drugs/DrugSafety/Postmarket DrugSafetyInformationforPatientsand Providers/UCM100190.

Acknowledgement

The work behind this chapter was sponsored by the Velux Foundation.

Chapter 16

Opioids

Dawn A. Sparks[1,3,4] & Gilbert Fanciullo[1,2,4]

[1] Dartmouth Medical School, Hanover, NH, USA
[2] Section of Pain Medicine, Department of Anesthesiology, Dartmouth-Hitchcock Medical Center, Lebanon, NH, USA
[3] Section of Anesthesiology and Pain Medicine, Children's Hospital at Dartmouth (CHaD), Lebanon, NH, USA
[4] Pain Clinic, Dartmouth-Hitchcock Medical Center, Lebanon, NH, USA

Pain is the experience, suffering is the interpretation (Dr. John Mizenko)

Introduction

In the last 40 years the pendulum has swung from underuse to increased use, and some would argue overuse, of opioids in management of chronic pain. With increasing use has come increased awareness of the risks associated with opioids, including drug misuse, abuse, addiction and diversion along with increases in prescription opioid-related deaths such that now government bodies are implementing strategies geared toward reducing the associated public health risk. In this context the scientific and clinical community have responded by creating guidelines based on the best evidence available [1]. Overall, the quality of evidence to support most recommendations in even the best guidelines is weak and further research is needed [2].

The aim of this chapter is to review molecular aspects, physiology and pharmacology of opioids, as well as to provide a substrate from which to base clinical decision-making when using opioids to treat patients with chronic pain.

Clinical Pain Management: A Practical Guide, 1st edition.
Edited by Mary E. Lynch, Kenneth D. Craig and Philip W.H. Peng.

Mechanism of action

There are several opioid receptor types: μ, δ and κ receptors. In addition, the opioid-receptor-like receptor 1 (ORL-1) has been identified. Receptors are named using the first letter of the first ligand that was found to bind to them. Morphine was the first chemical shown to bind to μ receptors, and ketocyclazocine was first shown to bind to κ receptors. μ receptors induce reactions principally at the suspraspinal level to mechanical, thermal and chemical stimuli. The μ receptor appears to be the chief receptor involved in analgesia. Receptors are found in the brain, spinal cord and in peripheral nociceptors in the gastrointestinal tract and other sites. The μ1 receptors are involved in mechanisms producing bradycardia, sedation and pruritus. μ2 receptors are involved in producing miosis, constipation, euphoria, orthostatic hypotension, venous dilatation and respiratory depression. The μ2 receptors, along with δ receptors, are thought to be involved in producing physical dependence. δ receptors, located primarily within the brain, modulate pain caused by inflammation and mechanical nociception. δ receptors also seem to potentiate the analgesia caused by the binding of the μ receptor through the endogenous ligands known as enkephalins. κ receptors located in the brain and the spinal cord act on pain related to visceral discomfort and can produce sedation. κ receptors also cause dysphoria, diuresis and meiosis. ORL-1 receptors are involved in in pain responses as well as having a major role in the development of tolerance to μ-opioid agonists [3]. σ and ε receptors are generally no longer considered as opioid receptors [4].

Opioid receptors and peptides coalesce to form an intricate neurotransmitter arrangement known as the endogenous opioid system. The endogenous opioids are dynorphins, enkephalins, endorphins and endomorphins which modify nociception in the same fashion as exogenous opioids. The opioid receptors are found within the cellular membranes and are comprised of numerous glycoproteins. Opioid receptors belong to a superfamily of guanine (G) protein-coupled receptors [5]. These G proteins act as second messengers and assist in regulating cell activities. All of these receptors coalesce with the G proteins and impede adenyl cyclase from acting on ion channels within the cellular membrane.

Opioid receptors vary widely in their distribution between individuals. On a cellular level, receptors are located in both presynaptic and postsynaptic positions. The dorsal horn of the spinal cord, medulla oblongata, thalamus and the cortex are involved in ascending pain transmission whereas the periaqueductal gray matter, nucleus raphe magnus and ventral medulla utilize the descending pain pathways, all of which possess opioid receptors. These receptors are activated by endogenous opioids as well as the opioids we prescribe and, in turn, modify nociceptive transmission, modulation and perception. Activated opioid receptors produce an influx of potassium ions into cells resulting in changes in transmembrane potential leading to alteration in action potentials. This change, along with the altering protein kinase C enzyme systems, results in decreased neurotransmitter release. This causes a closing of the voltage-gated calcium channel on presynaptic neuronal terminals. Furthermore, postsynaptic neurons become hyperpolarized by the increased potassium conductance. The voltage changes at the membrane level lead to augmented antinociceptive descending aminergic activity. This action also inhibits, at the spinal level, further processing of ascending nociceptive signals.

Clinical pharmacology

Most opioids can be classified by their action at the receptor [5]. A pure opioid agonist possesses affinity for binding sites as well as efficacy. Efficacy is defined as the ability to produce a desired amount of a desired effect. In contrast, a pure antagonist provides an affinity for binding; however, no efficacy. It blocks the capability of both endogenous and exogenous ligands from binding. A mixed agonist–antagonist produces an agonist effect at one receptor, usually κ, while it is generating an antagonistic result at a different receptor, μ. A partial agonist acquires affinity for binding only with low efficacy. κ agonists as well as partial μ agonists display a ceiling effect which limits their effectiveness. Most opioids used for management of chronic pain are μ opioid agonists such as codeine, morphine, oxycodone and hydromorphone and fentanyl.

The World Health Organization (WHO) divides opioids into two categories: weak and strong opioids. The most commonly used strong opioids include morphine, oxycodone, hydromorphone, fentanyl and methadone. Methadone also exhibits N-methyl-D-aspartate (NMDA) antagonist (Chapter 3) and monoaminergic mechanisms of action [6]. Among the weak opioids, codeine and tramadol are the most widely utilized. Tramadol may have lower abuse potential and is a dual action analgesic blocking reuptake of norepinephrine and serotonin as well as binding to μ receptors. Opioids can be delivered via many routes of administration: oral, rectal, sublingual, intranasal, inhalational, transdermal, subcutaneous, intravenous, intramuscular and neuraxial. The pharmacological properties and side effect profile assist clinicians in selection of the appropriate opioid. Table 16.1 lists most clinically available opioids along with equianalgesic doses, available routes of administration and duration of action. Table 16.2 provides morphine to fentanyl (in fentanyl transdermal delivery system) conversion guidelines. An easy rule of thumb for morphine to fentanyl conversion is that 25 μg/hour fentanyl is roughly equivalent to 1 mg/hour morphine intravenously. Methadone is unique not only in possessing three mechanisms

Table 16.1 Equianalgesic doses of opioids [7,9–11].

Drug (non-proprietary name)	Trade name	Route	Dose (mg)	Duration of action (hours)
Morphine		IV, IM, SC	10	4–6
		POIR	30–40	4
	MS Contin, Oramorph	POCR	30–40	8–12
	Kadian, Avinza	POSR	20–60	12–24
		PR	10	4–24
Codeine		IM, SC	110–130	4–6
		PO	200	4–6
Fentanyl	Sublimaze	IV	0.1	1
	Duragesic	Transdermal	See Table 16.2	
	Actiq, Fentora, Onsolis	SL	* Starting dose 200 μg/piece, only use in patients taking greater than 60 mg/day morphine	
Hydrocodone	Hydrocan	PO	20–30	4–6
Hydromorphone	Dilaudid	IM, SC	1.5	4–5
		PO	7.5	4–6
		PR	4.5	6–8
Heroin (diacetylmorphine)		IM, SC	5	4–5
		PO	60	4–6
Levorphanol	Levo-Dromoran	IM, SC	2	4–6
		PO	4	4–6
Oxymorphone	Numorphan	IM, SC	1	4–6
		PR	5–10	4–6
	Opana	PO	10	4–6
Propoxyphene	Darvon	PO	80–160	3–5
Oxycodone	Percocet, Roxicodone Tylox and others	PO	20	4–6
	OxyContin	POCR	5–10	12
Meperidine	Demerol	IM, SC	75	2–4
		PO	300	4–5
Tramadol	Ultram, Ultracet	PO	100*	4–6
Tapentadol†	Nucynta	PO	No equianalgesic dosing recommendations yet	
Buprenorphine	Buprenex	IV	0.2	4–6
		SL	0.8	5–6
Butorphanol	Stadol	IM	2	3–4
		Nasal	2	3–5
Nalbuphine	Nubain	IM, SC	10–20	3–6
Pentazocaine	Talwin	IM, SC	30–40	3–5
		PO	180	5–7
Morphine/Naltrexone	Embeda	PO	20–60	=

IM, intramuscular; IV, intravenous; PO, by mouth; POCR, by mouth, controlled release. Not specific regarding conversion from other opioids to Embeda. Usually restricted to POIR; POIR, by mouth, immediate release opioid tolerant patients due to life-threatening respiratory depression risks; POSR, by mouth, sustained release; PR, per rectum; SC, subcutaneous; SL, sublingual.

* Equianalgesic doses may vary and may be as high as 300 mg in patients with chronic pain.

†Tapentadol and tramadol also inhibit reuptake of norepinephrine and serotonin.

Table 16.2 Morphine to fentanyl patch conversion guidelines [12].

Oral morphine 24-hour dose (mg/day)	Duragesic® (μg/hour)
40–130	25
130–220	50
220–300	75
300–400	100
400–500	125
500–580	150
580–670	175
670–760	200

Table 16.3 Potential adverse effects of opioids.

Abuse, misuse, addiction, diversion
Overdose
Tolerance
Constipation
Nausea or vomiting
Sedation or clouded mentation
Hormonal changes (hypogonadism, hypocortisolism)
Immune modulation
Pruritus
Myoclonus
Respiratory depression
Abnormal pain sensitivity (hyperalgesia, allodynia)
Sphincter of Odi spasm

of analgesic action, but also with regard to elimination half-life which is close to 50 hours while its analgesic duration of action is approximately 6–8 hours as a result of high lipophilicity. Thus, it is important for the clinician to be familiar with the unique pharmacokinetics of methadone before using this agent. Also, when converting to methadone from another opioid the morphine : methadone conversion ratio fluctuates with increasing doses. Methadone is relatively more potent the higher the previous dose of conventional opioid. Thus, at morphine dosage of less than 100 mg/day the conversion ratio of morphine to methadone is 4 : 1; at dosage between 100 and 300 mg morphine equivalents per day it becomes 8 : 1 and at morphine dosage greater than 300 mg/day the ratio is between 12 : 1 and 20 : 1. The equianalgesic conversion table is intended only as a guideline. The unpredictability of opioid analgesia and side effect profile between individuals is still poorly understood and multifactorial [7]. Also of important note, repeated dosing and amassing of opioids at the receptor as well as their efficacy at the receptor can alter the analgesic interval and the dosing regimen needed.

Patient selection and risk stratification

Proper patient selection is critical and requires a thorough patient evaluation and a comprehensive risk–benefit assessment. This will include full

Table 16.4 Risk factors for abuse, misuse, addiction and diversion of opioids.

Poorly defined pain condition
Personal history of alcohol or drug abuse
Family history of alcohol or drug abuse
Presence of psychiatric illness
Current cigarette use
History of preadolescent sexual abuse
Prior history of aberrant drug-related behaviors
Age 45 years and younger
History of legal problems
Associates with others who abuse drugs

assessment and working diagnosis of the pain along with an assessment of risk of development of aberrant drug-related behaviors or addiction. Potential benefits such as reduction in pain and improvement in function should be methodologically weighed against risks. Defined therapeutic goals for each patient should be affirmed and enumerated prior to initiation of therapy. Potential risks and adverse effects of opioids are displayed in Table 16.3 [8]. Table 16.4 presents risk factors for abuse or misuse of opioids. Further discussion regarding risk stratification and management can be found in Chapter 40.

Initial treatment with opioids should be regarded as a clinical trial lasting several weeks to months to determine whether or not continued treatment is warranted. The decision to proceed with long-term opioid therapy should be made intentionally and only after careful deliberation. The clinical trial aspect of treatment should be a part of every patient's paradigm. The clinical trial model can be especially useful in helping patients define their goals of treatment before treatment and creating a measurable target on which to prospectively base continued use of opioids. Outcomes of the trial to consider include progress towards meeting agreed upon therapeutic goals, adverse effects, pain relief, improvement in function, changes in mental health conditions and the presence or absence of drug-related behaviors, addiction or diversion. If patients do not meet their predefined goals then the trial of opioid has not been therapeutic and the opioid should be decreased and discontinued. Figure 16.1 presents a treatment paradigm.

Opioid selection, dosing and titration should be individualized according to the patient's health status, age and previous exposure to opioids. Frail older patients and those with comorbid medical conditions should be treated with lower doses and titrated more slowly to avoid the risks of adverse effects. It has become almost dogmatic that using long-acting as opposed to short-acting opioids reduces the potential for abuse and eliminates the drug-use reinforcement model as opposed to helping patients develop other strategies to help control their pain. This has not yet been clearly demonstrated by research. Short-acting opioids may actually be safer for initiating treatment because of their shorter half-life and possibly lower risk of inadvertent overdose.

The treatment of pain including the use of opioids in patients with a past history or current risk of comorbid addiction or suspected of aberrant drug-related behaviors is discussed in Chapter 40.

Monitoring and management

Patients treated with opioids for non-terminal chronic pain should be monitored regularly. Regular repeated evaluations addressing many domains are likely to be more useful than infrequent, narrowly focused evaluations. It is reasonable practice to see most patients, with few exceptions, at least monthly. Patients at high risk may need to be seen as often as biweekly.

Monitoring should include an assessment and documentation of pain severity and functional ability. It should include a continuing confirmation that opioids have enabled the patient to achieve pre-established therapeutic goals without significant or unmanageable adverse effects. A thorough evaluation for the presence or absence of behaviors possibly indicative of a problem with drug use aberrancy should be conducted. The Pain Assessment and Documentation Tool (PADT) and Current Opioid Misuse Measure (COMM) are useful formal screening tools that can help identify aberrant drug abuse behaviors [1,8]. Because patient self-report of drug use can be unreliable, universal precautions should be considered and this is discussed in detail in Chapter 40.

Another group of patients who should be considered at "high risk" are those receiving "high-dose" opioid therapies. The American Pain Society and American Academy of Pain Medicine (APS/AAPM) guidelines committee has identified 200 mg/day oral morphine or its equivalent as the boundary for the line between usual doses and high dose. It must be recognized that this is a somewhat arbitrary number that was selected based on maximum opioid doses studied in randomized trials and average doses used in observational studies [8]. When doses reach these levels more intensive monitoring is indicated not only for abuse, misuse, addiction and diversion, but also for hyperalgesia, neuroendocrine dysfunction and possibly immunosuppression.

Patients who engage in repeated aberrant drug-related behaviors and/or patients whose urine toxicology specimens are inconsistent with reported use of drugs should have their opioids tapered off and should not be treated with opioids unless there are reliable and valid mitigating circumstances. This also applies to patients who do not meet therapeutic goals or who have serious adverse effects from their opioids. Symptoms from opioid withdrawal can be quite unpleasant but are only rarely life-threatening. A slow wean can mean a reduction of 10% of dosage every week and this is likely not to precipitate symptoms of withdrawal. A

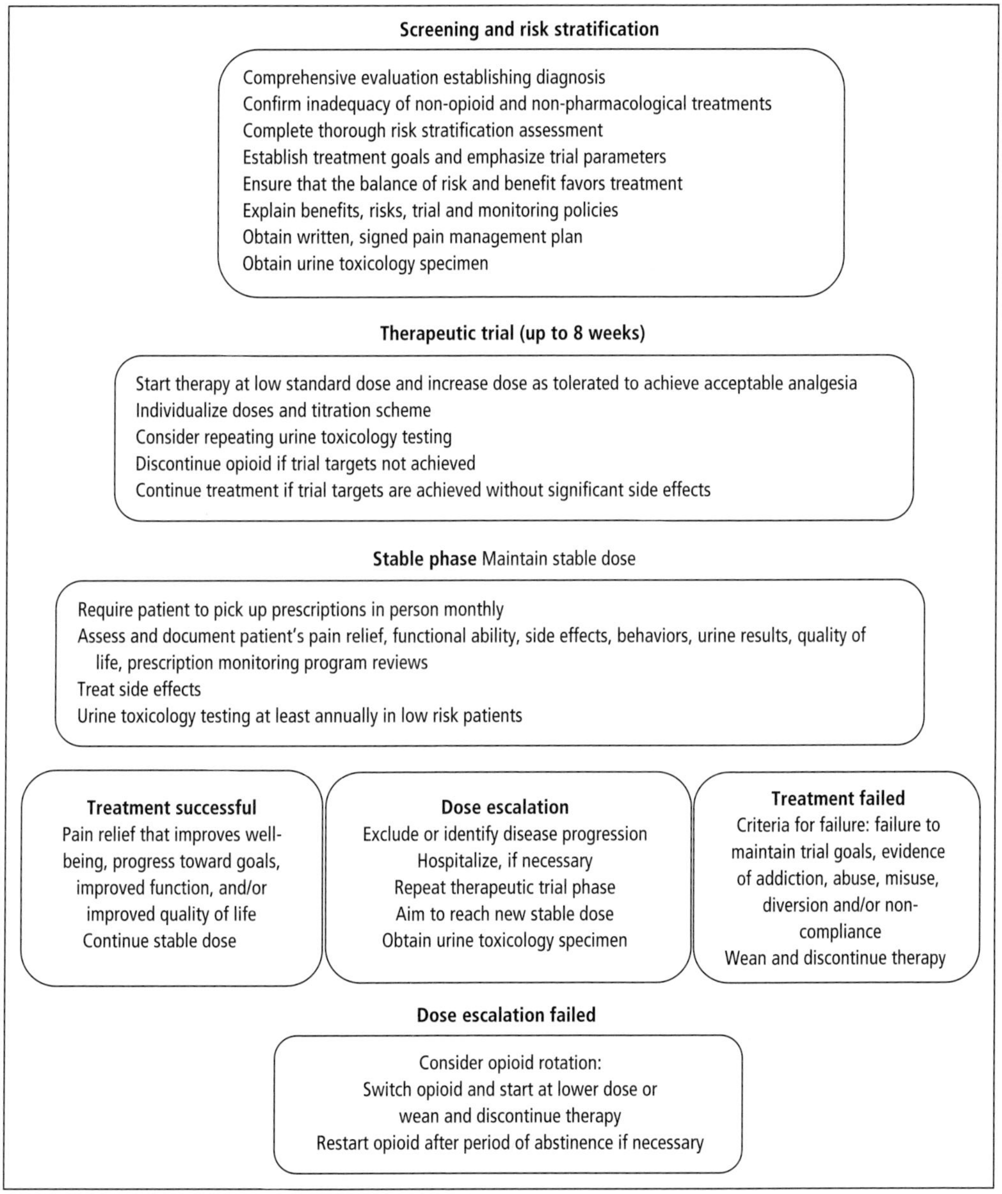

Figure 16.1 Opioid for chronic non-terminal pain treatment paradigm.

quick wean can mean a 25% reduction per week and even this rate will not likely precipitate severe symptoms of withdrawal. Concrete evidence to guide withdrawing opioids is lacking.

Similarly, there is little evidence to guide providers regarding counseling patients on the risk of driving using opioids. There may be transient or persistent cognitive impairment associated with the use of opioids. Patients should be counseled not to drive or perform potentially dangerous activities if they feel impaired. Somnolence, clouded thinking, difficulty concentrating and slower reflexes may occur more commonly with initiation of therapy or with dose adjustments as well as with concomitant use of other drugs or alcohol. In the absence of signs or symptoms of impairment, there is no evidence that patients maintained on opioids should be restricted from driving. It may be prudent to consider restricting driving when opioids are first begun or when doses are escalated for a period of approximately a week.

Opioids are not teratogenic. However, known risks to the neonate include opioid withdrawal syndrome and prolonged QT syndrome. There may be as yet unidentified risks of intrauterine exposure to opioids and clinicians should counsel minimal or no use of opioids during pregnancy whenever feasible.

Conclusions

This chapter reviews an approach for the clinician to safely prescribe controlled substances for chronic non-terminal pain. Proper patient selection including assessment of risk for development of aberrant drug-related behaviors or addiction, a good working knowledge of opioid pharmacology, and adverse effects and appropriate monitoring along with universal precautions are the key elements required.

References

1 Chou R, Fanciullo GJ, Fine PG *et al.* (2009) Clinical guidelines for the use of chronic opioid therapy in chronic noncancer pain. *J Pain* **10(2)**:113–30.

2 Chou R, Ballantyne JC, Fanciullo GJ *et al.* (2009) Research gaps on use of opioids for chronic noncancer pain: findings from a review of the evidence for an American Pain Society and American Academy of Pain Medicine clinical practice guideline. *J Pain* **10(2)**:147–59.

3 Trescot AM, Helm S, Hansen H *et al.* (2008) Opioids in the management of chronic non-cancer pain: an update of American Society of the Interventional Pain Physicians' (ASIPP) Guidelines. *Pain Physician* **11(2 Suppl)**:S5–S62.

4 Warfield CA, Zahid BH. (2004) Opioid pharmacotherapy. In: Warfield CA, Zahid BH, eds. *Principles and Practice of Pain Medicine.* McGraw-Hill, New York. pp. 268–72.

5 Stoelting H. (2006) Opioid agonists and antagonists. In: Stoelting H, ed. *Pharmacology and Physiology in Anesthetic Practice*, 4th edn. Lippincott, Williams & Wilkins, Philadelphia, PA. pp. 87–126.

6 Benzon HT, Rathmell JP, Wu CL *et al.* (2004) Major opioids. *Essentials of Pain Medicine and Regional Anethesia*, 4th edn. Mosby Elsevier, Philadelphia, PA. pp. 87–123.

7 Pereira J, Lawlor P, Vigano A *et al.* (2001) Equianalgesic dose ratios for opioids: a critical review and proposals for long-term dosing. *J Pain Symptom Manag* **22(2)**:672–87.

8 Chou R, Fanciullo GJ, Fine PG *et al.* (2009) Opioids for chronic noncancer pain: prediction and identification of aberrant drug-related behaviors: a review of the evidence for an American Pain Society and American Academy of Pain Medicine clinical practice guideline. *J Pain* **10(2)**:131–46.

9 Inturrisi CE. (2002) Clinical pharmacology of opioids for pain. *Clin J Pain* **18(4 Suppl)**:S3–13.

10 McMahon S, Koltzenburg M. (2006) In: Wall R, Melzack R, eds. *Wall and Melzack's Textbook of Pain*, 5th edn. Elsevier. pp. 444–48, and 453.

11 Scott LJ, Perry CM. (2000) Tramadol: a review of its use in perioperative pain. *Drugs* **60(1)**:139–76.

12 Patanwala AE, Duby J, Waters D, Erstad BL. (2007) Opioid conversions in acute care. *Ann Pharmacother* **41(2)**:255–66.

Chapter 17

Topical analgesics

Jana Sawynok

Department of Pharmacology, Dalhousie University, Halifax, Nova Scotia, Canada

Introduction

Topical analgesia generally refers to the localized delivery of drugs to the skin for the purpose of obtaining pain relief due to local drug actions on peripheral sensory nerves and adjacent tissues following dermal penetration of the active ingredient. Topical formulations typically consist of creams, gels, ointments, sprays and patches or plasters.[1] The skin is the largest organ of the body, and most topical applications involve delivery to somatic sites; in such cases innervation and central transmission occurs via projections to the spinal cord. Analgesia in the craniofacial region, where innervation occurs via the trigeminal system, also can occur following delivery to the skin of the head and neck region, as well and other surfaces such as the cornea and oral cavity.

[1]Drugs may also be applied to the skin as patches for the purpose of dermal absorption, systemic redistribution and systemic actions; this is referred to as transdermal drug delivery. Transdermal applications are often administered at sites remote from the intended site of action (e.g. nicotine and fentanyl patches) where the site of drug action is the central nervous system.

Clinical Pain Management: A Practical Guide, 1st edition.
Edited by Mary E. Lynch, Kenneth D. Craig and
Philip W.H. Peng.
© 2011 Blackwell Publishing Ltd.

As novel mechanisms involved in regulation of peripheral pain signaling are identified, there is a growing appreciation that drugs administered locally to sensory nerve endings may provide a valuable approach to pain management. Thus, topical analgesics provide therapeutic local drug concentrations but low systemic drug levels, and this leads to fewer adverse effects and potentially fewer drug interactions. A wider consideration of advantages and limitations of topical analgesics is presented in Table 17.1. It is also important to note that topical analgesics have the potential to be used either as single therapies or as an adjunct to oral analgesics which allows for recruitment of a wider range of actions for suppressing pain. This chapter considers the main classes of topical analgesics currently in clinical use, their place in treatment guidelines and the potential for the further development of novel topical analgesics.

Topical NSAIDs

Non-steroidal anti-inflammatory drugs (NSAIDs) act by inhibiting cyclo-oxygenase enzymes (both COX1 and COX2) involved in the production of prostanoids, and it is this action that leads to anti-inflammatory and analgesic properties. Prostaglandins sensitize sensory nerve endings and produce hyperalgesia by activating specific receptors; this leads to phosphorylation of ion channels

Table 17.1 Advantages and limitations of topical analgesics.

Advantages

Therapeutic tissue concentrations of drug with low systemic drug levels and avoidance of peak and trough concentrations in the blood

Avoids certain factors that affect bioavailability (e.g. first pass metabolism, influence of gastric pH and gastric emptying times)

Option when oral dosing not feasible (e.g. nauseated patients)

Improved patient acceptance and adherence to therapy

Limitations

Topical agents must have appropriate molecular size (small molecules) and physicochemical properties (aqueous/lipid solubility) for dermal and tissue penetration

Variations can occur in skin permeability and in the presence of tissue enzymes that metabolize drugs

Disease states may alter dermal absorption

Local dermal effects can occur in response to the drug or vehicle

and a shift in activation kinetics. There are a large number of topical NSAID formulations available [1,2].[2] Bioavailability and peak plasma concentrations via this approach are generally less than 10% compared to oral administration, while penetration studies indicate therapeutic concentrations below the site of application [1].

Several systematic reviews addressing the efficacy of topical NSAIDs in acute and chronic pain conditions have been written in the past decade, and a 2008 review provides a useful chronology of developments [2]. It cites a 2004 analysis revealing that when topical NSAIDs were compared with topical placebo (14 trials) using 2-week outcomes, 48% of patients achieved at least 50% pain relief compared to 26% with topical placebo, and topical NSAIDs had a number-needed-to-treat (NNT) of

[2]These include diclofenac, felbinac, flurbiprofen, ibuprofen, indometacin, ketoprofen, ketorolac, piroxicam, naproxen and nimesulide, as well as other NSAIDs.

4.6 (95% confidence interval [CI] 3.8–5.9) (Table 17.2). Higher quality trials (N = 10) had a NNT of 4.4 [2]. These NNT values were similar to those for topical NSAIDs for treating soft tissue injuries (strains, sprains) using 1-week outcomes (3.8, 95% CI 3.4–4.4) (Table 17.2). There was no difference between topical NSAID and topical placebo for local adverse events (rash, itching or stinging) or systemic adverse events (3–6%). Three trials directly compared topical NSAID with an oral NSAID (comparability trials) and found similar rates of treatment success with the two approaches (37%). However, the earlier dataset was largely limited to outcomes over 2 weeks, and the issue of longer-term efficacy remained unresolved.

Shortly after the 2004 review was published, six further high quality randomized trials evaluating topical NSAIDs for osteoarthritis of the knee were published – all involved diclofenac (four with dimethylsulfoxide [DMSO], Pennsaid®, one a gel and one a plaster) and, importantly, three trials extended to 6 or 12 weeks [2]. Five trials compared topical diclofenac with topical placebo, and one compared topical diclofenac with oral diclofenac. All trials comparing topical NSAID with placebo observed significantly better outcomes for pain, stiffness, physical function and patient global assessment. The trial comparing topical diclofenac with oral drug observed comparable efficacy with topical and oral routes of administration. Local adverse events (dry skin, rash, pruritus) were more common with topical diclofenac (about one-third of patients) than with topical placebo, and also compared to oral diclofenac. Gastrointestinal adverse events were no more common with topical diclofenac than placebo; however, such events (dyspepsia, abdominal pain, diarrhea) occurred significantly more often with oral than topical diclofenac. For oral treatment, the calculated number-needed-to-harm (NNH) for severe gastrointestinal effects over 12 weeks was 11 (95% CI 8–19). Overall, the evidence from the trials published between 2004 and 2006 indicates topical NSAIDs are consistently better than placebo, not inferior to oral NSAIDs, and have a better systemic adverse event profile than oral NSAIDs [2].

Table 17.2 Number-needed-to-treat (NNT) values for topical analgesics in several pain conditions.

Topical agent	Condition (number of trials)	NNT (95% CI)	Reference
NSAIDs	Osteoarthritis, musculoskeletal pain, rheumatism, back pain (14)	4.6 (3.8–5.9)	[2]
	Soft tissue injury (26) (strains, sprains)	3.8 (3.4–4.4)	[2]
Lidocaine 5% patch	Post-herpetic neuralgia (1)	4.4 (2.5–17.5)	[6]
Capsaicin	Neuropathic pain 0.075% (6)	5.7 (4.0–10)	[9]
	Musculoskeletal pain 0.015% (3)	8.1 (4.6–34)	[9]
Rubefacients	Acute pain (7)	Evidence not robust	[10]
(salicylates)	Chronic pain (9)	6.2 (4.0–13)	[10]

A recent study, published in 2009, compared topical diclofenac containing DMSO (Pennsaid®) to oral diclofenac over 12 weeks in 775 patients with knee osteoarthritis [3]. The five treatment groups were:

1 Topical diclofenac in DMSO (oral placebo);
2 Topical placebo (oral placebo);
3 Topical DMSO (oral placebo);
4 Oral diclofenac (topical placebo); and
5 Oral diclofenac (topical diclofenac).

Topical diclofenac was superior to both placebo and topical DMSO for pain, physical function, overall health and patient satisfaction, and topical DMSO had no significant effect alone. Topical diclofenac produced effects comparable to oral diclofenac, and the combination of topical diclofenac with oral diclofenac did not produce any further effect compared to either individual treatment with these outcomes. The most common adverse event with topical diclofenac was dry skin (18%), an effect also observed with topical DMSO (11%, compared to 3% with placebo); this was suggested to reflect dissolution of surface lipids. Fewer gastrointestinal effects and laboratory abnormalities were observed with topical diclofenac than with oral drug.

This study confirms findings from the 2004–06 series of trials with respect to efficacy of the topical diclofenac to 12 weeks, equivalence to oral drug and fewer systemically mediated adverse effects. It concluded that for patients initiating pharmacological therapy of osteoarthritis of the knee, topical diclofenac is a viable evidence-based treatment option. Topical NSAIDs for knee osteoarthritis are now recognized by several treatment guidelines [3,4].

Topical local anesthetics

Local anesthetics produce analgesia by blocking sodium channels on sensory nerve endings and diminishing activation of the nerve. Lidocaine 5% is available as a patch and is approved for use in the USA for treatment of post-herpetic neuralgia (PHN) [5]. Patch application (N = 3, up to 12 hours per day) leads to 3% systemic bioavailability. Three double-blind randomized trials examining efficacy in PHN were published between 1996 and 2002 [5]. In two trials, the lidocaine 5% patch provided a reduction in pain relief compared with vehicle patch when administered acutely (for 1 day) or chronically (for 21 days). The third trial used a time-to-exit design, and reported a mean time of > 14 days for the lidocaine patch compared to 3.8 days for the vehicle patch. A further controlled trial published in 2003 indicates that lidocaine 5% patch treatment reduces pain in focal peripheral neuropathic pain syndromes. In this latter trial, the NNT for the lidocaine patch was calculated to be 4.4 (95% CI 2.5–17.5) (Table 17.2). The most frequent adverse events seen with the lidocaine 5% patch were mild skin rash, redness and irritation at the site of application, which was also reported with the vehicle patch. A recent trial has compared the lidocaine 5% patch with oral pregabalin for PHN and diabetic polyneuropathy

(DPN) over 4 weeks; the topical treatment produced a comparable overall pain reduction compared to the oral treatment (62–65% responded with primary endpoints) but with fewer adverse events [6]. The lidocaine patch for treatment of PHN and focal neuropathic pain conditions has entered treatment algorithms as an early line treatment strategy [7].

Topical capsaicin

Capsaicin activates transient receptor potential vanilloid-1 (TRPV1) receptors on sensory nerve endings. This receptor is polymodal, responding to heat, protons, endogenous agents (e.g. anandamide) and exogenous agents (e.g. capsaicin, resiniferotoxin). It is regarded as a molecular integrator of noxious stimuli, and is receiving considerable attention with respect to the development of novel receptor antagonists as analgesics [8]. Following activation by capsaicin, the TRPV1 receptor desensitizes, leading to a refractoriness of the sensory nerve to subsequent activation; both this refractoriness and loss of fine sensory nerve branches (which is reversible) form the basis of the analgesic properties of topically administered capsaicin [9].

Topical creams with capsaicin have been examined for treatment of PHN and PDN (0.075% formulation) and osteoarthritis and rheumatoid arthritis (0.025% formulation) [9]. A systematic review of six trials of neuropathic pain, and three trials of musculoskeletal conditions produced NNT values of 5.7 (95% CI 4.0–10) and 8.1 (95% CI 4.6–34), respectively (Table 17.2). About one-third of patients experienced local adverse events, primarily a burning sensation (resulting from TRPV1 receptor activation); the presence of this can result in a lack of blinding, as well as a significant dropout rate. The NNH for an adverse local event was 2.5 (95% CI 2.1–3.1); for withdrawal from the trial, it was 9.8 (95% CI 7.3–15). Recommendations regarding topical capsaicin for these conditions indicate use where individuals are unresponsive to, or intolerant of, other treatments, and it is regarded as a third line medication in treatment algorithms for neuropathic pain [7].

Topical rubefacients

Rubefacients are traditional formulations containing salicylates and other natural products (e.g. clove oil, eucalyptus oil, menthol); capsaicin is considered separately [2]. These agents are also known as "counter-irritants" and are believed to counter pain by initiating a pattern of sensory activity that diminishes the pain sensation, and by affecting local blood flow. While salicylates are related to aspirin, their principal action is attributed to the counter-irritant effect and changes in local blood flow which leads to a sense of warmth [2]. The actions of other rubefacients are now better understood, as menthol (and eucalyptol) activates TRPM8 receptors, and camphor activates TRPV3 receptors, and their sensory actions may result from mechanisms similar to capsaicin (activation then desensitization of receptors on sensory nerves) [8]. However, given the limited efficacy of capsaicin noted above, the potential for such actions to significantly affect pain signaling is not clear. At present there is no evidence to support analgesic efficacy of topical rubefacients with components other than salicylates [10].

The effects of salicylate rubefacients have undergone recent systematic review [2,10]. Evidence in acute pain conditions (strains, sprains) (six studies) was not robust; while an overall NNT could be calculated (3.2, 95% CI 2.4–4.9), there was no effect in better quality studies. In chronic pain (musculoskeletal and rheumatic pain) (seven studies), the NNT was 6.2 (95% CI 4.0–13) (Table 17.2). This analysis noted that rubefacients were not recommended for treatment of osteoarthritis by national guidelines [10].

Peripheral and topical opioids

Since the early 1990s, it has been appreciated that opioid receptors are localized on sensory nerve endings, and that peripheral administration of exogenous opioids produces analgesia that is locally mediated [11]. The local action is validated by lack of effect when the drug is administered to the contralateral side, and by blockade with quaternary receptor antagonists that do not access the

Table 17.3 Peripheral targets being explored as potential novel topical analgesics [16].

Target	Comments
Na$^+$ channel	Na$_v$1.7, Na$_v$1.8 and Na$_v$1.9 most promising targets; much interest in isoform specific blockers and topicals
K$^+$ channels	Various K$^+$ channel subtypes implicated in analgesia by several drugs; no specific topical exploration
Ca^{2+} channels	ω-conotoxins and gabapentin/pregabalin interact with Ca^{2+} channels; limited topical exploration
Adenosine receptors	Peripheral A1 receptors inhibit pain; A1 receptor antagonists inhibit peripheral analgesia by amitriptyline; topical actions of amitriptyline being explored
Acid sensitive ion channels	ASICs selectively localized on sensory nerves and involved in several forms of pain; topical aspects not yet developed
Vanilloid and TRP receptors	TRPV1 activated then desensitized by capsaicin; at least 13 TRPV1 receptor antagonists in preclinical development as analgesics; antagonists could potentially be novel class of topical analgesics
Glutamate receptors	Ionotropic and metabotropic GluR antagonists being examined in preclinical studies; ketamine given topically in human neuropathic pain
Serotonin receptors	Peripheral 5-HT$_{1B}$ and 5-HT$_{1D}$ receptors inhibit pain; 5-HT$_2$, 5-HT$_3$, 5-HT$_4$ and 5-HT$_7$ receptors facilitate pain; analgesia occurs with ketanserin (5-HT$_{2A}$ antagonist) applied topically in preclinical studies
Adrenergic receptors	α1-, α2- and β-ARs implicated in pain facilitation; ARs involved in sympathetic-sensory coupling and interact with P2X$_3$ receptors; nerve injury produces complex effects on expression of AR subtypes; clinical studies have examined topical clonidine; interest in topical P2X$_3$ receptor antagonists
Cholinergic mechanisms	AChRs involved in peripheral pain; M4 mAChRs feasible target for analgesia; nAChRs also present on sensory afferents; nAChR agonists (epibatidine, ABT-594), and antagonist (α-conotoxin) explored as systemic analgesics; botulinum toxin (blocks ACh release) explored as analgesic; topicals not extensively explored
Cannabinoids	Peripheral CB1 and CB2 receptors involved in pain; mixed agonists given systemically for neuropathic pain; CB1 and CB2 agonists attractive targets for topical approaches
Opioids	Inflammatory pain reduced by peripherally acting morphine; effects in chronic inflammation may also reflect anti-inflammatory actions on immune cells; peripherally restricted μ- and κ-agonists are targets of interest; interest in topical development (skin, mucosa)
CGRP, substance P	Peptides present in sensory afferents involved in pain signaling in the spinal cord and role in neurogenic inflammation in periphery; antagonists explored as systemic analgesics but NK1 antagonists have not been successful clinically, no topical development
Somatostatin	Analogs exhibit systemic and spinal analgesia; peripheral analgesia occurs perhaps via opioid release from immune cells; intra-articular application of somatostatin relieves pain in rheumatoid arthritis; no topical development
Cytokines	Several cytokines involved in nociception; TNF ligands and IL-1 receptor antagonist used for rheumatoid arthritis; prostaglandin receptor antagonists are novel targets as topical analgesics (cf. topical NSAID efficacy)
Neurotrophic factors	NGF is pronociceptive; increased NGF levels occur in several inflammatory pain conditions; antagonism of NGF considered promising therapeutic target; no topical exploration

AchR, acetylcholine receptor (m, muscarinic; n, nicotinic); AR, adrenergic receptor; ASIC, acid-sensitive ion channel; CB, cannabinoid; CGRP, calcitonin gene-related peptide; GluR, glutamate receptor; 5-HT, 5-hydroxytryptamine; IL, interleukin; NGF, nerve growth factor; NK, neurokinin; TNF, tumor necrosis factor; TRPV1, transient receptor potential vanilloid-1.

central nervous system. Multiple opioid receptors (μ, δ, κ) are present on sensory afferents, but μ-opioid receptors have received the most attention. Peripheral opioid receptors are upregulated in inflammation, and mediate aspects of immune-neural communication [11].

In clinical settings, there is an extensive body of information on intra-articular morphine for arthroscopic knee surgery [12]. A rigorous analysis of the data revealed most positive studies reporting postsurgical analgesia used intra-articular doses of 3–5 mg morphine while negative studies used 1-mg doses. Postoperative pain relief lasted up to 24 hours. Analgesia following intra-articular morphine has also been reported when inflammation is chronic in knee osteoarthritis and rheumatoid arthritis; pain relief was long-lasting and similar to that observed with intra-articular dexamethasone [13]. Opioids also have been administered topically for painful skin and mucosal lesions; there are case reports and several trials reporting favorable clinical outcomes, but there is a need for primary studies to inform practice guidelines using this approach [14].

Investigational topical agents

Nitrates are used in the management of angina pectoris, and glyceryl trinitrate (GTN) is available as an ointment and transdermal patch [15]. Topical nitrates may also be useful as topical analgesics. GTN stimulates release of nitric oxide, and this has a variety of effects in endothelial cells and neural tissue, with the latter action leading to analgesia. Topical GTN reduces pain that is superficial and localized, such as chronic tendonitis, osteoarthritis and vascular disorders [15].

Tricyclic antidepressants exert multiple pharmacological actions including block of norepinephrine and serotonin uptake, block of sodium and calcium channels, block of adenosine uptake, and block of cholinergic, histamine and serotonin receptors, and many of these actions can contribute to the peripheral analgesia that has been demonstrated in preclinical inflammatory and neuropathic pain models [15]. There are several clinical studies reporting analgesia with topical

doxepin 3–5% (both alone and with capsaicin) in neuropathic pain, and potential peripheral analgesia by topical amitriptyline 1–4% in combination with ketamine 0.5–2% in neuropathic pain [15].

There is considerable current interest in the potential for development of novel analgesics that can act locally at peripheral nerve endings, and this reflects generalized advantages of the approach of topical administration (Table 17.1) [16]. There has been some clinical exploration with α_2-adrenergic agents (e.g. clonidine) and glutamate receptor antagonists (e.g. ketamine) [16]. The potential for novel targets to be developed as topical analgesics is indicated in the commentary in Table 17.3.

References

1 Heyneman CA, Lawless-Linday C, Wall GC. (2000) Oral versus topical NSAIDs in rheumatic diseases. *Drugs* **60**:555–74.
2 Moore RA, Derry S, McQuay HJ. (2008) Topical agents in the treatment of rheumatic pain. *Rheum Dis Clin North Am* **34**:415–32.
3 Simon LS, Grierson LM, Naseer Z et al. (2009) Efficacy and safety of topical diclofenac containing dimethylsulfoxide (DMSO) compared with those of topical placebo, DMSO vehicle and oral diclofenac for knee osteoarthritis. *Pain* **143**:238–45.
4 Zhang W, Moskowitz RW, Nuki G et al. (2008) OARSI recommendations for the management of hip and knee osteoarthritis. Part II: OARSI evidence-based, expert consensus guidelines. *Osteoarthritis Cartilage* **16**:137–62.
5 Davies PS, Galer BS. (2004) Review of lidocaine patch 5% studies in the treatment of postherpetic neuralgia. *Drugs* **64**:937–47.
6 Baron R, Mayoral V, Binder A et al. (2009) Efficacy and safety of 5% lidocaine (lignocaine) medicated plaster in comparison with pregabalin in patients with postherpetic neuralgia and diabetic polyneuropathy: interim analysis from an open-label, two-stage adaptive, randomized, controlled trial. *Clin Drug Invest* **29**:231–41.
7 Dworkin RH, O'Conner AB, Backonja M et al. (2007) Pharmacologic management of

neuropathic pain: evidence-based recommendations. *Pain* **132**:237–51.

8 Szallasi A, Cortright DN, Blum CA *et al.* (2007) The vanilloid receptor TRPV1: 10 years from channel cloning to antagonist proof-of-concept. *Nat Rev Drug Discov* **6**:357–72.

9 Mason L, Moore RA, Derry S *et al.* (2004) Systematic review of topical capsaicin for the treatment of chronic pain. *Br Med J* **328**:991–4.

10 Matthews P, Derry S, Moore RA *et al.* (2009) Topical rubefacients for acute and chronic pain in adults. *Cochrane Database Syst Rev* **3**:CD007403.

11 Stein C, Lang LJ. (2009) Peripheral mechanisms of opioid analgesia. *Curr Opin Pharmacol* **9**:3–8.

12 Kalso E, Smith L, McQuay HJ *et al.* (2002) No pain, no gain: clinical excellence and scientific rigour – lessons learned from IA morphine. *Pain* **98**:269–75.

13 Stein A, Yassouridis A, Szopko C *et al.* (1999) Intraarticular morphine versus dexamethasone in chronic arthritis. *Pain* **83**:525–32.

14 LeBon B, Zeppetella G, Higginson IJ. (2009) Effectiveness of topical administration of opioids in palliative care: a systematic review. *J Pain Symptom Manage* **37**:913–17.

15 McCleane G. (2007) Topical analgesics. *Anesthesiol Clin* **25**:825–39.

16 Cairns B. (2009) *Peripheral Receptor Targets for Analgesia: Novel Approaches to Pain Management.* John Wiley & Sons, Inc., Hoboken, NJ.

Chapter 18

Other pharmacological agents

Philip W.H. Peng[1] & Mary Lynch[2,3]

[1] Department of Anesthesia, University of Toronto, Toronto, Canada
[2] Pain Management Unit, Queen Elizabeth II Health Sciences Center, Halifax, Nova Scotia, Canada
[3] Department of Anesthesiology, Psychiatry and Pharmacology, Dalhousie University, Halifax, Nova Scotia, Canada

Introduction

This chapter reviews four classes of agents that have not been covered by other chapters: non-steroidal anti-inflammatory drugs (NSAIDs), acetaminophen, muscle relaxants and cannabinoids.

Non-steroidal anti-inflammatory drugs

NSAIDs have been prescribed widely for over a century and are the mainstay for managing chronic inflammatory conditions. There are at least 10 different drug classes represented within the NSAID group (Table 18.1). Most NSAIDs exhibit analgesic efficacy comparable with acetylsalicylic acid (ASA), and several exhibit superior efficacy [1].

NSAIDs have analgesic, anti-inflammatory and antipyretic properties. The anti-inflammatory effects work through the inhibition of cyclo-oxygenase (COX) enzymes, which are in two structurally distinct forms, COX 1 and COX 2. There is a poor correlation between the anti-inflammatory activity and analgesic efficacy of these agents. This probably reflects the multiple mechanisms that are involved in the analgesic action of NSAIDs such as central prostaglandin synthesis, and mechanisms involving serotonin and excitatory amino acids [1].

Given that there are many classes of NSAIDs it is reasonable to rotate from one class to another in an attempt to find the best option for an individual patient (Table 18.1). Although there is no risk of physiological tolerance there is a ceiling effect. In choosing the appropriate NSAID, a few factors may influence the clinician's choice: simplicity of dosing, tolerability, comparative toxicity, efficacy and the cost [1]. For chronic use, the lowest dose that provides a satisfactory response should be maintained. Elderly patients are at higher risk for adverse effects, therefore a lower dose should be used (gastrointestinal side effects may be dose-related), creatinine clearance should be checked and the adverse events should be monitored closely [2].

There are a number of side effects associated with the use of NSAIDs. Of particular importance are those associated with gastrointestinal, renal and cardiovascular adverse effects.

Gastrointestinal side effects

The risk of serious adverse gastrointestinal events is approximately three times greater for those using

Clinical Pain Management: A Practical Guide, 1st edition.
Edited by Mary E. Lynch, Kenneth D. Craig and Philip W.H. Peng.
© 2011 Blackwell Publishing Ltd.

Table 18.1 Commonly used non-steroidal anti-inflammatory drugs (NSAIDs).

Drug class	Drug name	Common trade name	Usual PO dose (mg)	Maximum daily dose (mg)
Salicylates	ASA	Aspirin	325–650 q4–6 h	4000
	Diflunasil	Dolobid	250–500 b.i.d.	1500
Propionic acid	Ibuprofen	Motrin, Advil	200–800 t.i.d.	3200
	Naproxen	Naprosyn	125–500 b.i.d.	1250
	Naproxen sodium	Anaprox	275–550 o.d./b.i.d.	1375
	Oxaprozin	Daypro	600–1800 o.d.	1800
	Ketoprofen	Actron, Orudis	25–100 t.i.d.	300
Indole acetic acids	Indometacin	Indocid	25–50 t.i.d.	200
	Sulindac	Clinoril	150–200 b.i.d.	400
Pyrolizine carboxylic acid	Ketorolac	Toradol	10 q6 h	40 (max. 7 days)
Pyranocarboxycolic acid	Etodolac*	Lodine	200–600 b.i.d.	1200
Phenylacetic acids	Diclofenac sodium	Voltaren	25–50 b.i.d.	150
	Diclofenac+misoprostol	Arthrotec 50 or 75	50 or 75 b.i.d.	150
Anthranilic acids	Mefamanic acid	Ponstan	250 q.i.d.	1500 (max. 7 days)
Oxicams	Piroxicam	Feldene	10 b.i.d., 20 o.d.	20
	Meloxicam*	Mobicox	7.5–15 o.d.	15
	Tenoxicam	Mobiflex	20–40 o.d.	40
Napthylalkanones	Nabumetone*	Relafen	1000–2000 o.d.	2000
COXIBs	Celecoxib*	Celebrex	100–200 b.i.d.	400

Not all preparations are available in every country. Some are available in sustained-released or injectable form. Only the oral preparations are listed above.
* NSAIDs with selective COX2 activity.
Source: Modified from Lynch & Watson [1].

NSAIDs than for non-users and the number of deaths associated with NSAID-induced gastrointestinal damage in the USA are comparable to those from AIDS and other terminal diseases (approximately 17,000 per year) [3]. Although only a relatively small proportion of NSAID users actually develop major gastrointestinal complications, the importance of these complications is magnified by the widespread use of these agents. NSAID-related gastrointestinal adverse events can be classified into three broad categories:

1 "Nuisance" symptoms such as heartburn, nausea, dyspepsia and abdominal pain (10–60%);

2 Mucosal lesions such as ulcers (15–30% with endoscopically detected ulcer but mostly asymptomatic); and

3 Serious gastrointestinal complications, such as perforated ulcers and catastrophic bleeding (1%) [3]. The greatest risk is during the first 3 months of therapy [3]. Several risk factors have been identi-

fied: a history of ulcer, presence of *Helicobacter pylori* infection, use of more than one NSAID (including aspirin), use of high-dose NSAIDs, concurrent anticoagulant or corticosteroid use, a serious underlying disease and age greater than 75 years [1–3]. In patients with gastrointestinal risk factors, use of an NSAID is better avoided and the clinician should consider the alternatives such as acetaminophen, antidepressant analgesics or a cannabinoid. Strategies that minimize the risk of gastrointestinal adverse events are the use of selective COX2 inhibitors and co-administration with a proton pump inhibitor (PPI) or the prostaglandin analog misoprostol (Table 18.2) [4]. Compared with NSAIDs, celecoxib (the only COXIB available in North America and Europe) had fewer symptomatic ulcers and bleeds, endoscopically detected ulcers, and discontinuations for adverse events or gastrointestinal adverse events [5].

Table 18.2 Canadian consensus guideline on long-term NSAIDs therapy and the need for gastroprotection: benefit vs. risk.

Recommendations
Patients with low GI and low CV risks should receive a traditional NSAID
Patients with low GI and high CV risks should receive naproxen
Patients with high GI and low CV risks should receive a cyclo-oxygenase 2 inhibitor plus a proton-pump inhibitor
Patients with high GI and high CV risks should receive a careful assessment to prioritize risks
NSAIDs should be prescribed at the lowest effective dose and for the shortest possible duration

* Although the members of the panel carefully evaluated the available evidence, the recommendations were based on clinical opinions. The proposed guidelines for NSAID use seem appropriate, but the best way to address the issue would be to conduct appropriate studies for each gastrointestinal (GI) and cardiovascular (CV) risk.
Source: Data from Rostom *et al.* [4].

Cardiovascular side effects

Cardiovascular adverse effects are also a concern. Meta-analysis clearly showed that selective COX2 inhibitors (exposure ≥ 4 weeks) increased serious vascular events, which were defined as non-fatal myocardial infarction, non-fatal stroke or vascular death, by 42% [6,7]. This corresponded to an excess of three persons with a vascular event per 1000 persons receiving a selective COX2 inhibitor per year. The risk of myocardial infarction was almost doubled, corresponding to an excess of three persons with myocardial infraction per 1000 persons receiving a selective COX2 inhibitor per year [6,7]. The risk of stroke was not increased [6,7].

Meta-analyses of case–control and cohort studies did not demonstrate an increase in cardiovascular risk of celecoxib at a dosage of 200 mg/day [6]. However, meta-analyses of randomized trials revealed an increased cardiovascular risk at dose 400 mg/day or higher [7]. Celecoxib did not increase the risk of myocardial infarction among those without a previous myocardial infarction (relative rate [RR] 1.03; 95% confidence interval

[CI] 0.88–1.20), but did increase the risk for those with a previous myocardial infarction (RR 1.40; 95% CI 1.06–1.84) [8–10].

Comparing traditional NSAIDs with selective COX2 inhibitors, the risk of a serious vascular event was similar. The overall risk for selective COX2 inhibitors and traditional NSAIDs was 1.0% and 0.9% per year, respectively [6,7]. This evidence resulted in the US Food and Drug Adminstration (FDA) warning that there is cardiovascular risk with all conventional NSAIDs. When compared directly with other NSAIDs (including diclofenac, indometacin, or both), naproxen was associated with a lower risk of cardiovascular complications [11].

An algorithmic approach was developed to help manage patients who require long-term NSAID therapy (Table 18.2) [4].

Renal side effects

In the USA, an estimated 2.5 million individuals experience adverse renal effects caused by the use of NSAIDs every year [12]. Recent evidence suggests that selective COX2 inhibitors cause a spectrum of renal effects similar to that caused by the NSAIDs [13,14]. Evidence supports that both COX1 and COX2 are constitutively expressed at substantial levels in the kidney [15]. The associated risk of renal dysfunction is low in most people and renal complications are usually reversible on timely withdrawal of the NSAIDs in individuals without previous renal disease [1]. Because a normal creatinine value does not guarantee normal kidney function, the Consensus Conference Group has recommended that a creatinine clearance should be checked both before and after initiating NSAIDs and selective COX2 inhibitors [2].

Summary

In managing patient with chronic pain, NSAIDs generally provide only mild relief (Table 18.3) and are associated with potentially serious adverse effects [2,16–22]. For these reasons their usefulness in assisting patients with moderate to severe chronic pain is limited [1].

Table 18.3 Analgesic effects (AE) of NSAID and acetaminophen in various clinical conditions.

Conditions	Agents	Comment	Remark	Reference
Acute low back pain	NSAIDs vs. placebo	↓ Pain, ↑ AE	WMD 8.39 (95% CI −12.68 to −4.10)	[16,17]
	NSAIDs vs. APAP	Similar analgesia, ↑ AE with NSAIDs		[16,17]
Acute back pain with sciatica	NSAID vs. placebo	No difference		[16]
Chronic low back pain	NSAID vs. placebo	↓ Pain, ↑ AE	WMD −12.40 (95% CI −15.53 to −9.26)	[16]
	NSAID vs. COX2I	Similar analgesia, ↓ AE with COX2I		[16]
Subacute/chronic neck pain	NSAID vs. placebo	No difference in analgesia		[18]
Osteoarthritis	APAP vs. placebo	↓ Pain, no ↑ AE	Only ~5% improvement	[19]
	NSAID vs. APAP	NSAID > APAP	Patients prefer NSAIDs	[2,20]
	NSAID vs. COX2I	Similar analgesia		[2]
	NSAIDs vs. placebo			[21]
Neuropathic pain	NSAID vs. placebo	Probably not		[22]

APAP, N-acetyl-p-aminophenol (acetaminophen); WMD, weighted mean difference.

Acetaminophen

Acetaminophen is widely available worldwide as an over-the-counter preparation or by prescription in combination with other drugs such as oxycodone. It is an antipyretic and analgesic but not an anti-inflammatory agent. It is equianalgesic with ASA in most types of pain except inflammatory arthritis; however, in head-to-head patient preference studies comparing acetaminophen with NSAIDs in osteoarthritis, patients preferred NSAIDs (Table 18.2) [1,23].

Recently the mechanism of action has been demonstrated to involve metabolism of acetaminophen into AM 404 which then reinforces activity in the endocannabinoid system through CB1 (cannabinoid 1) receptors which then reinforce activity of the bulbospinal serotonergic inhibitory pathways [24].

Acetaminophen is rapidly absorbed following the oral administration and the peak plasma level is reached at 30–60 minutes. Side effects such as abdominal pain and diarrhea are occasional and benign. Severe but rare side effects include liver toxicity [1], hypertension [25] and renal dysfunc-

tion [26]. Hepatotoxicity is a concern in acute overdose or in patients who are alcoholic or with pre-existing liver disease [23]. Although the maximum recommended dose is 4 gm, the FDA is considering revising this to a lower dose. The median daily dose of acetaminophen related to liver injury was 5–7.5 g/day, very near the current maximum daily dose [27]. Furthermore, chronic administration of acetaminophen at dose greater than 3 g was associated with a decrease in glomerular filtration rate 30 mL/min. Thus, the maximum daily dose should be less than 3 g and preferably closer to 2 g for chronic use [26].

Given its safety profile, acetaminophen is still considered a first-line drug for patients with osteoarthritis [2]. Other than osteoarthritis, the role of acetaminophen in the management of chronic pain is limited [1].

Skeletal muscle relaxants

Muscle relaxants are a heterogeneous group of medications commonly used to treat two different types of underlying conditions: spasticity from upper motor neuron syndromes (e.g. cerebral

Table 18.4 Muscle relaxants.

Drug	Common trade name	Recommended dose	Common side effects
Cyclobenzaprine	Flexeril	5–10 mg t.i.d.	Anti-ACh effect (drowsiness, dry mouth, urinary retention, increased intraocular pressure)
Methocarbamol	Robaxin	1,500 mg q.i.d. for first 3 days, then followed by 750 mg q.i.d.	Black, brown or green urine possible Cognition impairment
Tizanidine	Zanaflex	4 mg o.d. initially; titrate at increment of 2–4 mg up to 8 mg t.i.d. Although maximum daily limit is 36 mg, experience beyond 24 mg/day is very limited	Weakness, fatigue, drowsiness, dry mouth and dizziness; caution about hepatotoxicity and rebound hypertension from abrupt cessation from high dose
Metaxalone	Skelaxin	800 mg t.i.d. or q.i.d.	Drowsiness, dizziness, headache, nervousness

ACh, Anti-acetylcholinesterase.
* Not all drugs listed above available in all countries.

palsy, multiple sclerosis) and muscular pain or spasms from peripheral musculoskeletal conditions [28]. The FDA has approved a number of drugs for either spasticity (baclofen, dantrolene and tizanidine) or musculoskeletal conditions (carisoprodol, chlorzoxazone, cyclobenzaprine, metaxalone, methocarbamol and orphenadrine). The latter category of agents is composed of a diverse group of medications with different mechanisms of action for spasticity, the mechanism of action for analgesia is unknown (Table 18.4).

Although muscle relaxants are commonly used for peripheral musculoskeletal pain, the evidence supporting their use is limited [29,30]. Significant limitations of this literature include poorly designed studies and the fact that most trials were short term (2 weeks of treatment) and examined acute rather than chronic pain.

For most muscle relaxants the indication is for management of acute pain; however, in practice there are many patients who suffer with chronic pain who are using muscle relaxants in an attempt to find relief. Systematic reviews of controlled trials examining the use of muscle relaxants in non-specific low back pain [29,30] concluded that muscle relaxants are effective for short-term symptomatic relief in patients with acute and chronic low back pain. However, the incidence of drowsiness and dizziness and other side effects is high, caution was recommended and it was left to the discretion of the physician to review the risk–benefit analysis. It was acknowledged that large, high quality trials are necessary.

There are very limited or inconsistent data regarding the analgesic effectiveness of metaxalone, methocarbamol, chlorzoxazone, baclofen or dantrolene compared with placebo in patients with musculoskeletal conditions [29,30].

In summary, muscle relaxants have a limited role in the treatment of chronic pain and should be reserved for short-term use.

Cannabinoids

Cannabinoids are a group of substances that are structurally related to tetrahydrocannabinol or that bind to cannabinoid receptors that are naturally present in the nervous and immune systems of animals. There are several types of cannabinoids. Phytocannabinoids, also called natural or herbal cannabinoids, occur in the cannabis plant, endocannabinoids are naturally present in animals and there are a growing number of synthetic cannabinoids under development for therapeutic uses [23].

Table 18.5 Several cannabinoids that are currently available.

Agents	Trade name	Dose available	Route	Usual dose	Listed indication
Cannabis under the MMAR program*		14% THC in cannabis supplied by the program	Smoked or oral	3–5 g/day	
Nabilone Synthetic cannabinoids from CBN	Cesamet	0.25, 0.5, 1 mg capsule	PO	Initiate at 0.25–0.5 mg, ↑ by 0.25–0.5 mg q2–3 days to max. 3 mg b.i.d.	Antiemetic for chemotherapy
Dronabinol: Synthetic Δ-9-THC	Marinol	2.5, 5, 10 mg capsule	PO	Initiate at 2.5 mg, ↑ by 2.5 mg q2–3 days up to a max. 10 mg t.i.d.	Antiemetic for chemotherapy; appetite loss with AIDS
Extract of cannabis: THC, CBD 1 : 1 ratio	Sativex	THC 2.7 mg/CBD 2.5 mg/100 µL spray actuation	Buccal	Initiate at 1–2 spray, ↑ 1–2 spray q2–3 days up to a max. 12 sprays	Adjunctive Rx NeP with MS; Adjunctive therapy cancer pain

CBD, cannabidiol; CBN, cannabinol; MMAR, medical marihuana access regulations, a program for compassionate access available in Canada; MS, multiple sclerosis; NeP, neuropathic pain; PO, by mouth; THC, Delta 9-tetrahydrocannabinol.

Since the discovery of Δ-9-THC in 1964, two endogenous receptors have been identified, CB1 and CB2, primarily located in the central nervous and immune systems, respectively, along with several endogenous ligands such that a full endogenous cannabinoid system capable of endogenous pain modulation has been identified. The CB1 receptors are 10 times more abundant than opioid receptors in the brain but are present in very low levels in the cardiorespiratory centers in the brainstem, probably accounting for the high safety margin of these agents [31]. Cannabinoids are also present in the periphery with probable implications for peripheral analgesic potential (Chapter 17). The mechanism of analgesia is presented in more detail in key references for this chapter but essentially involves activation of CB1 receptors resulting in multiple levels of modulation of nociceptive and pain-related transmission via inhibitiory mechanisms similar to but independent of that by opioids.

Numerous randomized controlled trials examining cannabinoids in the treatment of pain have demonstrated a significant analgesic effect [23]. Cannabinoid agents tested included synthetic analogs as well as cannabis and cannabis-based extracts; these agents were tested in a number of pain conditions. The weight of evidence supports that cannabinoids exhibit a moderate analgesic effect in neuropathic pain and cancer pain with preliminary evidence for action in other types of pain such as spinal pain and headache [1,23].

There are four cannabinoid agents available in several countries (Table 18.5). These include a cannabis/cannabidiol buccal spray (Sativex®), nabilone (Cesamet®) and dronabinol (synthetic Δ-9-THC in sesame oil sold under the trade name Marinol®), as well as the naturally occurring agent cannabis which is available in some countries through special licensing procedures or used as a traditional folk remedy. Clinical practice guidelines have been established in Canada where there are four cannabinoids available [32]. Based on current evidence supporting that cannabinoids are analgesic and safe, these guidelines identify that it is reasonable to use a cannabinoid as a second or third line agent either as a single agent or in combination with other agents exhibiting a different mechanism of action [32]. In patients exhibiting a constellation of symptoms including nausea, anorexia or spasticity one might consider introducing a cannabinoid earlier as there is evidence cannabinoids exhibit antiemetic and antispasticity action [23,32].

Common adverse effects include euphoria ("high"), dizziness, drowsiness, dry mouth and nausea [1]. Cannabinoids are contraindicated in patients with uncontrolled hypertension, active ischemic heart disease and schizophrenia.

The guidelines for the use of cannabinoids are similar to those used for opioids [32]. To summarize the key points, one must carry out a full assessment, establish a working diagnosis, assess psychosocial issues including screening for risk of addiction, assure that traditional approaches have been tried or considered, discuss potential for adverse effects, and monitor and document treatment.

In summary, the NSAIDs and selective COX2 inhibitors may have a role in mild to moderate pain but are usually inadequate in more severe pain and it is important to consider serious adverse events associated with chronic use. Acetaminophen may also assist with mild to moderate pain, has a good safety profile and remains a first line agent for osteoarthritis. There is some support for the use of muscle relaxants for short-term use in acute and chronic low back pain and cannabinoids are emerging as a second and third line option in the management of chronic pain.

References

1 Lynch ME, Watson CPN (2006) The pharmaco-therapy of chronic pain: a review. *Pain Res Manage* **11**:11–38.

2 Tannenbaum H, Bombadier C, Davis P *et al.*, for the Third Canadian Consensus Conference Group. (2006) An evidence-based approach to prescribing nonsteroidal anti-inflammatory drugs. Third Canadian Consensus Conference. *J Rheumatol* **33**:140–57.

3 Peura DA, Goldkind L. (2005) Balancing the gastrointestinal benefits and risks of nonselective NSAIDs. *Arthritis Res Ther* **7(Suppl 4)**:S7–13.

4 Rostom A, Moayyed P, Hunt R, for the Canadian Association of Gastroenterology Consensus Group. (2009) Canadian consensus guidelines on long-term nonsteroidal anti-inflammatory drug therapy and the need for gastroprotection: benefits versus risks. *Aliment Pharmacol Ther* **29**:481–96.

5 Moore RA, Derry S, Makinson GT *et al.* (2005) Tolerability and adverse events in clinical trials of celecoxib in osteoarthritis and rheumatoid arthritis: systematic review and meta-analysis of information from company clinical trial reports. *Arthritis Res Ther* **7**:R644–65.

6 McGettigan P, Henry D. (2006) Cardiovascular risk and inhibition of cyclooxygenase: a systematic review of the observational studies of selective and nonselective inhibitors of cyclooxygenase 2. *JAMA* **296**:1633–44.

7 Kearney PM, Baigent C, Godwin J *et al.* (2006) Do selective cyclo-oxygenase-2 inhibitors and traditional non-steroidal anti-inflammatory drugs increase the risk of atherothrombosis? Meta-analysis of randomised trials. *Br Med J* **332**:1302–8.

8 Gislason GH, Jacobsen S, Rasmussen JN *et al.* (2006) Risk of death or reinfarction associated with the use of selective cyclooxygenase-2 inhibitors and nonselective nonsteroidal anti-inflammatory drugs after acute myocardial infarction. *Circulation* **113**:2906–13.

9 Hippisley-Cox J, Coupland C. (2005) Risk of myocardial infarction in patients taking cyclo-oxygenase-2 inhibitors or conventional non-steroidal anti-inflammatory drugs: population based nested case–control analysis. *Br Med J* **330**:1366–72.

10 Brophy JM, Levesque LE, Zhang B. (2007) The coronary risk of cyclo-oxygenase-2 inhibitors in patients with a previous myocardial infarction. *Heart* **93**:189–94.

11 Graham DJ. (2006) COX-2 inhibitors, other NSAIDs, and cardiovascular risk: the seduction of common sense. *JAMA* **296**:1653–6.

12 Sandhu GK, Heyneman CA. (2004) Nephrotoxic potential of selective cyclooxygenase-2 inhibitors. *Ann Pharmacother* **38**:700–4.

13 Perazella MA, Tray K. (2001) Selective cyclooxygenase-2 inhibitors: a pattern of nephrotoxicity similar to traditional nonsteroidal anti-inflammatory drugs. *Am J Med* **111**:64–7.

14 Zhang JJ, Ding EL, Song Y. (2006) Adverse effects of cyclooxygenase 2 inhibitors on renal and arrhythmia events: a class-wide meta-analysis. *JAMA* **296**:1619–32.

15 Breyer MD, Harris RC. (2001) Cyclooxygenase 2 and the kidney. *Curr Opin Nephrol Hypertens* **10**:89–98.

16 Roelofs PDDM, Deyo RA, Koes BW *et al.* (2008) Non-steroidal anti-inflammatory drugs for low back pain. *Cochrane Database Syst Rev* **1**:CD000396.

17 Chou R, Huffman LH. (2007) Medications for acute and chronic low back pain: a review of the evidence for an American Pain Society/American College of Physicians Clinical Practice Guideline. *Ann Intern Med* **147**: 505–14.

18 Peloso PMJ, Gross A, Haines T *et al.* Cervical Overview Group. (2007) Medicinal and injection therapies for mechanical neck disorders. *Cochrane Database Syst Rev* **3**:CD000319.

19 Towheed T, Maxwell L, Judd M *et al.* (2006) Acetaminophen for osteoarthritis. *Cochrane Database Syst Rev* **1**:CD004257.

20 Wegman A, van der Windt D, van Tulder M *et al.* (2004) Nonsteroidal antiinflammatory drugs or acetaminophen for osteoarthritis of the hip or knee? A systematic review of evidence and guidelines. *J Rheumatol* **31**:344–54.

21 Bjordal JM, Ljunggren AE, Klovning A *et al.* (2004) Non-steroidal anti-inflammator y drugs, including cyclo-oxygenase-2 inhibitors, in osteoarthritic knee pain: meta-analysis of randomised placebo controlled trials. *Br Med J* **329**:1317.

22 Vo T, Rice ASC, Dworkin RH. (2009) Non-steroidal anti-inflammatory drugs for neuropathic pain: how do we explain continued widespread use? *Pain* **143**:169–71.

23 Lynch ME. (2008) Drug treatment of chronic pain. Rashiq S, Schopflocher D, Taenzer P *et al.* eds. *Chronic Pain: A Health Policy Perspectives.*

Wiley Blackwell, Edmonton, Alberta. pp. 101–120.

24 Mallet C, Daulhac L *et al.* (2008) Endocannabinoid and serotonergic systems are needed for acetaminophen induced analgesia. *Pain* **139**:190–200.

25 Forman JP, Stampfer MJ, Curhan GC. (2005) Non-narcotic analgesic dose and risk of incident hypertension in US women. *Hypertension* **46**:500–7.

26 Curhan GC, Knight EL, Rosner B *et al.* (2004) Lifetime nonnarcotic analgesic use and decline in renal function in women. *Arch Intern Med* **164**:1519–24.

27 FDA Joint Meeting of the Drug Safety and Risk Management (June 29–30, 2009). http://www.fda.gov/AdvisoryCommittees/Calendar/ucm143083.htm. Accessed on September 15, 2009.

28 See S, Ginzburg R. (2008) Choosing a skeletal muscle relaxant. *Am Fam Physician* **78**:365–70.

29 van Tulder MW, Touray T, Furlan AD *et al.* (2003) Muscle relaxants for non-specific low-back pain. *Cochrane Database Syst Rev* **4**:CD004252.

30 Chou R, Peterson K, Helfand M. (2004) Comparative efficacy and safety of skeletal muscle relaxants for spasticity and musculoskeletal conditions: a systematic review. *J Pain Symptom Manage* **28**:140–75.

31 Lynch ME. (2005) Preclinical science regarding cannabinoids as analgesic: an overview. *Pain Res Manage* **10(Suppl A)**:7A–14A.

32 Clark AJ, Lynch ME, Ware M *et al.* (2005) Guidelines for the use of cannabinoids compounds in chronic pain. *Pain Res Manage* **10(Suppl A)**:44A–6A.

Part 5

Interventional

Chapter 19

Diagnostic and therapeutic blocks

Boris Spektor[1], Padma Gulur[2] & James P. Rathmell[2]

[1] Department of Anesthesiology, Emory University School of Medicine, Atlanta, USA
[2] Department of Anesthesia, Critical Care and Pain Medicine, Massachusetts General Hospital and Harvard Medical School, Boston, USA

Introduction

Local anesthetics block nerve conduction by binding to sodium channels and blocking generation of action potentials. When local anesthetics are deposited at the site where pain is generated, they eliminate the transmission of pain along the neuron, thereby temporarily eliminating input of pain signals to the central nervous system. Local anesthetics have proven beneficial in facilitating surgical procedures within the peripheral distribution of the nerve that has been blocked as well as providing several days of pain relief when used as short-term infusions around peripheral nerves. The usefulness of nerve blocks in diagnosing and treating chronic pain has been more limited. In this chapter, we review the use of local anesthetic blocks for diagnosing and treating specific chronic pain conditions.

Diagnostic blocks

Establishing the source of pain when it is not clearly evident can be done using diagnostic

Clinical Pain Management: A Practical Guide, 1st edition.
Edited by Mary E. Lynch, Kenneth D. Craig and Philip W.H. Peng.
© 2011 Blackwell Publishing Ltd.

blocks. Local anesthetics are infiltrated around the nerve supply of a structure and if it results in pain relief it is considered diagnostic of the source of pain. Diagnostic blocks include nerve blocks or intra-articular blocks. Diagnostic nerve blocks are usually performed on peripheral nerves that have a specific distribution. In order to remove confounders such as a placebo effect or malingering, many advocate the use of controls when performing diagnostic blocks. This usually involves the performance of more than one diagnostic block for the same structure. One method would be the use of placebo control where an inactive agent such as saline would be injected. More commonly, a comparative method is employed with the use of local anesthetics of varying durations of action in each block (e.g. lidocaine and bupivacaine). When interpreting the response, it is important to understand that the relative duration of the local anesthetics as opposed to the absolute duration is critical. Individuals vary in the duration of action of local anesthetics. While patients may have pain relief in excess of the expected 1–2 hours from lidocaine and 4–6 hours from bupivacaine for instance, all patients will have a longer duration of relief from bupivacaine than lidocaine. For an in-depth discussion of the optimal use of diagnostic nerve blocks, readers are encouraged to read the review by Bogduk [1].

Therapeutic blocks

For chronic pain states the use of nerve blocks for therapeutic purposes usually involves the use of neurolytic agents such as phenol and alcohol. When there are sympathetic mediators to a pain state (e.g. in complex regional pain syndrome), sympathetic nerve blocks have been employed but their value is more prognostic than therapeutic. Therapeutic blocks can be performed with intra-rticular steroids to reduce inflammatory mediators. Steroids have also been used with local anesthetics in nerve blocks to reduce inflammatory mediators associated with nerve entrapment syndromes.

Peripheral nerve blocks

Once a nerve can be accurately identified, virtually any nerve in the body can be blocked with the aid of local anesthetics. The accurate identification of nerves can be performed using landmarks, by eliciting a paresthesia with needle irritation, using nerve stimulators (for mixed motor and sensory nerves) and imaging techniques such as ultrasound guidance, fluoroscopy or even computed tomography (CT) guidance. Peripheral nerve blocks used commonly for chronic pain states include occipital nerve blocks for occipital headaches and lateral femoral cutaneous nerve blocks for meralgia paresthetica.

Occipital nerve blocks

Peripheral nerve blocks for headaches are commonly employed. However, the data to support these modalities are scarce. Greater occipital nerve blocks were first performed to evaluate headaches postulated to be secondary to compression of the greater occipital nerve between the posterior arch of the atlas and the lamina of C2 [2]. The greater occipital nerve is blocked where it emerges from the posterior neck muscles. Some occipital nerve blocks are performed for diagnostic reasons and employ only local anesthetics and others are performed for therapeutic response with the use of local anesthestics and steroids.

The greater occipital nerve emerges from beneath an aponeurotic sling, between the trapezius and sternocleidomastoid. This fibrous sling was theoretically thought to cause the nerve entrapment although no histological evidence of this has been cited in the literature. In addition, there is debate about the use of occipital nerve blocks as a diagnostic tool as it has been shown that their effect on the headache syndromes clearly outlasts the duration of the local anesthetic.

Lateral femoral cutaneous nerve block

Meralgia paresthetica is a painful mononeuropathy of the lateral femoral cutaneous nerve commonly caused by focal entrapment of this nerve as it passes beneath the inguinal ligament [3]. Other etiologies such as direct trauma or stretch-related injury of the nerve have also been implicated. The lateral femoral cutaneous nerve originates from the lumbar plexus with contribution from the L2 and L3 spinal nerves. The nerve runs through the pelvis along the lateral border of the psoas muscle to the lateral part of the inguinal ligament, where it passes to the thigh through a tunnel formed by the lateral attachment of the inguinal ligament and the anterior superior iliac spine. The most common site of entrapment is at the site where it crosses the inguinal ligament. Meralgia paresthetica presents with painful paresthesia and numbness of the upper lateral thigh area. Symptoms are typically unilateral with bilateral presentation in up to 20% of cases.

The lateral femoral cutaneous nerve can be blocked just inferior to the inguinal ligament, using either an ultrasound-guided or landmark-based technique (1 cm medial to the anterior superior iliac spine) administering a combination of local anesthetic and corticosteroid. At best, this provides temporary relief of painful symptoms. This nerve block has also been used as a prognostic tool for surgical decompression of the nerve. The success rate for surgical decompression has been a matter of some debate. The mainstay of treatment for this condition consists of weight loss, if appropriate, and lifestyle modification, including the elimination of triggers such as tight clothing or a heavy tool belt.

Sympathetic blocks

The presence of sympathetically maintained pain (SMP) serves as the rationale behind performing blockade of the sympathetic nervous system for pain relief. The true prevalence of this entity, whereby pain is thought to be sustained by sympathetic nervous system-mediated catecholamine release, remains unclear. Clinical findings suggestive of SMP include pain accompanied by edema, skin color changes, temperature fluctuation, alteration in hair growth and sweating. These symptoms are frequently manifested by patients with ischemic pain as well as complex regional pain syndrome (CRPS) Types I and II, and the latter is reviewed in Chapter 35. Classically, local anesthetic blockade of the sympathetic ganglia supply-

ing the painful region has been used to diagnose SMP in patients with CRPS as well as to provide analgesia in order to facilitate physical therapy, the mainstay of treatment.

Stellate ganglion block

Cervical sympathetic blockade (stellate ganglion block) has traditionally been used in the management of SMP involving the head and upper extremity. The stellate ganglion is a star-shaped neuronal cluster formed by the fusion of the inferior cervical and superior thoracic sympathetic ganglia and is typically located at or near the head of the first rib at the level of the first thoracic vertebra (Figure 19.1). Positioned adjacent to the origin of the vertebral artery just behind the dome of the lung, the stellate ganglion relays sympathetic fibers to and from the head, neck and arms. The most common approach to the ganglion involves blockade at the

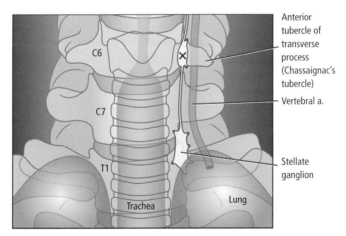

Figure 19.1 *Stellate ganglion block.* The stellate ganglion conveys sympathetic fibers to and from the upper extremities and the head and neck. The ganglion is comprised of the fused superior thoracic ganglion and the inferior cervical ganglion and is named for its fusiform shape (in many individuals, the two ganglia remain separate). The stellate ganglia lies over the the the head of the first rib at the junction of the transverse process and uncinate process of T1. The ganglion is just posteromedial to the cupola of the lung and medial to the vertebral artery. Stellate ganglion block is typically carried out at the C6 or C7 level to avoid pneumothorax, and a volume of solution that will spread along the prevertebral fascia inferiorly to the stellate ganglion is employed (usually 10 mL). When radiographic guidance is not used, the operator palpates the anterior tubercle of the transverse process of C6 (Chassaignac's tubercle), and a needle is seated in the location. With radiographic guidance it is simpler and safer to place a needle over the vertebral body just inferior the uncinate process of C6 (X) or C7. Particular care should be taken when performing the block at the C7 level to assure that the needle does not stray lateral to the uncinate process, as the vertebral artery courses anterior to transverse process at this level and is often not protected within a bony foramen transversarum. Reproduced with permission from [16].

C6 level using either palpation or fluoroscopic guidance and relying on caudal spread of local anesthetic along the prevertebral fascia. The scientific literature contains multiple favorable case reports and case series, but few randomized controlled trials assessing the efficacy of stellate ganglion blockade for CRPS of the upper extremity. Interestingly, placebo-controlled sympathetic blockade with normal saline versus lidocaine 1% showed no initial difference in pain relief at 30 minutes post-blockade; the median duration of pain relief, however, was significantly longer in patients receiving local anesthetic (6 hours with saline compared to 5.5 days with lidocaine). Usually, this nerve block is performed in a series in an effort to provide sustained pain relief. Unfortunately, despite a long history of widespread use, the duration and magnitude of pain relief are unpredictable, and there is little evidence that this is an effective approach [4]. Complications of stellate ganglion block include pneumothorax, somatic nerve block of the brachial plexus, phrenic nerve block and direct intra-arterial injection in to the vertebral artery with resultant seizure.

Lumbar sympathetic block

Lumbar sympathetic blockade (LSB) is the counterpart of SGB for the lower extremities, used primarily to diagnose and treat SMP of the legs in neuropathic conditions such as CRPS I and II, peripheral neuropathic pain and ischemic pain. The lumbar sympathetic chain is comprised of several paired ganglia lying along the anterolateral surface of the vertebral bodies generally between L2 and L4 (Figure 19.2), and can be blocked using a posterior percutaneous approach with fluoroscopic guidance. Similar to stellate ganglion block, the literature contains multiple retrospective case reports and case series, but few prospective randomized studies. The available randomized studies are flawed secondary to lack of any control group;

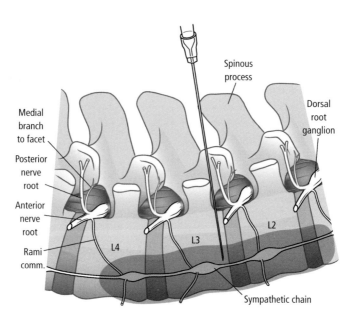

Figure 19.2 Lumbar sympathetic block. The lumbar sympathetic ganglia are variable in number and location from one individual to another. Most commonly, the ganglia lie over the anteromedial surface of the vertebral bodies between L2 and L4. Temporary lumbar sympathetic block using local anesthetic is best performed by advancing a single needle cephalad to the transverse process of L3 in order to avoid the exiting nerve root. The needle tip is placed adjacent to the superior portion of the anteromedial surface of the L3 vertebral body. Use of 15–20 mL of local anesthetic solution will spread to cover multiple vertebral levels (shaded region). Reproduced with permission from [16].

thus, efficacy of LSB is impossible to determine from these limited data. Complications of LSB include spinal or epidural spread of local anesthetic with resultant neuraxial blockade and hematuria from direct penetration of the kidney during needle placement.

Sympathetic blockade of the stellate ganglion or lumbar sympathetic chain may be a useful adjunct in a comprehensive multidisciplinary therapeutic approach to sympathetically maintained pain including physical therapy, oral neuropathic medications and cognitive behavioral therapy. Sympathetic blocks to the painful region in those with CRPS is used only when more conservative measures fail to provide effective pain relief; the use of repeated blocks is useful only to the extent that this approach provides enough pain relief to allow for more effective restoration through an ongoing and aggressive physical therapy program [5].

Celiac plexus block

The only sympathetic block to date with good support from multiple randomized controlled studies is the celiac plexus block (CPB). Indications for this block include pain arising from cancer of the abdominal viscera between the gastroesophageal junction and the splenic flexure of the colon. The most common application is for treatment of pain associated with pancreatic cancer, although limited case series support its use for chronic benign refractory abdominal pain secondary to chronic pancreatitis. The celiac plexus is comprised of a diffuse network of nerve fibers overlying the anterolateral surface of the aorta at the T12–L1 level near the origin of the celiac artery. The sympathetic nerve fibers to the proximal abdominal viscera originate from the T5–T12 levels of the spinal cord, progressing to the celiac plexus via the greater, lesser and least splanchnic nerves. Local anesthetic blockade typically results in short duration relief (days to weeks), whereas administration of a neurolytic agent (phenol or alcohol) yields long-term analgesia (months). While the majority of randomized controlled trials suggest statistically significant reduction in opioid consumption and opioid-related side effects in patients receiving

neurolytic CPB when compared with conservative management, quality of life and survival are generally unchanged [6]. There are multiple approaches to the celiac plexus including a posterior percutaneous approach with the aid of fluoroscopy or CT as well as a transgastric approach using endoscopy and ultrasound guidance. Notable side effects of CPB include hypotension secondary to visceral vasodilatation as well as diarrhea stemming from unopposed parasympathetic stimulation of the gut; potential complications include nerve injury, hemorrhage, pneumothorax and bowel injury. Sporadic case reports of paraplegia following neurolytic celiac plexus block have appeared; the proposed mechanism leading to paraplegia is direct injury or spasm of the artery of Adamkiewicz, leading to ischemic injury to the spinal cord.

Diagnostic and therapeutic blocks for neck and back pain

Neck and low back pain are among the most common painful conditions in adults of all ages. The degenerative cascade that effects all major bony structures with aging also affects the spine, leading to progressive loss of height of the intervertebral discs, disc herniation, as well as calcium deposition on the margins of the vertebra and the zygoapophyseal (facet) joints (termed spondylosis or facet arthropathy). The majority of episodes of acute low back pain with or without radicular pain (pain in the extremity due to spinal nerve irritation) will resolve without specific treatment. Overall, 60–70% of those affected recover by 6 weeks, and 80–90% recover by 12 weeks [7]. Epidural injection of steroids has been used for radicular pain in the upper or lower extremities due to disc herniation for many decades and is now in widespread use in many countries. In a subset of patients with chronic neck and low back pain without radicular pain, the pain can be related to facet arthropathy or previous whiplash injury.

Acute radicular pain: epidural steroid injection

Numerous randomized trials have examined the efficacy of this approach. The rationale behind injecting glucocorticoid into the epidural space adjacent to a spinal nerve is that it will combat the inflammatory response associated with acute disc herniation and will thus reduce pain. Systematic reviews of studies of epidural steroid injection appeared in the 1990s and yielded contradictory results: one suggested significant efficacy and one was inconclusive, citing the dearth of high-quality evidence [8,9]. Both are now significantly outdated and were conducted before the widespread adoption of fluoroscopic guidance and the increasing popularity of the X-ray guided transforaminal technique (use of epidural steroid injection directed to the affected spinal nerve) over the conventional interlaminar approach to the epidural space.

One of the most widely cited studies examined the effectiveness of epidural steroid injections compared with saline for treating acute radicular pain due to disc herniation and concluded that there were no long-term benefits of epidural steroid injection [10]. In this randomized controlled trial, although there were no demonstrable differences between epidural steroid and placebo treatment groups at 3 months after injection, there was significantly earlier reduction in pain and decrease in sensory deficits (3 weeks after treatment) in those receiving epidural steroid injections. The WEST trial, a large multicenter trial of epidural corticosteroid injections for sciatica, appeared in 2005 [11]. At 3 weeks, those receiving epidural steroids demonstrated a significantly greater reduction in pain, but no difference between groups was seen from 6 to 52 weeks of follow-up monitoring. The authors concluded that epidural steroid injections afforded patients earlier relief of pain but no long-term decrease in pain or the need for surgery. When earlier studies are re-examined, similar early reduction in pain can be seen despite the lack of long-term benefit from epidural steroid injections.

Injection route has also been much debated recently. The transforaminal approach to placing epidural steroids has been advocated as a means of delivering the steroid in high concentration directly to the inflammation site near the spinal nerve within the lateral epidural space. A recent small randomized controlled trial compared the efficacy of transforaminal versus interlaminar corticosteroid injection in treating radicular pain and found significantly better pain reduction in the transforaminal group at 30 days [12]. Results of a mailed questionnaire also revealed significantly better pain relief and increased daily activity levels 6 months after injection. This small study warrants further validation by a larger controlled trial. We are still lacking studies that compare the transforaminal route with the interlaminar route.

Collectively, numerous studies examining the usefulness of epidural steroids for treating acute radicular pain due to herniated nucleus pulposus have failed to show that injection reduces long-term pain or obviates the need for surgery. Similarly, there is scant evidence to suggest that epidural steroids have any beneficial effect in those with acute low back pain without leg pain or in those who have chronic low back or leg pain. However, most studies have demonstrated more rapid resolution of pain in those who received epidural steroid injections versus those who did not. Thus, the role of epidural steroid injections in the conservative management of radicular pain is simply to facilitate earlier pain relief, allowing return to full function [13].

Chronic neck and low back pain: facet joint injections, medial branch blocks and radiofrequency treatment

A subset of patients with chronic neck or low back pain will respond to targeted blocks of the facet joints [14]. The sensory innervation of the facet joints is supplied by the medial branch of the posterior primary ramus of each spinal nerve, and the anatomic location of the medial branch nerves is relatively invariable, allowing for reliable blockade. The first approach employed for treating facet-related pain was to place a combination of local anesthetic and steroid directly in to the joint at the level suspected to be symptomatic. Controlled trials in patients with both neck and low back pain demonstrated that this produced only short-term pain relief in most individuals, lasting days to weeks.

In recent decades, a reliable technique for denervating the facet joints using radiofrequency neurolysis has evolved. Radiofrequency neurolysis is a precise means of producing a small area of tissue destruction at a depth via a small gauge needle. Patients suspected of having facet-mediated pain first undergo a series of comparative local anesthetic blocks of the medial branch nerves at the level of pain. Those who report brief duration of pain relief after blocks with lidocaine and longer duration of pain relief after bupivacaine are then treated with radiofrequency facet neurolysis. Well-controlled trials have demonstrated that this approach can produce intermediate duration pain relief lasting, on average, 3–6 months after treatment. The procedure can be repeated with similar duration of pain relief following subsequent treatment. Complications are rare, although transient exacerbation of pain for several days after treatment is common.

Chronic low back pain: sacroiliac joint blocks

Pain arising from the sacroiliac joint is thought to be a common cause of axial low back pain, affecting 15–25% of low back pain patients using controlled analgesic response to injection as a diagnostic criterion [15]. The sacroiliac joints are paired synovial joints formed at the junction of the sacrum medially and pelvic ilium laterally. Functionally, the sacroiliac joints serve as the principal weight-bearing structures connecting the spine with the pelvis and lower extremities. Sacroiliac joint pain typically presents over the lower back or upper buttock in the vicinity of the posterior superior iliac spine with occasional radiation to the proximal lower extremity, rarely below the knee level. Neither medical history nor physical examination findings are consistently able to isolate the sacroiliac joint as the pain generator. The two most commonly used diagnostic distraction maneuvers include Patrick's test, also known as the FABER test (hip *f*lexion, *ab*duction and *e*xternal *r*otation with pain repro-

duction over the axial low back or buttock) and Gaenslen's test (extension of the ipsilateral hip joint over the edge of an examining table with stabilization of the contralateral hip to reproduce pain), each with approximately 75% sensitivity and specificity. Imaging is rarely helpful. Resolution of pain following intra-articular injection of local anesthetic serves as the best diagnostic tool available. As with other diagnostic blocks, comparative local anesthetic blocks with duration-appropriate relief are the most diagnostically specific approach. In clinical practice, the initial injection is typically combined with corticosteroid in efforts to produce more durable pain relief, rendering it a combined diagnostic and therapeutic intervention. Small randomized controlled trials have suggested that fluoroscopically guided sacroiliac joint injections provide good to excellent analgesia lasting up to 6 months [15]. In those patients receiving only transient relief from therapeutic blocks, longer lasting relief has been sought utilizing percutaneous radiofrequency treatment of the joint nerve supply; however, the efficacy of newer percutaneous techniques for sacroiliac joint radiofrequency treatment is currently being investigated.

Conclusions

Overall, local anesthetic blocks have limited value in diagnosing and treating chronic pain; however, peripheral nerve blocks have shown some utility in treating occipital neuralgia and meralgia paresthetica. Sympathetic blocks of the upper and lower extremities can provide pain relief to facilitate functional restoration in patients with complex regional pain syndrome. Neurolytic celiac plexus block can provide effective pain relief in those with cancer-related pain of the abdominal viscera. Epidural injection of steroids has proven beneficial for reducing the severity and duration of acute radicular pain associated with intervertebral disc herniation. In patients with chronic neck or low back pain related to facet arthropathy, diagnostic blocks of the medial branch nerves can identify those patients who are most likely to attain durable pain relief with radiofrequency neurolysis.

References

1 Bogduk N. Diagnostic blocks: a truth serum for malingering. *Clin J Pain* (2004) **20(6)**:409–14.

2 Bogduk N. (2004) Role of anesthesiologic blockade in headache management. *Curr Pain Headache Rep* **8(5)**:399–403.

3 Grossman MG, Ducey SA, Nadler SS *et al.* (2001) Meralgia paresthetica: diagnosis and treatment. *J Am Acad Orthop Surg* **9(5)**:336–44.

4 Cepeda MS, Carr DB, Lau J. (2005) Local anesthetic sympathetic blockade for complex regional pain syndrome. *Cochrane Database Syst Rev* **4**:CD004598.

5 Day M. (2008) Sympathetic blocks: the evidence. *Pain Pract* **8(2)**:98–109.

6 Yan BM, Myers RP. (2007) Neurolytic celiac plexus block for pain control in unresectable pancreatic cancer. *Am J Gastroenterol* **102(2)**: 430–8.

7 Rathmell JP. (2008) A 50-year-old man with chronic low back pain. *JAMA* **299(17)**: 2066–77.

8 Koes BW, Scholten RJ, Mens JM *et al.* (1995) Efficacy of epidural steroid injections for low-back pain and sciatica: a systematic review of randomized clinical trials. *Pain* **63(3)**:279–88.

9 Nelemans PJ, de Bie RA, de Vet HC *et al.* (2000) Injection therapy for subacute and chronic benign low back pain. *Cochrane Database Syst Rev* **2**:CD001824.

10 Carette S, Leclaire R, Marcoux S *et al.* (1997) Epidural corticosteroid injections for sciatica due to herniated nucleus pulposus. *N Engl J Med* **336(23)**:1634–40.

11 Arden NK, Price C, Reading I *et al.* (2005) A multicentre randomized controlled trial of epidural corticosteroid injections for sciatica: the WEST study. *Rheumatology (Oxford)* **44(11)**:1399–406.

12 Thomas E, Cyteval C, Abiad L *et al.* (2003) Efficacy of transforaminal versus interspinous corticosteroid injection in discal radiculalgia: a prospective, randomised, double-blind study. *Clin Rheumatol* **22(4–5)**:299–304.

13 Sethee J, Rathmell JP. (2009) Epidural steroid injections are useful for the treatment of low back pain and radicular symptoms: pro. *Curr Pain Headache Rep* **13(1)**:31–4.

14 Bogduk N, Dreyfuss P, Govind J. (2009) A narrative review of lumbar medial branch neurotomy for the treatment of back pain. *Pain Med* **10(6)**:1035–45.

15 Cohen SP. (2005) Sacroiliac joint pain: a comprehensive review of anatomy, diagnosis, and treatment. *Anesth Analg* **101(5)**:1440–53.

16 Rathmell JP. (2006) *Atlas of image-guided intervention in regional anesthesia and pain medicine.* Lippincott Williams & Wilkins, Philadelphia.

Chapter 20

Neuromodulation therapy

Krishna Kumar & Sharon Bishop

Department of Neurosurgery, Regina General Hospital, Regina, Canada

Introduction

Neuromodulation utilizes implantable devices discharging electricity or chemical substances that modify signal transmission in order to achieve inhibition, excitation or modulation of the activity of neuronal groups and networks. Neuromodulation is a reversible therapy that is used to treat various types of pain (non-cancer and cancer), as well as conditions such as spasticity, epilepsy, cardiac or limb ischemia, alterations in the motility of the intestine and bladder, movement disorders and has growing indications within the field of psychiatry. Results are dependent on the precise placement of the neuromodulatory system as well as the underlying pathology being treated. The field of neuromodulation has developed over the last 30 years as a viable and highly effective option for the management of chronic pain.

Types of neuromodulation therapy

Neuromodulation devices can be implanted within the brain, spinal cord or along the peripheral nerves.

Cranial

Deep brain stimulation (DBS) is used for the management of pain, cluster headaches, movement disorders and recently for psychiatric disorders

such as obsessive compulsive disorder, refractory depression, Tourette's syndrome and eating disorders. Alternatively, motor cortex stimulation (MCS) is used predominantly for facial pain, post-stroke thalamic pain, brachial plexus avulsion pain or deafferentation pain. For further discussion of DBS and MCS see Chapter 21.

Spinal cord stimulation

Historical overview

Shealy inserted the first dorsal column stimulator in 1967. Initially, electrodes were unipolar, with the first percutaneous quadripolar electrode being introduced in 1980. Currently, 8-contact percutaneous leads and 16-contact surgical leads have been developed that allow for superior programming and steering capabilities, thus improving outcomes (Figure 20.1).

Originally, only radio frequency-driven receivers were available with an external transmitter. In the mid-1970s, the first fully implantable pulse generator (IPG) was introduced and was powered by a non-rechargeable primary cell battery. The disadvantage of this system is the battery life of 2–5 years. When battery exhaustion occurs a surgical procedure is required for replacement. As the technology continued to "mushroom," a transcutaneously rechargeable and programmable IPG was developed. The first rechargeable IPG was approved by the US Food and Drug Administration (FDA) in 2004. Bench testing anticipates that these IPGs could last 10–25 years, and hence will need fewer replacements, resulting in reduced morbidity and cost savings [1].

Clinical Pain Management: A Practical Guide, 1st edition.
Edited by Mary E. Lynch, Kenneth D. Craig and
Philip W.H. Peng.
© 2011 Blackwell Publishing Ltd.

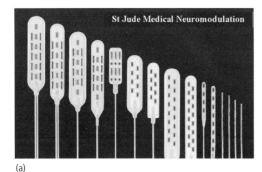

(a)

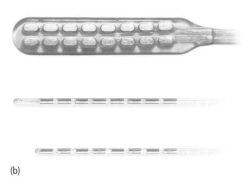

(b)

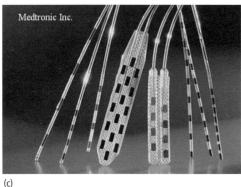

(c)

Figure 20.1 Leads currently available through various vendors. Images provided courtesy of St. Jude Medical Neuromodulation, Boston Scientific, Medtronic Inc.

Mechanism of action

It is likely that the mechanism of analgesic action of spinal cord stimulation (SCS) is a result of a complex interplay between both electrical and chemical changes that occur along the whole segment of the spinal cord being stimulated. The mechanism of action for control of neuropathic pain can be subdivided into either electrical and/or chemical. SCS is thought to modulate pain through several mechanisms including:

1 Suppression of the hyperexcitability of wide dynamic range neurons in the dorsal horn;

2 Suppression of high threshold on nociceptive-specific spinothalamic neurons by dorsal column stimulation [2];

3 Activation of interneuron networks near or in substantia gelatinosa, which in turn inhibit the deeper lamina III–V in the dorsal horn [3]; and

4 Supraspinal mechanisms are also activated – the anterior pretectal nucleus can be excited which causes analgesia by inhibiting the nociceptive dorsal horn neurons.

The long-lasting effects are thought to be mediated via the dorsolateral funiculus because sectioning of this tract abolishes the long-lasting effect [4]. In addition, SCS is theorized to induce release of gamma-aminobutyric acid (GABA) and activate GABA$_B$ receptors, which suppress the excitatory amino acids in the dorsal horn cells; and induce the release of neurotransmitters such as glycine, adenosine and 5-hydroxytrytamine (5-HT) [5].

For ischemic pain the mechanism of action differs, the most popular theory being that SCS suppresses efferent sympathetic activity, especially that relayed via nicotinic ganglionic receptors and peripheral 1-adrenoreceptors, resulting in diminished peripheral vasoconstriction and secondarily in relief of pain. However, recent evidence indicates that antidromic mechanisms may also be activated by SCS intensities far below the motor threshold and that this may result in peripheral calcitonin gene-related peptide and nitric oxide release with subsequent peripheral vasodilatation [6].

While in recent years solid evidence underlying the physiological mechanisms of SCS has emerged, the exact mechanism of action is still only partially understood and further research is required.

Indications and patient selection

SCS has been used for a variety of pain conditions such as failed back surgery syndrome [7,8], complex regional pain syndrome (CRPS) Types I and II [9–10], intractable angina [11–14], lower extremity ischemic pain [15–17], phantom limb and stump pain, spinal cord injury pain, peripheral neuropathies, interstitial cystitis and, recently, intractable abdominal and visceral pain.

Considerations with regards to patient selection include non-cancer pain; failure of conventional treatment for at least 6 months; remedial surgery inadvisable; no major psychiatric disorder, including somatization; willingness to stop inappropriate drug use before implantation; no secondary gain or litigation involved; and ability to give informed consent for the procedure and operate equipment. Once the patient is deemed a suitable candidate, psychological testing is desirable.

Failed back surgery syndrome

Failed back surgery syndrome (FBSS) is the most common indication for SCS and constitutes approximately 70% of the caseload. While several case series and meta-analyses have been reported, two randomized controlled trials (RCTs) have been published. The PROCESS Study recruited 100 patients with FBSS, comparing SCS in combination with conventional medical management (CMM) (52 patients) with CMM alone (48 patients) [7] with follow-up at 6, 12 and 24 months. North et al. [8] randomized 60 patients and compared SCS (30 patients) with repeated lumbosacral spine surgery (30 patients), with results reported at 6 months and a mean of 2.9 years. The primary outcome in both studies was the proportion of people who had 50% or greater pain relief. Table 20.1 presents the results of both trials. In summary, there is strong evidence to support the finding that SCS may benefit appropriately selected patients with FBSS.

Complex regional pain syndrome Type I

Kemler et al. [9] investigated the effect of SCS in combination with physical therapy (SCS + PT) compared with physical therapy (PT) alone. This trial reported that SCS + PT was more effective than PT alone in reducing pain at 6 months and at 2 years. At 5 years, SCS + PT produced results similar to those following PT for pain relief and all other measured variables. The reduced effectiveness of SCS over time is unknown but may have been

Table 20.1 Efficacy and cost effectiveness of spinal cord stimulation in failed back surgery syndrome randomized controlled trials (RCTs).

Author	Study design	Follow-up period/no. patient, treatment	Results and outcome measures
Kumar et al. [28]	RCT Consecutive	5 years/60 SCS, 44 CMM	27% improvement in QoL for the SCS, compared with 12% improvement for CMM. After 2.5 years SCS becomes cost effective
North et al. [8]	RCT	3 years/19 SCS, 26 reoperation	Significant pain relief (39%) and reduced opioid consumption (87%) in SCS when compared with repeat operation (12% and 58%)
North et al. [29]	RCT	3 years/19 SCS, 21 reoperation	SCS was less expensive (SCS $48,357 versus reoperation $105,928). SCS should be considered as the initial therapy of choice
Kumar et al. [30]	RCT, Multicenter	1 year/52 SCS, 48 CMM	48% of SCS and 9% of CMM patients (p < 0.001) achieved > 50% pain relief
Kumar et al. [7]	RCT, Multicenter	2 years/42 SCS, 41 CMM	In "per treatment analysis" 47% of SCS and 7% of CMM patients achieved > 50% pain relief. (In "intention-to-treat analysis": SCS 37% and CMM patients 2%)

CMM, conventional medical management; FBSS, failed back surgery syndrome; QoL, quality of life; SCS, spinal cord stimulation.

related to a number of factors including disease progression with pain increase in the SCS group; exaggeration of pain relief in the trial period; or the possibility that the PT group may have shown some spontaneous improvement. Further research is required. Kemler & Furnee [10] have shown that SCS remains a cost-effective viable option with high patient satisfaction.

Refractory angina pectoris

SCS is one of the most promising treatment options for this disease. Prospective RCTs of SCS showed benefits both in quality of life and cardiac indices [11,12]. Specifically, exercise duration and time to angina increased in the SCS group compared with controls. Nitrate consumption, ischemic episodes at rest and with exercise decreased. SCS was also found to be cost effective in this population [13]. An important finding is that SCS does not mask the pain associated with myocardial infarction [14].

Peripheral vascular disease

Peripheral vascular disease can lead to critical limb ischemia which is manifested by rest pain, ulcers, gangrene in the toes and claudication. Several pre-clinical and clinical studies using SCS have been performed to investigate potential beneficial effects such as reduction in amputation rate, pain relief, and healing of ulcers [15,16]. The most desired effect is limb salvage. The best parameter used to predict the percentage of limb salvage is a baseline transcutaneous PO2 (TcPO2) of 10 to 30 mm Hg. Improvement in pain control, combined with an increase in TcPO2 values that was greater than 10 mm Hg from baseline, are early predictors of long-term success. Similarly, an initial increase in peak blood flow velocities (measured in Doppler studies) of greater than 10 mm also signified a good long-term outcome [17].

Technique

The procedure is performed in two steps. The first step involves a trial period, using either a cylindri-cal or surgical lead. The trial is important to determine effectiveness. Different pathologies have varying rates of failure on trial; cumulatively the range is 18–20%. The second step involves implantation of a permanent lead with subsequent internalization.

Cylindrical leads are used more commonly and implanted percutaneously via a Tuohy needle under fluoroscopic guidance. Once the lead is in the desired anatomic position, intraoperative testing for concordancy of paresthesia to the patient's pain is performed. This is done by attaching the lead to an external stimulator outside of the sterile field. The final position will be dictated by the patient's area of pain and the overlapping stimulation-induced paresthesia. If the overlap is less than 80% the results are less than satisfactory.

For lower limb pain the superior electrode should be positioned between T8–T11. For cervical pain, entry point at T4–5 is preferred. The electrode is positioned guided by the patient's dermatomal pain pattern and is commonly positioned between C4 and C7. For angina, best results are achieved when the electrode is situated at the C7–T1 level.

Implantation of a surgical lead requires a small laminotomy, either at T10–11 or T11–12, performed using local anesthesia, supplemented by conscious sedation, general anesthesia or spinal anesthesia [18]. The surgical lead is inserted into the epidural space. As with implantation of a cylin-drical lead, intraoperative testing for concordancy of paresthesia to the patient's pain is performed.

Contrary to popular belief that spinal anesthesia produces complete motor and sensory block, it has been shown that it does not block all sensory transmission in the superficial layers of the spinal dorsal columns, thus permitting intraoperative testing and proper lead positioning. If general anesthesia is used, X-ray position or somatosensory evoked potentials will be necessary to ascertain proper placement.

The system is then externalized and a trial period of stimulation commences lasting approximately 5–10 days. If more than 50% pain relief is achieved on trial, the lead is then internalized and attached to either a non-rechargeable or rechargeable pulse generator (IPG). The placement of the IPG can be either in the buttock region or, preferably, the anterior abdominal wall.

Complications

Complication rates are variable, ranging 34–36%. Complications can be divided into three categories:

1 Hardware-related (27–30%);
2 Biological (3–5%); and
3 Other (3–4%).

The most common hardware-related complications are lead migration (13%) and fracture (9%) or hardware malfunction (3%). Biological complications are related to infection (3–5%), cerebrospinal fluid leak (0.3%), symptomatic hematoma (0.3%) or pain located at the incision, electrode or IPG site. Battery exhaustion is not a real complication per se, but a non-rechargeable battery will need to be replaced every 3–4 years depending upon usage.

Cost effectiveness

Despite the initial high costs of hardware, SCS has been shown to be cost-effective in the treatment of FBSS when compared with the costs of repeated lumbosacral spine surgery, CRPS and intractable angina. From an economic perspective the high costs of SCS are recouped within 2.5 years in cases with FBSS (Table 20.1).

Peripheral nerve

The indication for peripheral nerve stimulation (PNS) is rapidly evolving. It is used for occipital nerve stimulation for chronic headaches such as migraine. In these cases, under local anesthesia supplemented by conscious sedation, cylindrical electrodes are placed under the skin and over the deep fascia in the back of the head at the level of C2. If successful pain relief is achieved after a brief trial, the electrodes are internalized [19]. Similarly, for incisional pain following thoracotomy or herniorraphy, electrodes can be placed along the incision line under the skin, followed by a trial period of stimulation with internalization if successful. Success rates run as high as 70%. PNS has also been used for sacral nerve stimulation for

pelvic pain and bowel and bladder dysfunction [20]. Vagus nerve stimulation is gaining popularity for uncontrolled epilepsy and depression [21].

Intrathecal drug therapy

Overview

Intrathecal drug therapy (IDT) has emerged as a therapeutic option for treatment of pain, either non-cancer or secondary to malignancy. It also has an important role in the management of spasticity secondary to cerebral palsy, spinal cord injury or demyelinating diseases such as multiple sclerosis. For the purposes of this chapter we confine our discussion to IDT for non-cancer pain.

IDT is an indication in the management of patients who have failed other conventional treatment modalities, or those who suffer intolerable side effects related to high doses of oral or parental therapy. Practice guidelines published in 2007 [22] have concluded that evidence for IDT is strong for the short-term and moderate for the long-term management of neuropathic and mixed pain. Morphine, hydromorphone and zinconotide are now first-line treatments in intrathecal drug therapy. The highest incidence of granuloma formation has been reported with the use of morphine and hydromorphone, and none with zinconotide. Zinconotide is most useful in cases that prove refractory to other drugs. To reduce the incidence of granuloma formation, it has been recommended that both the concentration and total daily dose of morphine or hydromorphone are decreased. Future promising drugs for use in IDT are gabapentin and other conotoxins which are currently undergoing research.

Indications and patient selection

IDT may be considered in cases where the patient has obtained inadequate management of pain after maximizing conventional treatment modalities such as self-management approaches, interdisciplinary therapies and full trials of combination pharmacotherapy. In addition, the patient should not have an active medical or psychiatric condition that might compromise the patient's safety or ability to benefit from IDT. Similarly, IDT may be considered for patients who have found partial relief of their pain with the use of oral or parenteral drug therapy, but which has been limited by intolerable side effects. It is very important that the patient and their family have realistic expectations of the treatment goals and that appropriate pharmacy and medical support is available for this technology.

IDT should not be considered until patients have mastered basic self-management skills for pain and psychosocial stress. IDT should be avoided in patients where there is no established diagnosis, where there are inconsistencies between symptoms and physical findings, or where there are concerns about addiction, frequent emergency room visits or unresolved litigation.

Trial period

The purpose of a screening trial is to determine the patient's response to the medication to ensure effectiveness and to make certain that no intolerable side effects are experienced. The trial involves the insertion of a temporary or permanent catheter that can be placed in either the intrathecal or epidural space. The duration of the trial may vary from 1 day to several weeks, with the average being 3–5 days. It can be conducted using continuous infusion or bolus dosing. For a continuous infusion trial the catheter is connected to an external ambulatory drug delivery system.

According to the national outcomes registry for low back pain the success rate of trial screening in appropriately selected patients with chronic low back pain is 93%, with an implantation rate of 82% [23]. The pathology causing the pain dictates the length and the outcome of the trial. A very thorough assessment is required in order to maximize success and once the intrathecal pump is implanted there needs to be appropriate follow-up and monitoring of this technology.

Complications

Procedural

1 *Postdural puncture headache* The incidence during trial has been reported to be as high as 30%, which

reduces to 5–6% following permanent implantation. The headache is usually short-lived and responds to oral analgesics although a blood patch may be necessary in some refractory cases. Surgery is rarely needed.

2 *Paralysis* The incidence of producing a neurological deficit while introducing an intrathecal catheter is < 1%. In the rare circumstance where a lumbar puncture has been performed at L1–2 or higher level, injury to the conus has been reported.

3 *Infection* Most infections occur within 3–4 months of implantation and are caused by organisms such as *Staphylococcus aureus* or *Staphylococcus epidermidis*. The reported infection rate varies 1–10%. Once recognized, the infection must be treated aggressively, usually with cephalosporin or vancomycin. The incidence of infection that may warrant explantation and reimplantation is 2–3%. While the incidence of meningitis is low, one must be vigilant in early detection.

Mechanical

The annual rate of device-related complication requiring surgical intervention is reported to be 10.5%, with 35% being pump-related and 65% being catheter-related [24]. Catheter-related mechanical problems consist of catheter leakage 13%, catheter migration 11%, disconnection or fracture at the pump nozzle 9% and catheter occlusion 4%. All these circumstances require surgical intervention for correction. Mechanical pump malfunction is rare and if suspected requires confirmation by X-ray. Battery exhaustion usually occurs within 55–60 months and requires surgical replacement of the pump.

Drug-related

1 *Inadvertent drug overdose* Drug overdose can result because of programming errors or if there is an error in refilling the pump reservoir. If refilling of the reservoir is accidentally done via the catheter access port a massive overdose will occur with respiratory arrest and even death.

2 *Granuloma formation* The incidence reportedly increases over time: 0.4% after 2 years, 1.6% after 6 years; however, it has been reported as early as

27 days. All drugs, except ziconotide, have been reported to cause granuloma, the most frequent culprits being morphine and hydromorphone. Granuloma formation is influenced by drug concentration and daily dose. A high level of suspicion should be aroused when for no apparent reason pain control starts to decline. The patient may or may not exhibit neurological signs. Magnetic resonance imaging (MRI) is the preferred method of investigation. To treat when there is no neurological deficit, pulling the catheter down 2–3 cm will restore pain control and the granuloma will resolve without further intervention. Conversely, if neurological deficit is present surgical excision of the granuloma is necessary. In order to prevent further reoccurrence, revision of drug dosage and concentration is advised.

3 *Endocrine effects* Endocrine side effects are common and are secondary to hypothalamic-pituitary axis suppression causing hypogonadism (86%), growth hormone deficiency (17%) and reduced libido (4.9%) [25]. Hormonal effects are most commonly seen with the use of morphine/hydromorphone (possibly because of the lipophylic properties) and are least likely with ziconatide. For sexual dysfunction supplemental testosterone is indicated. Weight gain and/or edema may also be related to hormonal changes.

Polyanalgesic drug admixtures

It has been noted that 11% of patients with neuropathic pain fail the initial trial with IDT morphine alone and that 35–40% of patients become refractory to the opioid over time, with a success rate of only 50% at 1 year. To improve efficacy of IDT, it has become important to consider polyanalgesia. The aim of polyanalgesia is to prolong analgesic duration, enhance or optimize analgesic efficacy (e.g. analgesic synergy), diminish or minimize adverse effects, reduce opioid tolerance/opioid-induced hyperalgesia (OIH) and to combat dependency issues/addiction potential/craving sensations. The 2007 polyanalgesic algorithm (Figure 20.2) is a

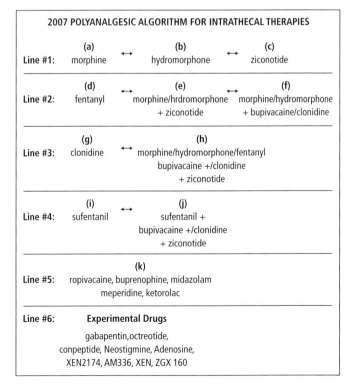

Figure 20.2 2007 Polyanalgesic consensus algorithm. Reproduced with permission from [22].

useful tool to guide physicians in choosing various drug admixtures [22].

Morphine is the gold standard for IDT therapy. Morphine and ziconotide are the two drugs approved by the FDA for the IDT management of pain. Morphine is the only opioid analgesic drug that is approved by the FDA for long-term IDT administration. The use of other drugs such as hydromorphone, bupivacaine, clonidine, fentanyl, sufentanil, midazolam, buprenorphine, meperidine and ketorolac are considered off label. Experimental drugs in the pipeline include gabapentin, octreotide, conopeptide, neostigmine and adenosine.

Cost effectiveness

IDT has proven to be cost effective over time. IDT becomes cost effective, when compared with conventional medical treatment, within 2–2.5 years [26,27].

Conclusions

In summary, there is good support that SCS is effective in appropriately selected patients with chronic pain caused by FBSS and refractory angina. There is initial support that SCS is also helpful in patients with CRPS Type 1. To get the maximum benefit and improve function, SCS should be started within the first year of onset of pain, and in younger patients with stage I disease.

In patients with chronic non-cancer pain who have failed maximal conventional treatments, it may be reasonable to consider a trial of intrathecal drug therapy. The evidence for implantable IDT is strong for short-term improvement in pain of malignancy or neuropathic pain. The evidence is moderate for long-term management of persistent pain. Reasonably strong evidence exists for use of IDT in alleviation of cancer pain; however, the evidence supporting long-term efficacy in persistant non-cancer pain is less convincing. Further research into long-term IDT for persistent non-cancer pain is necessary, especially with respect to new drugs or combination of drugs to treat specific etiologies of pain.

References

1 Hornberger J, Kumar K, Verhulst E et al. (2008) Rechargeable spinal cord stimulation versus non-rechargeable system for patients with failed back surgery syndrome: a cost–consequence analysis. Clin J Pain 24:244–52.

2 Chandler MJ, Brenman TJ, Garrison DW et al. (1993) Mechanism of cardiac pain suppression by spinal cord stimulation: indications for patients with angina pectoris. Eur Heart J 14: 96–105.

3 Dubuisson D. (1989) Effect of dorsal column stimulation on gelatinosa and marginal neurons of cat spinal cord. J Neurosurg 70:257–65.

4 Roberts MH, Rees H. (1994) Physiological basis of spinal cord stimulation. Pain Review 1:184–98.

5 Linderoth B, Meyerson B. (2002) Spinal cord stimulation; mechanism of action. In: Burchiel K, ed. Surgical Management of Pain. Thieme, New York. pp. 505–26.

6 Linderoth B, Foreman RD, Meyerson BA. (2009) Mechanisms of spinal cord stimulation in neuropathic and ischemic pain syndromes. In: Krames E, Peckham PH, Rezai A, eds. Neuromodulation. Academic Press/Elsevier, London. pp. 345–54.

7 Kumar K, Taylor RS, Jacques L et al. (2008) The effects of spinal cord stimulation in neuropathic pain are sustained: a 24-month follow-up of the prospective randomized controlled multicenter trial of the effectiveness of spinal cord stimulation. Neurosurgery 63:762–70.

8 North RB, Kidd DH, Farrokhi F et al. (2005) Spinal cord stimulation versus repeated lumbosacral spine surgery for chronic pain: a randomized, controlled trial. Neurosurgery 56:98–106.

9 Kemler MA, De Vet HCW, Barendse GAM et al. (2008) Effect of spinal cord stimulation for chronic complex regional pain syndrome Type I: five-year final follow-up of patients in a randomized controlled trial. J Neurosurgery 108:292–8.

10 Kemler MA, Furnee CA. (2002) Economic evaluation of spinal cord stimulation for chronic reflex sympathetic dystrophy. Neurology 59(8): 1203–9.

11 Mannheimer C, Augustinsoson LE, Carlsson CA *et al.* (1988) Epidural spinal cord electrical stimulation in severe angina pectoris. *Br Heart J* **59**:56–61.

12 Sanderson JE, Brooksby P, Waterhouse D *et al.* (1992) Epidural spinal electrical stimulation for severe angina: a study of its effect on symptoms, exercise tolerance and degree or ischemia. *Eur Heart J* **15**:810–14.

13 Taylor RS, De Vries J, Buchser E *et al.* (2009) Spinal cord stimulation in the treatment of refractory angina: systematic review and meta-analysis of randomised controlled trials. *BMC Cardiovasc Disord* **9**:13.

14 Anderson C, Hole P, Oxhoj H. (1994) Does pain relief with spinal cord stimulation for angina conceal myocardial infarction? *Br Heart J* **71**:419–21.

15 Cameron T. (2004) Safety and efficacy of spinal cord stimulation for the treatment of chronic pain: a 20-year literature review. *J Neurosurg Spine* **100(3)**:254–67.

16 Klomp HM, Spincemaille GH, Steyerberg EW. (1999) Spinal-cord stimulation in critical limb ischemia: a randomized trial. *Lancet* **353**:1040–4.

17 Kumar K, Toth C, Nath RK *et al.* (1997) Improvement of limb circulation in peripheral vascular disease using epidural spinal cord stimulation: a prospective study. *J Neurosurg* **86(4)**:662–9.

18 Kumar K, Lind G, Winter J *et al.* (2009) Spinal cord stimulation: placement of surgical leads via laminotomy-techniques and benefits. In: Krames ES, Peckham PH, Rezai AR, eds. *Neuromodulation*, Vol. II. Elsevier, New York. pp. 1005–12.

19 Weiner RL, Alo' KM (2009) Occipital neurostimulation for treatment of intractable headache syndromes. In: Krames ES, Peckham PH, Rezai AR, eds. *Neuromodulation*. Elsevier, London. pp. 409–16.

20 Al-Kaisy AA, Khan KR. (2009) Sacral nerve root stimulation for painful bladder syndrome/interstitial cystitis. In: Krames ES, Peckham PH, Rezai AR, eds. *Neuromodulation*. Elsevier, London. pp. 931–44.

21 Amar AP. (2007) Vagus nerve stimulation for the treatment of intractable epilepsy. *Expert Rev Neurother* **7(12)**:1763–73.

22 Deer T, Krames ES, Hassenbusch SJ *et al.* (2007) Polyanalgesic Consensus Conference 2007. Recommendations for management of pain by intrathecal (intraspinal) drug delivery: report of an interdisciplinary expert panel. *Neuromodulation* **10**:300–28.

23 Deer T, Chapple I, Classen A *et al.* (2004) Intrathecal drug delivery for treatment of chronic low back pain: report from the national outcomes registry for low back pain. *Pain Med* **5(1)**:6–13.

24 Fluckiger B, Knecht H, Grossmann S *et al.* (2008) Device-related complications of long-term intrathecal drug therapy via implanted pumps. *Spinal Cord* **46**:639–43.

25 Naumann C, Erdine S, Koulousakis A *et al.* (1999) Drug adverse events and system complications of intrathecal opioid delivery for pain: origins, detection, manifestations, and management. *Neuromodulation* **2(2)**:92–107.

26 Kumar K, Hunter G, Demeria D. (2004) Treatment of chronic pain by using intrathecal drug therapy compared with conventional pain therapies: a cost-effectiveness analysis. *J Neurosurg* **97**:803–10.

27 De Lissovoy G. Brown R, Halpern M *et al.* (1997) Cost-effectiveness of long-term intrathecal morphine therapy for pain associated with failed back surgery syndrome. *Clin Ther* **19(1)**:96–112.

28 Kumar K, Malik S, Demeria D. (2002) Treatment of chronic pain with spinal cord stimulation versus alternative therapies: cost-effectiveness analysis. *Neurosurgery* **51**:106–16.

29 North RB, Kidd D, Shipley J *et al.* (2007) Spinal cord stimulation versus reoperation for failed back surgery syndrome: a cost effectiveness and cost utility analysis based on a randomized, controlled trial. *Neurosurgery* **61**:361–8.

30 Kumar K, Taylor RS, Jacques L *et al.* (2007) Spinal cord stimulation versus conventional medical management for neuropathic pain: a multicentre randomised controlled trial in patients with failed back surgery syndrome. *Pain* **132**:179–88.

Chapter 21

Neurosurgical management of pain

Diaa Bahgat, Ashwin Viswanathan & Kim J. Burchiel

Department of Neurological Surgery, Oregon Health & Science University, Portland, USA

Introduction

Pain is the most common reason for patients to seek the care of a neurosurgeon. Neurosurgical interventions for the management of pain can broadly be categorized as anatomic, neuromodulatory and neuroablative. Anatomic procedures for the treatment of pain seek to correct structural abnormalities leading to pain, as in the case of spondylolysis with spondylolisthesis or in entrapment neuropathies. Neuromodulatory procedures include both drug infusion therapies and neurostimulation procedures such as peripheral nerve stimulation, spinal cord stimulation, motor cortex stimulation and deep brain stimulation. In contrast, neuroablative procedures seek to interrupt the pathways of pain transmission and may be directed towards the peripheral nerve, root entry zone, spinal cord or brain. To the degree that evidence to support the particular procedure can be classified, it will be listed according to contemporary standards. In general, Class I evidence derives from randomized controlled trials, Class II from well-constructed prospective cohort trials, or in some cases high-quality meta-analysis, and Class

III evidence pertains to case series, case reports or expert opinion.

Anatomic

Most patients who consult neurosurgeons do so to understand the etiology of, and to relieve, a pain problem. In the subset of patients in whom an anatomic etiology for the pain can be identified, neurosurgical intervention may prove an effective intervention.

Spinal disorders

The most common pain problems neurosurgeons deal with are related to the spine. A full discussion of indications and surgical strategies for spinal surgery are beyond the scope of this chapter. In general, radicular pain is tractable to neurosurgical intervention, while axial pain in the absence of a structural abnormality is more difficult to treat and outcome from surgery uncertain. Indications for spinal surgery include the relatively straightforward removal of a herniated disk producing a clearcut radicular syndrome, to stabilization of spondylolisthesis associated with spondylolysis. Our understanding of the indications for spinal fusion in the setting of degenerative disease of the cervical and lumbar spine are still developing; recent reviews seek to clarify patient selection and outcomes [1,2].

Clinical Pain Management: A Practical Guide, 1st edition.
Edited by Mary E. Lynch, Kenneth D. Craig and Philip W.H. Peng.
© 2011 Blackwell Publishing Ltd.

Trigeminal neuralgia

In selected cases of trigeminal neuralgia (TN) surgery is indicated (for clinical presentation see Chapter 30) [3]. Before considering surgical therapy for patients with TN, patients must have had an adequate trial of one or more oral medications such as carbamazepine, oxcarbazepine or a gabapentinoid and have become either intolerant of, or refractory to, the medications. Microvascular decompression is a surgical option that can lead to long-term pain relief. This surgical therapy addresses what is thought to be the anatomic correlate of TN – arterial compression of the root entry zone (REZ) of the trigeminal nerve. High resolution magnetic resonance imaging aimed at delineating the arterial and neural anatomy can demonstrate compression at the REZ. Microvascular decompression is associated with a 0.2% mortality and<5% morbidity, which includes hearing loss in 1%, cerebrospinal fluid leakage in 2–3% and rare (<1%) cranial nerve deficits. Use of microvascular decompression for TN is supported by Class III evidence, but no Class I–II studies have been completed.

Entrapment neuropathies

A number of peripheral nerve compression syndromes exist that can be improved through surgical decompression. The most common entrapment neuropathy is compression of the median nerve by the transverse carpal ligament at the wrist (carpal tunnel syndrome). Patients may present with diffuse aching of the arm and forearm, associated with numbness and weakness of the hands. Symptoms are typically worse at night. Physical examination may reveal weakness of thumb abduction or opposition and provocative tests such as tapping the median nerve over wrist may induce paresthesias. In a recent updated Cochrane review it was found that surgery for carpal tunnel syndrome relieved symptoms significantly better than splinting. The author concluded that further research is needed in order to determine whether this applies to people with mild symptoms and whether surgical treatment is better than steroid injections [4].

Neuromodulatory

Deep brain stimulation

The mechanism of pain relief from deep brain stimulation (DBS) is hypothesized to involve activation of descending inhibitory pain pathways. Two targets for neurostimulation have been proposed: the thalamic ventralis caudalis (Vc) nucleus and the periaqueductal gray/periventricular gray matter. DBS should only be considered for patients in whom all other treatment modalities have not shown adequate improvement. Symptoms should have been present for more than 6 months, and the patient should have been evaluated by a multidisciplinary pain center first [5].

A frame-based stereotactic approach is generally used in placing DBS electrodes. Following implantation, patients undergo an externalized trial period of 3–7 days. During this time, patients maintain a pain diary and various stimulation parameters are used. If a patient has a successful stimulation trial, they undergo implantation of the generator. If the trial is unsuccessful, the electrodes are then removed. Surgical complications associated with DBS include infection (5%), stroke (3%), asymptomatic intracerebral bleeding (4%) and other hardware related complications (7%).

Only case series, and case reports (Class III) support the use of DBS for chronic pain. Chronic pain conditions that have been treated with DBS include failed back syndrome, cancer pain, anesthesia dolorosa, stroke pain, thalamic syndromes and others. Published series report better long-term outcomes for nociceptive pain than for neuropathic pain [6].

Motor cortex stimulation

Motor cortex stimulation (MCS) was introduced as a treatment modality for central deafferentation pain in the early 1990s. Investigators noted that stimulation of the motor cortex led to inhibition of thalamic hyperactivity associated with deafferentation. Epidural electrodes for MCS may be placed through either burr holes or craniotomy. The surgical target can be adjusted based upon the

171

location of the pain. Placement of the epidural electrodes is typically followed by a 5–10 day trial period. Patients who have a successful trial are then implanted with a generator [7].

Case series evidence (Class III) indicates that MCS *may* provide benefit for patients with neuropathic pain. In contrast, there is no evidence to support the use of MCS in patients with nociceptive pain. MCS has been applied to various neuropathic pain syndromes including facial pain, central pain secondary to stroke and peripheral deafferentation pain including phantom limb pain. Overall, approximately 40–70% of appropriately selected patients may have a successful trial period of MCS, warranting implantation of a generator. Patients with TN pain form a subgroup of patients in whom generally positive results have been reported. Despite these promising initial results, MCS is still a treatment modality in development. Given our current understanding, the best candidates for MCS are patients with unilateral neuropathic facial pain that has been resistant to best multidisciplinary medical management.

Spinal cord stimulation

Spinal cord stimulation (SCS) was first used as treatment modality for cancer pain in the 1960s. The surgical technique evolved from subdural electrode placement, to intradural placement to epidural placement today. A more detailed discussion of SCS is presented in Chapter 20.

Other neuromodulatory interventions

As with SCS, intrathecal opiates have significantly expanded the treatment options available to the pain management physician. This therapy is discussed further in Chapter 20. Intracerebroventricular opioids have been shown to be an effective intervention in patients with malignant pain unresponsive to other therapies. This route of administration may be particularly useful in patients with malignancy involving the head and neck, or in whom respiratory depression may be a risk with high spinal administration. The surgical technique involves implantation of a ventricular catheter into the lateral ventricle for delivery of opiates near target receptors around the aqueductal wall of the midbrain [8]. Side effects from intraventricular administration of opioids can include somnolence, nausea and respiratory depression.

Neuroablation

The increased use of SCS and intrathecal drug delivery has led to a decrease in the use of neuroablative procedures to manage pain. A recent systematic review identified that destructive techniques for the treatment of pain have had a long and important history with 146 studies examining the use of neuroablative procedures in non-cancer pain [9]. This review found the majority of studies constituted Class III evidence with the majority of Level I and II studies focused on radiofrequency rhizotomies (Table 21.1). Further research is needed, but in the meantime this review identifies that there is a wealth of experience to date and for the appropriately selected patient with pain unresponsive to other interventions, neuroablative procedures can serve as an invaluable therapy (Table 21.2).

Neuroablative lesions can be created mechanically by surgical scalpel, chemically, thermally by radiofrequency lesioning and through radiation

Table 21.1 Number of studies by class of evidence assessing ablative procedures for non-malignant pain.

Procedure	Class I	Class II	Class III
Cingulotomy	0	0	13
Cordotomy	0	0	11
DREZ lesioning	0	0	26
Ganglionectomy	2	0	15
Mesencephalotomy	0	0	9
Myelotomy	0	0	3
Rhizotomy for:			
trigeminal neuralgia	0	2	18
lumbar facet syndrome	4	1	9
discogenic back pain	1	0	0
cervical pain	4	1	4
cluster headache	0	0	3
Thalamotomy	0	0	12

DREZ, dorsal root entry zone.

Table 21.2 Ablative procedures, appropriate clinical application and pitfall application.

Ablative procedure	Clinical application	Pitfall application
Neurectomy	Stump or traumatic neuroma Meralgia paresthetica Post-herniorrhaphy pain	Phantom limb pain Post-herpetic neuralgia
Dorsal rhizotomy and dorsal root ganglionectomy	Chest wall pain Post-thoracotomy syndrome Occipital neuralgia	Lumbar radiculopathy Low back pain Post-herpetic neuralgia
Sympathectomy	Causalgia* Reflex sympathetic dystrophy* Abdominal cancer pain	Non-sympathetically mediated pain

Trigeminal system procedures:
  radiofrequency
  balloon compression
  glycerol rhizolysis
	Classic trigeminal neuralgia
	Facial pain due to multiple sclerosis
		Neuropathic trigeminal
		  pain

DREZ	Nerve root avulsion (brachial plexus injury) Local segmental pain after spinal cord injury Localized cancer pain	Post-herpetic neuralgia Facial pain

Cordotomy	Unilateral cancer pain below C5
	Paroxysmal neuropathic pain after
	  traumatic spinal cord injury
		Caution with midline
		  and central pain

Myelotomy	Pelvic and sacral cancer pain Midline cancer pain	
Mesencephalotomy	Head and neck cancer pain Central, post stroke pain	Facial pain
Thalamotomy	Cancer pain Central pain	Deafferentation pain
Cingulotomy	Diffuse cancer pain Failed back syndrome Best in patients with depressive symptoms	

DREZ, dorsal root entry zone.
* Based on limited evidence.

therapy. Figures 21.1 and 21.2 illustrate spinal and cerebral neuroablative and neuromodulatory procedures, respectively.

Peripheral nervous system

Neurectomy

Neurectomy is the surgical sectioning of a nerve [10,11]. Application is limited because it involves sacrifice of a nerve, which may carry motor and sensory fibers. In the long-term, intact sensory neurons, which are adjacent to the denervated area, can sprout axons, leading to a smaller region

of denervation and denervation hypersensitivity. Local anesthetic blockade should always be performed diagnostically and to demonstrate the expected postoperative deficit that may be incurred from sectioning the nerve. Indications are listed in Table 21.2.

Dorsal rhizotomy and dorsal root ganglionectomy

Dorsal rhizotomy involves sectioning the dorsal nerve root. Evidence suggesting that up to one-third of axons in the ventral nerve root are derived from the dorsal root ganglion, led surgeons to

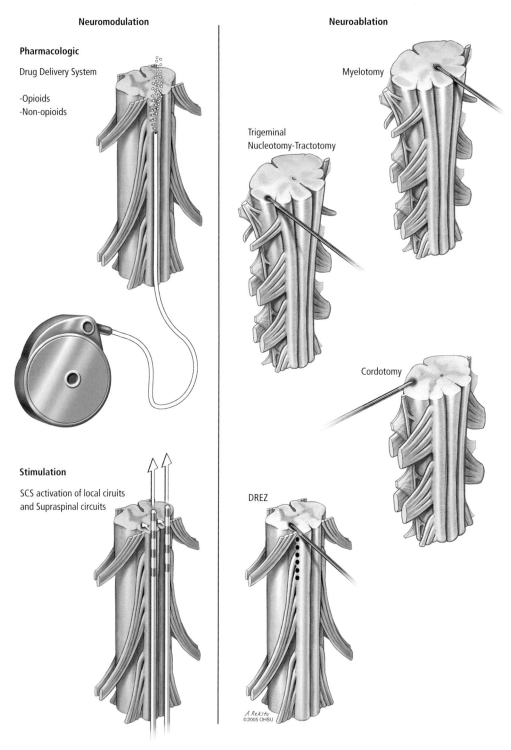

Neuromodulation

Pharmacologic

Drug Delivery System

-Opioids
-Non-opioids

Stimulation

SCS activation of local ciruits
and Supraspinal circuits

Neuroablation

Myelotomy

Trigeminal
Nucleotomy-Tractotomy

Cordotomy

DREZ

A.Rekito
©2005 OHSU

Figure 21.1 Diagrammatic representation of spinal neuromodulation and neuroablation procedures. Reproduced with permission from Raslan AM, McCartney S, Burchiel KJ. (2007) Management of chronic severe pain: spinal neuromodulatory and neuroablative approaches. In: Sakas DE, Simpson B, Krames ES, eds. *Acta Neurochir Suppl*, Springer-Verlag, pp. 33–41.

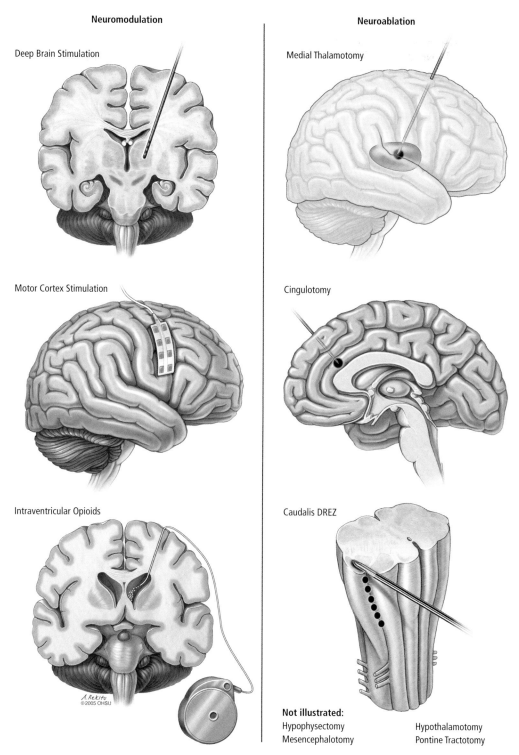

Neuromodulation

Deep Brain Stimulation

Motor Cortex Stimulation

Intraventricular Opioids

A. Rekito
© 2005 OHSU

Neuroablation

Medial Thalamotomy

Cingulotomy

Caudalis DREZ

Not illustrated:
Hypophysectomy   Hypothalamotomy
Mesencephalotomy   Pontine Tractotomy

Figure 21.2 Diagrammatic representation of cerebral neuromodulation and neuroablation procedures. Reproduced with permission from Raslan AM, McCartney S, Burchiel KJ. (2007) Management of chronic severe pain: cerebral neuromodulatory and neuroablative approaches. In: Sakas DE, Simpson B, Krames ES, eds. *Acta Neurochir Suppl*, Springer-Verlag, pp.17–26.

consider resection of the dorsal root ganglion as an alternative procedure. Both rhizotomy and ganglionectomy lead to the loss of proprioception and, consequently, the procedure is not appropriate for extremity pain. Despite these drawbacks, long-term pain relief can be achieved when treating chest wall pain, post-thoracotomy syndrome and occipital neuralgia through sectioning of the C2 ganglion [12]. Application of rhizotomy and ganglionectomy to lumbar radiculopathy, lower back pain and post-herpetic neuralgia have shown disappointing results, with fewer than 30% of patients obtaining pain relief [13].

As with neurectomy, sprouting of adjacent sensory axons can limit the long-term effectiveness of this procedure. In the long-term, patients may also develop deafferentation pain, which can lead to significant disability. Rhizotomy and ganglionectomy lead to denervation, which further limits the future use of neurostimulation.

Sympathectomy

Recent reviews have identified that treating neuropathic pain by sympathectomy is based on very limited evidence [9,14–16]. Sympathetically maintained pain and complex regional pain syndrome are presented in Chapter 35.

Spinal cord

Dorsal root entry zone lesioning

The dorsal root entry zone (DREZ) includes the central portion of the dorsal or sensory root, Lissauer's tract and the most superficial Rexed layers of the dorsal horn of the spinal cord. These areas are involved in the processing of nociceptive information. Altered peripheral input to these areas can result in hyperactivity of this region, leading to pain syndromes. By lesioning the DREZ, the area of hyperactivity can be eliminated, leading to pain relief [17].

In a recent systematic review, a total of 26 case series were included. All studies reported more than 50% relief in pain in a majority of patients and the results were durable. Patients with brachial

plexus avulsion and traumatic spinal cord injury tended to have the best response [9]. Results of DREZ lesioning for post-herpetic neuralgia or for post-amputation pain have not been favorable. For these indications, patients with paroxysmal electric shooting pain respond better than those with continuous aching pain.

Cordotomy

Cordotomy targets the lateral spinothalamic tract located in the anterolateral quadrant of the spinal cord. As the spinothalamic tract carries information regarding pain and temperature sensation from the contralateral body, the goal of cordotomy is abolishing pain sensation contralateral to and below the level of the lesion.

Lancinating, paroxysmal, neuropathic and allodynic pain secondary to cancer or spinal cord injury and lateral rather than midline pain tend to respond well to cordotomy. Treatment of continuous neuropathic pain has been less successful. The treatment of midline pain may require bilateral cordotomy, which carries a higher risk of weakness, sexual dysfunction and respiratory depression. The highest level of analgesia that can be reliably produced by cordotomy is at the C5 dermatome, thus cordotomy is not indicated for head and neck pain.

Class III evidence supports the use of cordotomy for appropriately selected patients with malignant and non-malignant pain, with best results in cancer pain. The efficacy of cordotomy, however, reduces with time, with less than 50% of patients still having pain relief after 1 year. The level of analgesia produced by cordotomy also falls with increasing time from procedure. The introduction of the percutaneous approach for cordotomy has reduced the morbidity associated with this procedure. Complications of cordotomy include sleep apnea, post cordotomy dysesthesia and mirror-image pain [18].

Myelotomy

Commissural midline myelotomy seeks to interrupt the crossing fibers of the spinothalamic tract within the anterior commissure. The effectiveness of this procedure in patients with visceral pain led to the recognition of a visceral pain pathway at the midline of the dorsal columns. Compared with other neuroablative procedures, myelotomy has the advantages of providing bilateral pain relief with a single procedure, and is effective in treating visceral pain, which is difficult to treat with other interventions [19].

Class III evidence supports the use of midline myelotomy in patients with pelvic pain related to cancer unresponsive to other interventions. Case series have demonstrated satisfactory pain relief in 60–80% of cancer patients who underwent myelotomy [20]. Surgical complications include bladder and bowel dysfunction, diminished proprioception and gait disturbances.

Brainstem

Brainstem lesioning is indicated in the treatment of pain involving the head, face and neck, carried by fibers of the trigeminal, glossopharyngeal, vagus, nervus intermedius and upper cervical nerves. Neuroablative procedures targeting the brainstem include mesencephalotomy, trigeminal tractotomy and caudalis DREZ.

Mesencephalotomy

When applied to face and head pain, mesencephalotomy targets the trigeminothalamic and reticulothalamic tracts contralateral to the patient's pain. If a patient has bilateral pain, a lesion placed contralateral to the more painful side can provide bilateral pain relief. Series of mesencephalotomy for cancer pain report 85% of patients having complete or good pain relief, and 60% with good results in the long-term. Mesencephalotomy for central post-stroke pain has not proven as efficacious with 60% of patients reporting acceptable pain relief but with poor long-term benefit. Other indications, including facial pain, have not shown promising results.

Complications associated with mesencephalotomy include changes in ocular motility, which are usually mild and asymptomatic. Use of a stereotac-

tic approach to mesencephalotomy has reduced the incidence of dysesthesia to less than 15%; an open technique has been associated with a 50% or greater risk of postoperative dysesthesias [21].

Intracranial

The introduction of stereotaxis and the ability to target deep brain structures has led to the development of several intracranial targets for pain management. Ablative procedures for the management of pain have been directed towards the thalamus, pulvinar, pituitary, cinglate gyrus and the precentral and postcentral gyrus [5]. However, the exact mechanisms through which these procedures relieve pain are not fully understood. The limited number of patients who have undergone these procedures and few published series make treatment recommendations difficult.

Thalamotomy

Because of the wide involvement of thalamic nuclei in pain processing, the thalamus has been a target of interest for both neuroablative and neurostimulative procedures for pain management. The main sensory nucleus, Vc nucleus, was the first target for neuroablation. However, targeting of the Vc nucleus was associated with the development of significant deafferentation pain. The medial thalamus including the centralis lateralis, centrum medianum and parafascicularis have become the more common target for thalamotomy. Medial thalamotomy is thought to influence pain transmission through the non-specific spinoreticulothalamic tract.

Outcome after thalamotomy is difficult to ascertain because of the lack of controlled studies. Although thalamotomy is thought to be more effective in the treatment of nociceptive, rather than neuropathic pain, it has been applied to a variety of pain syndromes including cancer pain, central and peripheral deafferentation pain, spinal cord injury pain and arthritis [22]. Medial thalamotomy has been shown to provide good short-term pain relief in more than 50% of patients, but the long-term success rate is only 30%.

Consequently, thalamotomy is most appropriate for the treatment of cancer pain in selected patients with a short life expectancy.

Cingulotomy

The goal of cingulotomy is to disrupt the anterior cingulate gyrus, usually bilaterally. Cingulotomy is thought to alter the patient's emotional reaction to pain through interruption of the Papez circuit of the limbic system. The major indication for cingulotomy is in the terminally ill cancer patient with widely metastatic disease, whose pain has not responded to other therapeutic modalities. Success rates of up to 68% have been reported but efficacy decreases with time, reaching 50% by 6-month follow-up. Cingulotomy has also been applied to non-malignant chronic pain, with failed back syndrome being the dominant indication. In a series of 18 patients with a median follow-up of 6 years, 72% of patients reported useful pain relief, with 70% patients having improved social function and 25% of patients returning to work. Postoperative seizures can occur and should be managed medically with antiepileptic medicines [23].

Conclusions

Neurosurgical techniques for the management of pain include a wide array of interventions. Correction of an anatomic abnormality where clearly identified in spinal pain is reasonable to consider in appropriately selected patients. Neuromodulation is a rapidly developing field and is discussed in more detail in Chapter 20. For some procedures, including DBS and MCS, the indications are still being developed, and further studies are necessary to determine the most appropriate candidates for these therapies. With regards to neuroablative techniques there is a long history with significant clinical experience but most support for ablative procedures in chronic non-cancer pain is based on Class III evidence. Further research is needed. In the meantime this chapter provides guidance into situations where an ablative procedure may be considered.

References

1 Mummaneni PV, Kaiser MG, Matz PG *et al.* (2009) Cervical Surgical techniques for the treatment of cervical spondylotic myelopathy. *J Neurosurg: Spine* **11**(**2**):130–41.

2 Gibson JN, Waddell G (2005) Surgery for degenerative lumbar spondylosis. *Cochrane Database Syst Rev* **4**:CD001352.

3 Miller JP, Acar F, Burchiel KJ. (2009) Classification of trigeminal neuralgia: clinical, therapeutic, and prognostic implications in a series of 144 patients undergoing microvascular decompression. *J Neurosurg* **111**(**6**):1231–4.

4 Verdugo RJ, Salinas RA, Castillo JL *et al.* (2008) Surgical versus non-surgical treatment for carpal tunnel syndrome. *Cochrane Database Syst Rev* **4**:CD001552.

5 Raslan AM, McCartney S, Burchiel KJ. (2007) Management of chronic severe pain: cerebral neuromodulatory and neuroablative approaches. *Acta Neurochir Suppl* **97**(**Part 2**):17–26.

6 Whitworth L, Fernandez J, Feler C. (2005) Deep brain stimulation for chronic pain. In: Fisher W, Burchiel KJ, eds. *Seminars in Neurosurgery Pain Management for the Neurosurgeon*. Thieme, New York. pp. 183–93.

7 Fontaine D, Hamani C, Lozano A. (2009) Efficacy and safety of motor cortex stimulation for chronic neuropathic pain: critical review of the literature. *J Neurosurg* **110**(**2**):251–6.

8 Lazorthes YR, Sallerin BA, Verdie JC. (1995) Intracerebroventricular administration of morphine for control of irreducible cancer pain. *Neurosurgery* **37**(**3**):422–8.

9 Cetas JS, Saedi T, Burchiel KJ. (2008) Destructive procedures for the treatment of nonmalignant pain: a structured literature review. *J Neurosurg* **109**(**3**):389–404.

10 Burchiel KJ, Johans TJ, Ochoa J. (1993) The surgical treatment of painful traumatic neuromas. *J Neurosurg* **78**(**5**):714–9.

11 Williams PH, Trzil KP. (1991) Management of meralgia paresthetica. *J Neurosurg* **74**(**1**):76–80.

12 Acar F, Miller J, Golshani KJ *et al.* (2008) Pain relief after cervical ganglionectomy (C2 and

C3) for the treatment of medically intractable occipital neuralgia. *Stereotact Funct Neurosurg* **86(2)**:106–12.

13 North RB, Kidd DH, Campbell JN *et al.* (1991) Dorsal root ganglionectomy for failed back surgery syndrome: a 5-year follow-up study. *J Neurosurg* **74(2)**:236–42.

14 Mailis A, Furlan A. (2003) Sympathectomy for neuropathic pain. *Cochrane Database Syst Rev* **2**:CD002918.

15 Sweet W. (1990) Sympathectomy for pain. In: Youmans J, ed. *Youmans Neurological Surgery*, 3rd edn. W.B. Saunders, Philadelphia, PA. pp. 4086–107;

16 Furlan AD, Mailis A, Papagapiou M. (2000) Are we paying a high price for surgical sympathectomy? A systematic literature review of late complications. *J Pain* **1(4)**:245–57.

17 Sindou MP, Blondet E, Emery E *et al.* (2005) Microsurgical lesioning in the dorsal root entry zone for pain due to brachial plexus avulsion: a prospective series of 55 patients. *J Neurosurg* **102(6)**:1018–28.

18 Kanpolat Y, Ugur HC, Ayten M *et al.* (2009) Computed tomography-guided percutaneous cordotomy for intractable pain in malignancy. *Neurosurgery* **64(3 Suppl)**:187–93.

19 Nauta HJ, Soukup VM, Fabian RH *et al.* (2000) Punctate midline myelotomy for the relief of visceral cancer pain. *J Neurosurg* **92(2 Suppl)**: 125–30.

20 Nauta H, Westlund K, Willis W. (2002) Midline myelotomy. In: Burchiel KJ, ed. *Surgical Management of Pain*. Thieme Medical, New York. pp. 714–31.

21 Shieff C, Nashold BS Jr. (1990) Stereotactic mesencephalotomy. *Neurosurg Clin North Am* **1(4)**:825–39.

22 Gybels J, Kupers R, Nuttin B. (1993) Therapeutic stereotactic procedures on the thalamus for pain. *Acta Neurochir (Wien)* **124(1)**:19–22.

23 Wilkinson HA, Davidson KM, Davidson RI. (1999) Bilateral anterior cingulotomy for chronic noncancer pain. *Neurosurgery* **45(5)**: 1129–34.

Acknowledgment

We thank Shirley McCartney, PhD, for editorial assistance.

Part 6

Physical Therapy and Rehabilitation

Chapter 22

Physical therapy and rehabilitation

Maureen J. Simmonds[1] & Timothy Wideman[2]

[1] School of Physical and Occupational Therapy, McGill UniversityMontreal, Canada
[2] Department of Psychology, McGill University, Montreal, Canada

Chronic pain and rehabilitation

Pain and the impact of pain are complex multidimensional problems that are central to rehabilitation. Knowledge of this complexity has had a profound influence on rehabilitation approaches. The contemporary rehabilitation approach is conceptually expanded and based on the International Classification of Functioning, Disability, and Health (ICF) framework [1]. Rehabilitation is outcome oriented, biopsychosocially based, person focused and empowered, and best-evidence and activity driven. This approach also recognizes that the therapist, and the therapeutic relationship, have important non-specific effects on outcome. Indeed, in some instances, the quality of the therapeutic relationship may be the single most important factor for improving function, promoting well-being and enabling self-management of chronic pain.

The ICF model recognizes that disablement and pain are influenced by sets of variables such as predisposing risk factors, intra-individual factors (e.g. lifestyle), psychosocial attributes (e.g. anxieties and coping skills) and extra-individual physical and social factors that can affect the presence or severity of disability (Figure 22.1). For example, a similar back injury (pathology) can be a minor inconvenience for someone with good coping skills in a flexible relatively sedentary work environment (minimal disability). The same type of injury can lead to a downward spiral of distress and disability in an individual who is very anxious about the injury, tends towards catastrophic thinking and who has a heavy manual occupation with few employment options (major disability).

The model also addresses the bidirectional "causal" links between pathological processes (e.g. osteoarthrosis) and pathological consequences (e.g. disability). For example, joint stiffness and muscle weakness were long thought to be disease expressions of osteoarthritis – the condition. Obesity was thought to be a predictor of osteoarthritis or at least a comorbid problem. It is now known that these problems are consequences of the inactivity which is secondary to arthritis rather than part of the disease process per se [2]. Inactivity may also be due to inadequately managed pain and inaccurate beliefs about the harmful effects of exercise on arthritic joints. Research has shown that judicious exercise and activity is not harmful to joints and conversely promotes health and wellness of the person with the arthritic joints [3,4].

Clinical Pain Management: A Practical Guide, 1st edition.
Edited by Mary E. Lynch, Kenneth D. Craig and
Philip W.H. Peng.
© 2011 Blackwell Publishing Ltd.

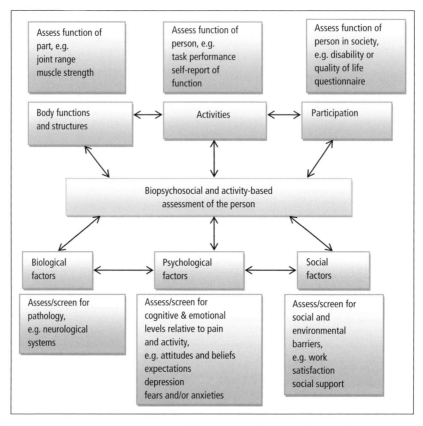

Figure 22.1 An example of assessment test areas applied to the International Classification of Functioning, Disability, and Health (ICF) and biopsychosocial activity-based model of rehabilitation.

Clinical assessment

Successful rehabilitation is based on a sound understanding of the person with pain, their beliefs, their physical abilities, their expectations and their environment. This information must be explicitly obtained through questions, questionnaires and tests of physical function. This knowledge provides the therapist with an understanding of what modifiable factors (physical, psychological or social) should be targeted in order to positively impact function and social participation.

Patient self-reports

A plethora of standardized self-report assessment measures are used in clinical settings to measure pain, pain beliefs, disability and quality of life. The measures range from simple one-dimensional or global questionnaires that are specific and take a few seconds or minutes to complete, to complex multidimensional questionnaires that can sample a wide range of activities, thoughts and interference with social roles, and which are useful for patients with a range of conditions (Chapter 10). Measures in common use include the Brief Pain Inventory (BPI) [5] and Brief Fatigue Inventory (BFI) [6]. These measures assess the magnitude of a symptom and also how much that symptom interferes with activity. Unfortunately, activity interference questions are very general and are not judged against a standard criterion. For example, using the BPI, patients may report that pain interferes with walking, and they may score this as a "5" on a 0–10 scale. However, this "5" does not differentiate between the walking ability of patients who can walk between the bed and bathroom, who walk minimally in the community or those who take long walks for pleasure. Self-reports of function are also often inaccurate because individuals are inaccurate in their estimates of time and distance [7] and use idiosyncratic criteria to make judgments on their compromised functional ability or perceived difficulties. Thus, there is a need for self-report to be complemented by physical tests of function.

Physical performance tests

In contrast, physical performance measures use standard criteria (time and/or distance) and measure rather than judge performance ability. Simple quick measures of performance complement self-reports of function and provide a more comprehensive understanding of the patient, their movement abilities and difficulties, thereby guiding treatment decisions [8,9].

Table 22.1 presents examples of performance test batteries that are simple for the therapist to administer and interpret and for the patient to do. The tests have strong psychometric properties and have been evaluated in individuals with different conditions. Clinicians and researchers can use the whole battery or select specific tasks based on the patient's movement problems. The tasks are basic activities (or components of activities) that are done many times throughout the day. Thus, it is relatively easy to determine the impact (i.e. burden of the health-related condition) on the patient.

Treatment approaches

In treating individuals with acute pain, therapists usually focus on facilitating tissue healing. As healing progresses, pain is expected to resolve and the emphasis of treatment shifts toward improving function. However, in treating individuals with chronic pain, this treatment approach can prove problematic. In these cases, the original injury has typically healed, but pain persists. As a result, therapists are faced with the dilemma of

how to improve function, despite elevated levels of pain.

To overcome this challenge, unique goals and therapeutic approaches must be developed and therapy approached from a biopsychosocial perspective in which the development of constructive coping strategies, disability reduction and increased social engagement are the principal goals of treatment [10,11]. Numerous factors influence chronic pain and chronic pain outcomes and thus no single intervention will resolve the suffering and disability associated with chronic pain [10]. Treatment should focus on integrating key principles into the treatment for the individual. Guiding therapeutic principles include aiming for long-term changes in beliefs and behaviors; focusing on increasing activity; limiting passive interventions; promoting education and self-management; and facilitating social support from peers and employers [10,11].

Reassurance, activity-encouragement and education

Advice and education about chronic pain are essential components of effective treatment. These messages should aim to demystify and demedicalize the patient's condition, dissociate pain from tissue damage, encourage participation in physical activity and explain the biological mechanisms underlying chronic pain [12,13]. In addition, research suggests that reassurance, activity-encouragement and education are effective in reducing the risk for disability, decreasing sick leave, increasing return to work and improving function [13]. The means of educational information includes information booklets, one-to-one sessions, group classes and online forums.

Reassurance is an effective method for helping patients with chronic pain overcome some of the distress associated with their condition and sets the stage for increasing physical activity. The key messages communicated through reassurance interventions are that hurt does not equal harm, that the pain condition is not life-threatening or permanently disabling, and that it is safe to engage in physical activity [14]. Care must be taken to

Table 22.1 Performance batteries (Simmonds *et al.* 1998; Simmonds 2002).

Condition	Task	Procedure	Measure
Back pain	Repeated sit-to-stand	Subjects rise to standing and return to sitting as quickly as possible five times. After a brief pause the task is repeated	The average of the two task times is recorded
	Repeated trunk flexion	The subject is timed as they bend forward to the limit of their range and return to the upright position as fast as tolerated five times. After a brief pause the task is repeated	The average of the two task times is recorded
	Loaded reach	Subjects stand next to a wall on which a meter rule is mounted horizontally at shoulder height. They hold a weight that is 5% of their body weight (up to maximum of 5 kg) at shoulder height and close to the body and then reach forward	Maximum distance reached in centimeter is recorded
	50-foot walk	Subjects walk 25 feet, turn around and walk back to start as fast as they can	Time taken is recorded
	Five-minute walk	Subjects walk as far and as fast as they can for 5 minutes	Distance walked is recorded
	360° rollover	Subjects lie supine on a treatment bed. They roll over 360° as fast as they can. After a brief pause, they roll 360° in the opposite direction	The time to complete a rollover in both directions is summed and recorded
Cancers and HIV/AIDS	Coin test	Subjects sit at a table. They are timed as they pick up four coins and place them in a cup. (They are required to pick up each coin individually)	Time taken is recorded
	Belt tie	Subjects sit in a standard chair. They are timed as they wrap a bandage (approximately 4 feet long) around their waists and tie it in front of them	Time taken is recorded
	Sock test	Subjects sit in a standard chair. They are timed as they put on one loose-fitting sock	Time taken is recorded
	Repeated sit-to-stand	Subjects rise to standing and return to sitting as quickly as possible twice. After a brief pause the task is repeated	The average of the two task times is recorded
	Repeated reach-up	Subjects stand facing a wall and reach up as high as they can with both hands. A mark is placed on the wall at the reach distance. Subjects then reach up and return their hands to their sides three times, as fast as they can. After a brief pause the task is repeated	The average of the two task times is recorded
	Forward reach	Subjects stand sideways next to a wall on which a meter rule is mounted horizontally at shoulder height. They then reach forward as far as they can	Maximum distance reached in centimeter is recorded
	Pen pick up from floor	Subjects stand and a pen is placed on the floor directly in front of the subject's feet. They are timed as they bend down and pick up the pen as fast as they can	Time taken is recorded
	50-foot walk	Subjects walk 25 feet, turn around and walk back to start as fast as they can	Time taken is recorded
	Six-minute walk	Subjects walk as far and as fast as they can for 6 minutes. (They are allowed to sit and rest if and as necessary during the 6-minute period)	Distance walked is recorded

avoid patients interpreting reassurance as dismissive or patronizing [15].

Activity encouragement is arguably the most important step in reducing disability. Early on the therapist should explicitly address patients' beliefs and expectations and discuss how they relate to increasing physical activity. This discussion will require additional patience and persistence for patients who have strong convictions that pain signifies tissue damage, that pain reduction is a prerequisite to re-engaging in normal activities or that passive interventions are required for pain reduction. Most patients require support in shifting their focus from searching for a diagnosis and cure to returning to their normal activities despite persistent pain. Patient resources such as the Back Book can facilitate this process [16]. However, the therapist should resist the expectation that one conversation or an information booklet will resolve this transition [17]. Encouraging activity and reassuring the patient are strategies that should permeate the therapeutic process. Therapists should also be mindful of their personal beliefs and biases and how these influence the therapeutic relationship. Therapists with elevated fear-avoidance beliefs tend to recommend passive coping strategies and rest for pain reduction [18]. Recognition of personal pain-related beliefs can help ensure that messages delivered to patients are consistent with evidence-based practice.

Brief educational interventions are commonly incorporated into therapy but their content and effectiveness varies. Traditional patient education interventions focus on the musculoskeletal anatomy and biomechanics of the "damaged" tissue (e.g. information provided in "back schools"). More recently, educational interventions have shifted their focus to psychosocial factors that influence disability and the mechanisms of chronic pain neurophysiology [17]. Growing evidence suggests that the latter interventions are significantly more effective in improving clinical outcomes [12,14]. Therapists must consider how patients perceive the explanation of their pain condition. An increased focus on the anatomy and biomechanics of the pain condition may reinforce the belief that pain results from damaged tissue, undermining the goals of increasing physical activity [12]. Effective educational interventions focus on current evidence-based explanations of pain, the factors that influence it and the importance of physical activity. Therapists should therefore present information on anatomy and biomechanics in the context of improving movement and function, rather than as an explanation of the underlying cause of pain.

Biophysical modalities

Biophysical modalities are typically passive interventions that involve the application of various forms of energy (e.g. heat, cold, electrical current, sound) to targeted tissues. Their intended therapeutic effects are varied, but commonly involve one or more of the following: pain reduction, muscle relaxation, increased soft-tissue extensibility, increased blood circulation, inflammation reduction and stimulation of tissue healing. Commonly used biophysical agents include interferential therapy, laser therapy, shortwave diathermy, therapeutic ultrasound, thermotherapy and transcutaneous electrical nerve stimulation (TENS).

Overall, there is very little support in the literature for the use of biophysical agents in the treatment of individuals with chronic pain. Several reasons account for the lack of support including, the paucity of high quality placebo-controlled clinical studies. Although some studies have shown equivocal evidence with a small or modest effect, others show no clinical effect. For these reasons, current clinical practice guidelines do not recommend the use of biophysical agents for chronic pain [10,11].

Despite the lack of support by research and some practice guidelines, biophysical modalities are still commonly used by therapists to treat chronic pain conditions. In part because patients expect such treatments and in part because clinicians believe that these interventions have at least a placebo effect with minimal risk of harm. Unfortunately, integrating these modalities into chronic pain treatments is associated with risk of harm. Passive modalities aimed at tissue-level impairments reinforce patients' beliefs that tissue damage is at the root of their pain condition and that pain reduction is a prerequisite for reducing their levels of disability. Patients that experience positive effects related to these interventions may also develop an increased dependence on therapy and therapists. It could be argued that the psychological risk of dependency on specific therapies is as potentially harmful as dependence on specific medications given that it can add to the economic costs of chronic pain and can disrupt a patient's return to work and their independent self-management. That said, there can be strong and specific justification for their limited use in clinical practice.

For example, certain patients may expect the application of a modality and be unwilling to engage in treatments that focus exclusively on self-management strategies. In such situations, therapists can introduce biophysical agents as a means for facilitating exercise. The therapist can also select modalities that can be readily integrated into home-based self-management strategies. For example, a home TENS unit or a hot pack can be a useful self-management strategy that empowers patients to self-manage their pain and increase their daily physical activity. In general, therapists should use modalities judiciously and only as part of a long-term self-management strategy that increases activity.

Spinal manual therapy

Manual therapy is a commonly used intervention in chronic pain treatments which can be associated with some beneficial short-term outcomes. In clinical settings, "manual therapy" consists of a variety of hands-on interventions. However, the definition commonly used in the literature (and in this chapter) involves either spinal manipulations (high velocity, low amplitude thrust) or spinal mobilizations (relatively low velocity movements that are limited to the joint's physiological range, e.g. Maitland technique) or a combination of the two. Most research fails to differentiate between these two types of interventions, making it difficult to distinguish their effects [19]. While the

mechanisms of manual therapy are unclear, these interventions aim to reduce pain, improve movement and restore function through spinal movements. The clinical effectiveness of manual therapy for low back pain is a controversial issue [19]. The most recent clinical practice guidelines for chronic low back pain suggest that a short course of manual therapy is better than sham or other "ineffective, control treatments" at improving short-term levels of pain and function [19]. However, manual therapy is no more or less effective than GP care with analgesics or exercise-based physical therapy. As with other passive treatments, there are risks associated with increased dependency and reinforcement of fear-avoidance beliefs. However, more specific to this intervention, spinal manipulations have been associated with negative physical side effects of varying intensity. Neck manipulations, for example, have been associated with an increased occurrence of serious consequences (e.g. vertebobasilar accidents, disc herniation, cauda equina symptoms), while roughly half of manipulations, regardless of the spinal level, typically result in up to 2 days of local discomfort, headache or fatigue[19]. Patients with chronic pain who agree to these interventions with the expectation of pain reduction may be distressed when their pain temporarily increases, and thus may be less willing to engage in active interventions. In sum, if manual therapy is considered it should be a short-term intervention that is contextualized within an activity-augmentation framework, and weighed against risks.

Physical activity

Good evidence supports participation in physical activity for chronic pain [10]. The content of activity programs can be quite diverse and include strengthening, flexibility and/or cardiovascular activities. More specific programs such as core stabilization exercises, or McKenzie exercises, are commonly used in clinical settings. While past research suggests that participation in an activity program can result in significant short and long-term reductions in pain and disability [11], it remains unclear whether the specific activity performed, or the prescribed dosage, contributes any unique variance to these positive outcomes. A recent systematic review suggests that programs that are individually designed and supervised, and that aim to improve strength and flexibility are the most effective in improving function [20]. However, the mechanism of action of such activity programs is unclear given that exercise-based interventions that lead to disability reductions do not always improve range of motion or strength [10,21]. It seems that participation in any physical activity is more important than performing specific exercises.

The greater therapeutic challenge is facilitating and maintaining participation in activity rather than establishing parameters of exercise prescription. Numerous factors influence patients' participation (e.g. pain levels, social support, time and financial resources and readiness for change), as well as the specific activity program. Previously described strategies that relate to reassurance, activity encouragement and education can help facilitate participation and adherence to activity programs, as can cognitive behavioral techniques described below. Unfortunately, therapists attempting to use the literature to navigate these complex issues are confronted with a lack of research that specifically addresses adherence to rehabilitation programs for individuals with chronic pain [22]. Indeed, as the emphasis in the literature shifts to more active self-management interventions, a deeper understanding of adherence and motivational issues will be required.

Cognitive behavioral approaches in physical therapy

Emerging research suggests that cognitive behavioral interventions delivered by therapists improve chronic pain outcomes. In the broadest sense, cognitive behavioral interventions focus on using structured techniques to change maladaptive thoughts, feelings and behaviors. Cognitive behavioral techniques are described in Chapter 24. These interventions can effectively reduce pain-related anxiety and disability, and facilitate return to work [22]. Psychologists have used these interventions

for patients with chronic pain for decades and there is compelling literature that suggests therapists can improve their treatment efficacy by using similar approaches [16,23]. Graded activity, graded exposure to feared activities and thought monitoring are three specific cognitive behavioral interventions shown to improve therapists' outcomes [16,23].

Social reintegration

Despite the need for chronic pain interventions that target social barriers to recovery, a dearth of research has addressed these issues [24]. A central goal of rehabilitation is to facilitate reintegration into preinjury social roles. Resuming life roles at home and in the workplace often involve factors that are external to the individual with chronic pain (e.g. the attitudes and level of support from employers, coworkers, family and friends). Past research has provided little guidance for therapists on avenues for intervention. Incorporating family and significant others into treatment where possible and close communication with employers regarding modified work schedules and activities are general strategies that can address these factors. However, research in this area is essential to help shape the interventions of therapists who are working independently of a multidisciplinary team.

References

1 World Health Organization. (2001) *ICF-International Classification of Functioning, Disability and Health*. World Health Organization, Geneva.

2 Jordan J, Kington R, Lane N *et al.* (2000) Systemic risk factors for osteoarthritis. In: Felson DT, conference chair. Osteoarthritis: New insights. Part 1: The disease and its risk factors. *Ann Intern Med* **133**:637–9.

3 Minor M, Kay D, eds. (1997) *Arthritis*. Human Kinetics, Champaign, IL.

4 Thomas K, Muir K, Doherty M *et al.* (2002) Home based exercise programme for knee pain

and knee osteoarthritis: randomised controlled trial. *Br Med J* **325(7367)**:752.

5 Cleeland C. (1989) Measurement of pain by subjective report. In: Chapman C, Loeser J, eds. *Issues in Pain Measurement*. Raven Press, New York. pp. 391–403.

6 Mendoza TR, Wang SX, Cleeland CS *et al.* (1999) The rapid assessment of fatigue severity in cancer patients. *Cance* **85**:1186–96.

7 Sharrack B, Hughes R. (1997) Reliability of distance estimation by doctors and patients: cross-sectional study. *Br Med J* **315**:1652–4.

8 Simmonds M. (2002) Physical function in patients with cancer: psychometric characteristics and clinical usefulness of a physical performance test battery. *J Pain Symp Manage* **24**:404–14.

9 Lee C, Simmonds M, Novy D *et al.* (2000) A comparison of self-report and clinician measured physical function among patients with low back pain. *Arch Phys Med Rehabil* **82**:227–31.

10 Airaksinen O, Brox JI, Cedraschi C *et al.* (2006) European guidelines for the management of chronic nonspecific low back pain. *Eur Spine J* **15(Suppl 2)**:S192–300.

11 Chou R, Huffman LH, American Pain Society, American College of Physicians. (2007) Nonpharmacologic therapies for acute and chronic low back pain: a review of the evidence for an American Pain Society/American College of Physicians clinical practice guideline. *Ann Intern Med* **147(7)**:492–504.

12 Moseley GL, Nicholas MK, Hodges PW. (2004) A randomized controlled trial of intensive neurophysiology education in chronic low back pain. *Clin J Pain* **20(5)**:324–30.

13 Brox JI, Storheim K, Grotle M *et al.* (2007) Systematic review of back schools, brief education, and fear-avoidance training for chronic low back pain. *Spine J* Nov 13.

14 Burton AK, Waddell G, Tillotson KM *et al.* (1999) Information and advice to patients with back pain can have a positive effect: a randomized controlled trial of a novel educational booklet in primary care. *Spine* **24(23)**: 2484–91.

15 Linton SJ, McCracken LM, Vlaeyen JW. (2008) Reassurance: help or hinder in the treatment of pain. *Pain* **134(1–2)**:5–8.

16 George SZ, Fritz JM, Bialosky JE *et al.* (2003) The effect of a fear-avoidance-based physical therapy intervention for patients with acute low back pain: results of a randomized clinical trial. *Spine* **28(23)**:2551–60.

17 Liddle SD, Gracey JH, Baxter GD. (2007) Advice for the management of low back pain: a systematic review of randomised controlled trials. *Man Ther* **12(4)**:310–27.

18 Linton SJ, Vlaeyen J, Ostelo R. (2002) The back pain beliefs of health care providers: are we fear-avoidant? *J Occup Rehabil* **12(4)**:223–32.

19 Assendelft WJ, Morton SC, Yu EI *et al.* (2004) Spinal manipulative therapy for low back pain. *Cochrane Database Syst Rev* **1**:CD000447.

20 Hayden JA, van Tulder MW, Tomlinson G. (2005) Systematic review: strategies for using exercise therapy to improve outcomes in chronic low back pain. *Ann Intern Med* **142(9)**: 776–85.

21 Mannion AF, Taimela S, Müntener M *et al.* (2001) Active therapy for chronic low back pain. Part 1. Effects on back muscle activation, fatigability, and strength. *Spine* **26(8)**:897–908.

22 Turk DC, Okifuji A. (2002) Psychological factors in chronic pain: evolution and revolution. *J Consult Clin Psychol* **70(3)**:678–90.

23 Sullivan MJ, Adams H, Rhodenizer T *et al.* (2006) A psychosocial risk factor: targeted intervention for the prevention of chronic pain and disability following whiplash injury. *Phys Ther* **86(1)**:8–18.

24 Sullivan MJ, Feuerstein M, Gatchel R *et al.* (2005) Integrating psychosocial and behavioral interventions to achieve optimal rehabilitation outcomes. *J Occup Rehabil* **15(4)**:475–89.

Part 7

Psychological

Chapter 23

Pain self-management: theory and process for clinicians

Michael McGillion[1], Sandra M. LeFort[2], Karen Webber[2]
& Jennifer N. Stinson[1,3]

[1] Lawrence S. Bloomberg Faculty of Nursing, University of Toronto, Toronto, Canada
[2] School of Nursing, Memorial University of Newfoundland, St. John's, Canada
[3] Child Health Evaluative Sciences, Chronic Pain Program, The Hospital for Sick Children, Toronto, Canada

Introduction

Chronic non-cancer pain remains an important public health problem that seriously affects people's everyday lives including their family, social and working lives. Chronic pain, defined as pain lasting 6 months or longer, affects 19% of Europeans and 25% of Canadians [1,2]. The burden of chronic pain on individuals includes functional limitations and high rates of depression, sleep problems, low self-esteem as well as significant job change or job loss [1,3].

Because prevalence rates are so high, access to appropriate care is a problem. While there has been an increase in the number and types of pain treatment centers, it is estimated that only 2% of Europeans and 1.1% of Americans with chronic pain are treated by specialist healthcare providers [1,4] and that wait times for pain care are unacceptably long [5]. While the onus is on primary care providers (most of whom are generalists) to fill the gap in care, most have had little training in the effective management of chronic pain [6].

One approach to improving patient care at the primary care level is self-management education [7]. Traditional patient education provides information and teaches technical skills about how to manage the condition itself. By contrast, self-management education is broader in scope, emphasizing problem solving, action planning for behavior change and confidence building to enable people to deal better with everyday problems that result from chronic conditions [8]. In other words, self-management education helps people with a chronic condition better manage their lives. Evidence is mounting from studies conducted in the USA, Canada, the UK and Australia that low cost community-based self-management programs as an adjunct to usual care are effective in improving health outcomes and quality of life for individuals with a variety of chronic health conditions including chronic pain [8–14].

This chapter provides an overview of key self-management principles, successful program models, critical process elements and their impact on patient outcomes, and practical tips for program start-up.

What is self-management?

Active self-managers are people who are willing to learn about and take responsibility for the daily

Clinical Pain Management: A Practical Guide, 1st edition.
Edited by Mary E. Lynch, Kenneth D. Craig and
Philip W.H. Peng.
© 2011 Blackwell Publishing Ltd.

management of their chronic condition and its consequences. The goal of self-management is to maintain a wellness focus in the foreground, even in the midst of a chronic health problem, to improve overall quality of life. The daily tasks that need self-management are threefold:

1 Taking care of one's overall health (e.g. healthy eating, being physically active, relaxing and reducing stress, learning about one's condition, treatments and medications);

2 Carrying on with normal activities and roles in life (e.g. maintaining healthy social relationships and staying involved in home, social and work activities); and

3 Managing the emotional changes that are inherent in the chronic illness experience such as anger, fear, frustration, depression, etc. [15].

To manage these tasks successfully, people need a set of core self-management skills: problem-solving skills; decision-making skills; how to find, evaluate and utilize appropriate resources; how to work effectively in partnership with healthcare providers; and how to take action to change behavior [15]. Like other chronic conditions, managing chronic pain on a daily basis requires the acquisition and use of these five core self-management skills. But many people with pain have not had the opportunity to learn these skills in a constructive and supportive environment; rather, they have been told that they will have to "learn to live with the pain." This is where a pain self-management education program can help at the primary care level. These programs have been developed to provide patients with the skills to live an active and meaningful life even with a complex and difficult problem such as chronic pain.

Background: Stanford self-management program model

The Chronic Pain Self-Management Program (CPSMP) [9,10] and the Chronic Angina Self-Management Program (CASMP) [10] are derived from the Stanford University Patient Education Research Center model of self-management. By all accounts, the Stanford self-management programs developed by Dr. Kate Lorig and colleagues have

been the most rigorously developed and evaluated over the last 30 years with over 64 research publications from this research group alone [16]. The first such program was the Arthritis Self-Management Program (ASMP) developed in 1978 which was built with "bits and pieces taken from theory, accepted practice and good intentions" [17, p. 356]. However, over time, it evolved to become a program grounded in Albert Bandura's concept of self-efficacy, defined as "the exercise of human agency through people's beliefs in their capabilities to produce desired effects by their actions" [18, p. 3]. This is referred to as a sense of control.

The program design of the ASMP was fully revised in 1989 to incorporate strategies known to enhance self-efficacy. The four confidence-building strategies are skills mastery, modeling, reinterpretation of symptoms and social persuasion [18]. Subsequently, all the Stanford-based self-management programs including the CPSMP and the CASMP have maintained these important self-efficacy enhancing strategies.

Content, process and strategies to enhance self-efficacy

Self-management education is, by definition, problem-based and is designed to address the common problems and difficulties that arise for a given chronic health problem [15]. Using the CPSMP as an example, the program content, delivered to groups of participants over 2.5 hours per week for 6 weeks, includes the following topics: self-management principles; debunking myths about pain; differences between acute and chronic pain; balancing activity and rest; exercise and physical activity; relaxation; depression; nutrition; evaluating non-traditional treatments; problem solving; communication skills with family, friends and healthcare providers; medications and medication responsibilities; fatigue and sleep; and action planning and goal setting to change behavior [19].

As part of the program, participants are introduced to the idea of a "self-management tool box" and that, like a carpenter's tool box, different tools work best for different types of problems (Figure 23.1). Hence, over the 6 weeks of the program,

Self-Management Tool Box	
Physical Activity/Exercise	Problem-Solving
Managing Fatigue	Using your Mind
Pacing & Planning	Healthy Eating
Relaxation & Better Breathing	Communication
Medications	Understanding Emotions
Working with Health Professionals	Finding Resources

Figure 23.1 Self-management tool box.

participants practice these different techniques and begin to use problem-solving and decision-making skills about which types of tools work best for them given their day-to-day circumstances. They begin to understand that there is no "magic bullet" that will take the pain away, but that working at managing their overall health and their pain and other symptoms by using these tools can improve their enjoyment of life.

Self-management programs are structured to maximize active involvement of group participants. They are not the passive receivers of information. Therefore, the critical process components of the program are also standardized and include the following components:

• *Mini-lectures*: provide an opportunity for brief information sharing about all topics.

• *Self-reflection*: sharing feelings provides an opportunity for participants to discuss what chronic pain means to them and what kinds of difficult emotions are associated with their chronic pain.

• *Quiz*: group activity that helps to debunk myths about chronic pain.

• *Brainstorming*: allows group members to discuss the benefits of exercise, good nutrition, symptoms of depression, etc.

• *Setting weekly action plans*: learning the process of setting achievable short-term goals each week.

• *Feedback*: participants report back to the group each week about how they did with their action plan and receive feedback from the group.

• *Group problem solving*: allows opportunities to problem solve a variety of common problems.

• *Support*: telephone or e-mail support mid-week from a peer in the group.

The confidence-building strategies are embedded in the processes of the program. Opportunities for skills mastery or taking action are provided at every session of the 6-week program and participants are encouraged to try new techniques each week at home. In the Stanford model of self-management, action planning is the key element to skills mastery [15]. Modeling is a key strategy to enhance self-efficacy and is accomplished in a number of ways including the use of appropriate materials, the use of peers (not always healthcare professionals) as facilitators for the program, and program participants acting as models for each other. It is powerful for people with chronic pain to see others like themselves problem solve and achieve desired goals; they begin to see that "if they can do it, I can do it." The reinterpretation of physiologic symptoms as having multiple causes rather than just one cause helps participants realize that many of the tools in their toolbox might be useful. Finally, social persuasion, by being involved in a group that provides gentle support and encouragement to change behaviors, can be a powerful tool to enhance confidence.

Effectiveness of pain self-management programs: main findings

The CPSMP [9] was adapted from the Stanford ASMP and later the Chronic Diseases Self-Management Program (CDSMP) in order to make it more directly applicable to people with chronic non-cancer pain. Specific modifications were made with regard to content but all process elements remained the same. In a first randomized controlled trial (n = 110), LeFort *et al.* [9] found that the CPSMP significantly improved pain outcomes, dependency on others, aspects of role functioning, sense of vitality and life-satisfaction, and self-efficacy and resourcefulness to self-manage pain. Building on the results of this single-site trial, LeFort *et al.* [10] conducted a larger scale (n = 279) multisite effectiveness trial with longer-term follow-up. This trial found that the positive effects of the CPSMP on aspects of mental health and resourcefulness were retained up to 12 months

Table 23.1 Key resources.

Websites
Stanford University Patient Education Research Center http://patienteducation.stanford.edu/ Chronic Pain Self-Management Program Modules Online http://www.medschoolforyou.com/
Agencies currently offering the Chronic Pain Self-Management Program (CPSMP) in Canada
British Columbia Center on Aging, University of Victoria, Ladner, B.C. Fraser Health, Maple Ridge, B.C. Interior Health Authority, Shuswap Health Services, Salmon Arm, B.C.
Alberta Alberta Health Services, Capital Health, Edmonton, AB Alberta Health Services, Chronic Disease, Edmonton, AB
Ontario* Bridgepoint Health, Toronto, ON Central East Local Health Integrated Network, Scarborough, Ontario CPM Centers, Toronto and other Ontario sites Yee Hong Center for Geriatric Care, Scarborough, ON Kingston YM/YWCA, Kingston, Ontario Minto Mapleton Family Health Team, Drayton, Ontario Providence Health Care, Toronto, ON Upper Grand Family Health Team, Fergus, Ontario Wasser Pain Management Center, Mt. Sinai Hospital, Toronto, ON
Nova Scotia South Shore Health, Lunenburg, N.S.

* Other centers in Ontario have taken the CPSMP training but have not yet mounted a program.

post-intervention when delivered by generic healthcare providers [10]. The CPSMP is now available in several provinces across Canada (for a list of agencies offering the program see Table 23.1).

The CASMP was developed by McGillion *et al.* [11] in 2006. Like the CPSMP, adaptations were made from the CDSMP to address issues specific to living with persistent cardiac pain arising from chronic stable angina (CSA) including fear and anxiety management, chest pain symptom monitoring, decision making about seeking emergency medical assistance, correct use of antianginal medications, heart healthy diet and communicating

with life partners and healthcare professionals about cardiac pain [11]. In a recent RCT (n = 130), McGillion *et al.* [11] found that the CASMP was effective for improving angina pain, self-efficacy, physical functioning and general health status in the short-term; the sustainability of these observed improvements for CSA patients is yet to be tested.

In addition to group-based models, recent advancements have been made in distance-based pain self-management. Stinson *et al.* [20] have developed an Internet-based self-management program for children living with juvenile idiopathic arthritis (JIA) entitled Teens Taking Charge: Managing Arthritis Online. This is a 12-week program consisting of disease-related information, self-management skills and social support to address pain and quality of life; trained non-healthcare professionals provide brief weekly telephone support to help participants tailor online information to their needs and review weekly assignments. A recent pilot randomized controlled trial (n = 46) was conducted to test the feasibility (acceptability and compliance) and obtain estimates of effectiveness [20]. Those in the intervention group had significantly higher disease knowledge and lower average weekly pain intensity ratings compared with those in the control group [20]. Initial program usage patterns and feasibility data also indicated that participants completed the program as instructed and were actively engaged in self-management goal-setting and completion; plans for a larger-scale effectiveness trial are now underway.

Getting started: conducting a needs assessment

A critical first step in launching a pain self-management program is conducting a comprehensive needs assessment. Many patient education programs in the past have fallen short because their content has been driven by the input of clinicians alone [21]. This is problematic because clinicians often have particular beliefs about priorities for patient pain-related education that differ from those of patients. Moreover, aside from potential discrepancies between clinicians' and patients' views, there may be other stakeholder viewpoints to consider that will have implications for program success (e.g. family, institutional administrators, non-governmental agencies) [22,23]. The following are a list of key questions that can assist in deciding which key stakeholder representatives to involve in a needs assessment:

- Who should give input into development of the program and why?
- Who will deliver it and who will support its ongoing implementation?
- Where will it take place?
- How will it be advertised and who will pay for this?
- What are the cost and resource implications for day-to-day program delivery?
- Are there public policies, guidelines or practice standards that should be considered in the approach?

In addition to learning needs, it is also critically important to examine the salient pain-related beliefs of those involved. Understanding these beliefs can have major implications for optimizing program adherence and benefits. Maladaptive or incorrect pain-related beliefs are common and have been increasingly recognized as key factors in treatment and education program failure [24,25]. Inclusion of questions about pain-related beliefs will help to ensure that common underlying assumptions are targeted and related cognitions associated with the particular pain problem that the program will be designed to address.

Focus groups

A convenient way of collecting needs assessment data is to run focus groups. Focus groups involve hosting a group of participants to have a focused discussion and share ideas. Cumulative evidence has demonstrated that the ideal number of participants in order to foster productive discussion is between 8 and 12 [26,27]. For depth and clarity, participants should also be from similar cohorts, so it is usually best practice to hold separate groups for patients and other stakeholder representatives (e.g. family members, clinicians, administrators) [21].

Like the discussion on pain-related beliefs, the steps involved in executing focus groups are best explained by example; we will refer to the development of the CASMP program. McGillion et al. [28] held four focus groups to identify CSA patients' pain self-management learning needs; two groups involved patients and two involved clinicians and administrator stakeholders. Each group lasted approximately 1.5 hours and utilized a semi-structured interview format. Questions were developed for each group to generate thinking and discussion about: (a) key angina-related beliefs; (b) the day-to-day problems that patients with CSA face; and (c) the corresponding self-management learning needs. Each participant was asked to provide input and the discussion format remained as open as possible. All of the discussions were audio taped and transcribed; an assistant also made note of key discussion points. The data were then coded for major themes via content analysis [28].

There are a couple of caveats worth mentioning. It is important to remember that clinicians inevitably have preconceived ideas of the learning priorities for patients and so having an impartial third party conduct the process, when possible, is ideal. Also, focus groups typically generate quite a lot of data and thematic content analyses of these data require some methodological expertise. If this is an unfamiliar practice, it is a good idea to consult with a methods expert in order to plan an organized and comprehensive approach. There are several ways to conduct a needs assessment and the use of focus groups is an example of one method we have found helpful. Choice of method ultimately depends on individual preferences, institutional program goals, depth and breadth of information required, and suitability to the particular patient population.

Conclusions and resources

This chapter provides background and an overview of the concept of self-management, key strategies for enhancing self-efficacy to self-manage pain and practical suggestions for getting started. Considerable progress has been made in the field of pain self-management but work remains to be done. While much of our work has been focused on adaptations of the group-based Stanford University model, alternative approaches, such as individual pain self-management training, require attention. Online-based pain self-management also remains a burgeoning field. For those interested in developing online programs, we suggest that processes similar to those we have reviewed (assessment of beliefs, identification of key learning priorities, program development and testing) could be followed.

We conclude this chapter by referring those wishing to incorporate pain self-management into their practices to helpful websites and a list of agencies currently offering the CPSMP in Canada (Table 23.1).

References

1 Breivik H, Collett B, Ventafridda V et al. (2006) Survey of chronic pain in Europe: prevalence, impact on daily life, and treatment. Eur J Pain **10**:287–333.

2 Boulanger A, Clark, AJ, Squire P et al. (2007) Chronic pain in Canada: have we improved our management of chronic noncancer pain? Pain Res Manag **12**:39–47.

3 Meana M, Cho R, DesMeules M. (2004) Chronic pain: the extra burden on Canadian women. BMC Womens Health **4(Suppl 1)**:S17.

4 Turk D, McCarberg B. (2005) Non-pharmacological treatments for chronic pain: a disease management context. Dis Manag Health Outcomes **13**:19–30.

5 Lynch M, Campbell F, Clark AJ et al (2008). A systematic review of the effect of waiting for treatment for chronic pain. Pain **136**:97–116.

6 Hunter J, Watt-Watson J, McGillion M et al. (2008) An Interfaculty Pain Curriculum: Lessons learned from six years' experience. Pain **140**:74–86.

7 Smith BH, Elliott, AM. (2005) Active self-management of chronic pain in the community. Pain **113**:249–50.

8 Bodenheimer T, Lorig K, Holman H et al. (2002) Patient self-management of chronic disease in primary care. JAMA **288**:2469–75.

9 LeFort SM, Gray-Donald K, Rowat KM et al. (1998) Randomized controlled trial of a community-based psychoeducation program for the self-management of chronic pain. Pain **74**:297–306.

10 LeFort S, Watt-Watson J, Webber K. (2003) Results of a randomized trial of the chronic pain self-management program in three Canadian provinces. Pain Res Manag **8(Suppl B)**:73.

11 McGillion M, Watt-Watson J, Stevens B et al. (2008) Randomized controlled trial of a psychoeducation program for the self-management of chronic cardiac pain. J Pain Symptom Manag **36**:126–40.

12 Newman S, Steed L, Mulligan K. (2004) Self-management interventions for chronic illness. Lancet **364**:1523–37.

13 King-Vanvlack C, Di Rienzo G, Kinlin M et al. (2007) Education and exercise program for chronic pain patients. Pract Pain Manag **7**: 17–27.

14 Harris MF, Williams AM, Dennis SM et al. (2008) Chronic disease self-management: implementation with and within Australian general practice. Med J Aust **189**:S17–S20.

15 Lorig KR, Holman H. (2003) Self-management education: history, definition, outcomes, and mechanisms. Ann Behav Med **26**:1–7.

16 http://patienteducation.stanford.edu/bibliog.html (last accessed October 10, 2009).

17 Lorig KR, Gonzalez V. (1992) The integration of theory with practice: a 12-year case study. Health Educ Q **20**:17–28.

18 Bandura A. (2000) Self-Efficacy: The Exercise of Control. W.H. Freeman, New York.

19 LeFort SM. (2009) Chronic Pain Self-Management Program Leader's Manual. Stanford, Palo Alto, CA.

20 Stinson JN, McGrath PJ, Hodnett E et al. (2009) Feasibility testing of an online self-management program for adolescents with juvenile idiopathic arthritis (JIA): a pilot randomized controlled trial. Arthritis Rheum **60**:S87.

21 Lorig K. (2000) How do I know what patients want and need? Needs assessment. In: Lorig K, and Associates, eds. Patient Education: A Practical Approach, 3rd edn. Sage, London. pp. 1–20.

22 McGillion M, LeFort SM, Stinson J. (2008) Chronic pain self-management. In: Rashiq S, Schopflocher D, Taenzer P *et al*. *Chronic Pain: A Health Policy Perspective*. Wiley-Blackwell, Weinheim. pp. 167–181.

23 Horvath AO, Greenberg LS. (1989) Development and validation of the working alliance inventory. *J Couns Psychol* **36**:223–33.

24 DeGrood DE, Tait RC. (2001) Assessment of pain beliefs and pain coping. In: Turk DC, Melzack R, eds. *Handbook of Pain Assessment*, 2nd edn. Guilford Press, New York. pp. 320–345.

25 Watt-Watson J. (1992) Misbeliefs about pain. In: Watt-Watson J, Donovan M, eds. *Pain Management: Nursing Perspective*. Mosby, St. Louis, MO. pp. 36–58.

26 Madriz E. (2000) Focus groups in feminist research. In: Denzin KN, Lincoln YS, eds. *Handbook of Qualitative Research*, 2nd edn. Sage, London. pp. 835–50.

27 Morgan DL. (1997) *Focus Groups as Qualitative Research*, 2nd edn. Sage, Thousand Oaks, CA.

28 McGillion M, Watt-Watson J, Kim J *et al*. (2004) Learning by heart: a focused groups study to determine the psychoeducational needs of chronic angina patients. *Can J Cardiovasc Nurs* **14**:12–22.

Acknowledgments

Portions of the Chronic Pain Self-Management Program first appeared in or are derived from the Arthritis Self-Help Program Leader's Guide (1995). These portions are Copyright 1995, Stanford University. Portions of the Chronic Angina Self-Management Program first appeared in or are derived from the Chronic Disease Self-Management Program Leader's Master Trainer's Guide (1999). Those portions are Copyright 1999, Stanford University.

Chapter 24

Psychological interventions: cognitive behavioral and stress management approaches

Heather D. Hadjistavropoulos[1], Amanda C. de C. Williams[2] & Kenneth D. Craig[3]

[1] Department of Psychology, University of Regina, Regina, Canada
[2] Research Department of Clinical, Educational and Health Psychology, University College London, London, UK
[3] Department of Psychology, University of British Columbia, Vancouver, Canada

Introduction

Psychosocial interventions have demonstrable effectiveness in diminishing painful distress and pain-related disability [1]. At the level of subjective experience, they can influence somatosensory, affective and cognitive features; at the level of behavior, they may reduce avoidance of valued or necessary activities, and interpersonal stress and conflict. Because psychosocial factors are important contributors to individual differences in pain [2], psychological interventions must be considered from the outset for patients for whom there is an uncertain diagnosis (such as chronic low back pain) [1], and also among patients with identifiable underlying pathophysiology with significant impact on quality of life (such as arthritic or cancer-related pain) [3,4]. Where pain is construed – by

Clinical Pain Management: A Practical Guide, 1st edition.
Edited by Mary E. Lynch, Kenneth D. Craig and Philip W.H. Peng.
© 2011 Blackwell Publishing Ltd.

patients or by the medical team – solely as a biomedical phenomenon, psychosocial factors will be neglected, to the detriment of treatment outcome.

At present, it is desirable to combine psychological interventions with contributions of other professionals with appropriate pain training, particularly physicians, nurses, physiotherapists or physical therapists, exercise therapists, occupational therapists and therapists with focus on vocational concerns. Less commonly, but also effective, psychological treatments are delivered separately. Treatment may occur in inpatient or outpatient settings, individually or in a group, and with or without the involvement of family members or significant others.

This chapter aims to provide a succinct overview of evidence for the most important psychological mechanisms involved in pain followed by presentation of specific psychological techniques supported by evidence and commonly used with people with chronic pain. Reference is provided for efficacy (comparison of outcomes between intervention and a control condition) and effectiveness (examination of social, economic and clinical benefits in naturalistic settings) where possible.

Mechanisms underlying and evidence supporting psychological interventions

Psychologically based pain treatment interventions have developed considerably over the past 50 years, as have treatment targets. The operant approach focused on overt behavior [5]; the respondent and stress management approaches which followed tended to emphasize muscle tension [6]. Cognitive approaches (often within cognitive behavioral therapy [CBT]) shifted attention to the central role of dysfunctional thinking [7]; family and system therapies addressed interpersonal processes and conflict [8]; and, most recently, Acceptance and Commitment Therapy (ACT) uses mindfulness and values-based action [9].

Behavioral dysfunction

Fordyce [5] proposed that observable behaviors, such as medication consumption, limping, grimacing and resting, can come to be governed by their contingent consequences, even though precipitated by an antecedent event, usually injury or disease. The contingent consequences maintained or strengthened those behaviors by positive reinforcement (e.g. social attention or financial gain), negative reinforcement (e.g. use of analgesic drugs reducing pain) and/or avoidance of negative consequences (e.g. unpleasant work). The operant approach capitalizes upon the potent impact of reinforcement, and opportunities to avoid negative consequences, by making these contingent on healthy behavior (e.g. providing adequate analgesia on a non-demand basis, or social reinforcement for increased activity). At present, few clinicians would set out to identify specific well and illness behaviors or engage in systematic control of reinforcement contingencies, but routinely work with patients on increasing certain behaviors that are assumed to be desirable and incompatible with pain (e.g. exercising, distraction) while working to reduce others that are assumed to be negative or maintain pain and disability (e.g. guarding, avoidance of activity, high levels of complaint).

Evaluations of the efficacy and effectiveness of specific forms of psychological interventions for pain are rare; therapeutic components are almost invariably combined. Reviews of operant therapy for heterogeneous chronic pain patients, however, have been encouraging [10].

Somatosensory issues

Where pain is narrowly conceptualized as a sensory experience, there is an assumption that diminishing pain severity will automatically produce secondary reductions in emotional distress and disability, hence the long-standing search for the magical pharmacological bullet (effective analgesic drugs that do not have destructive side effects) or for non-pharmacological methods to activate the same endogenous systems. Respondent theory takes a broader formulation of somatosensory features of pain, identifying automatic or habitual reactions to painful threat that prepare the individual for urgent escape or avoidance of further painful insult [11]. The related non-pharmacological pain management approach largely focuses upon musculoskeletal reactions, with pain-tension construed as central to pain experience and reduction of muscle tension as the major goal of treatment [6].

Reviews of the effects of relaxation therapy and biofeedback are largely supportive [12], although studies are often difficult to interpret because of differences in procedures, patient groups and characteristics of treatment. It is also unclear whether reducing muscle tension is essential, or whether interventions work by improving sleep, increasing well-being and, perhaps most importantly, enhancing a sense of control.

Cognitive features of painful experience

Given the important contribution of thoughts to distress and unhelpful behavior, psychosocial interventions often focus on cognitive content or habits of processing, of which one of the most important is catastrophizing [13]. Another, self-efficacy, describes the belief that one can initiate strategies to achieve personal goals, despite continuing pain and is also important in any active intervention [14]. Coping, although poorly defined and difficult to measure in context, is also often a clinical focus. In this case, emotion-focused coping (e.g. wishful thinking, self-blame, withdrawing from others) has been found to predict greater emotional distress and pain-related disability than a problem-solving approach [15].

Several systematic reviews [10,16] have demonstrated the efficacy of CBT. These typically have been qualified by concerns about study designs, generalizability of findings, sample size, etc. In the most recent systematic review and meta-analysis [17], the evidence was that CBT only had weak effects in improving pain, minimal effects on pain-related disability, but importantly large effects in altering mood outcomes of chronic pain, with changes maintained at 6 months. While trial methodology has improved in recent years, treatment remains of variable quality, and some trials are very brief. If there is any dose–response effect, it is likely that many fall below minimum dose requirements.

Emotional difficulties

The fear avoidance model of pain [18] proposes that widespread fear of increased pain or of injury or reinjury, with related avoidance of any activity significantly contributes to disability among individuals with chronic pain. Following from this, many clinicians have turned to treating fear of pain and reinjury with gradual exposure to the avoided activity. Although the treatment model of gradual exposure to the avoided activities is proving effective [19], the parallels between fear of pain and phobia are limited. Most recently, a model of ruminative worry as an attempt to solve the problem of pain has been proposed [20]. As a consequence, treatment is now focusing on reframing the problem from pain to how to realize personal values despite pain, as specifically addressed in ACT. Preliminary findings suggest that over 75% of patients experience improvements using this approach [9].

Interpersonal targets

Patients do not experience pain in isolation: pain and disability affect work, family, leisure, health-care and other environments. These in turn influence the thoughts, feelings and behavior of the individual. Vocational concerns (job stress, job dissatisfaction, vocational uncertainty) and family concerns all feed into the complexities of pain and related disability. Ideally, psychological interventions extend into these environments.

The operant approach was the first to emphasize that pain occurs in a social context [5]. Nevertheless, characterizing financial and social consequences of pain and disability as reinforcers led to the unfortunate myth that "secondary gain" often consciously or unconsciously maintained the disability. This supported a pejorative understanding of pain wherein the absence of a physiological basis for pain was taken as evidence that patients were malingering, coinciding with derisive perspectives on pain patients adopted by some healthcare practitioners and others in disability, rehabilitation and insurance industries. It is now recognized that the social relationships of pain patients are substantially more complicated, with relationships promoting health as well as contributing to disability.

While the potential scope for treating chronic pain patients through attention to the social environment is broad (potentially including employers and the workplace, the community, health service providers and public policy), the primary treatment focus has been upon family or marital therapy as an adjunct to the treatment of chronic pain [8]. The family represents a primary social environment that could be enlisted to facilitate treatment changes, and the introduction of models of marital interaction is promising [21].

Best clinical practice

Psychological treatment goals are important determinants of treatment targets, and follow careful psychological assessment (Chapter 10). Both patient objectives and the interests of referral sources can be diverse and poorly specified, and patient goals may diverge or conflict with those specified by the referrer or by treatment staff. In the sections that follow, attention is directed to common targets of psychosocial intervention, although interventions may have multiple effects.

Behavior change

The essential elements of the operant approach were described by Sanders [22]. This approach begins with functional behavioral analysis which identifies relevant overt pain and well behaviors, along with, as far as possible, antecedent stimuli and contingent consequences. Operant treatment then uses: (a) response prevention for escape/avoidance behaviors; (b) positive and negative reinforcement (e.g. encouragement, social attention) to increase the probability of well behaviors (e.g. physical exercise, uptime), with subsequent shifts to an "intermittent" reinforcement schedule to maintain; (c) shaping or reinforcement of gradual changes in well behaviors, including exercising to levels of activity below pain tolerance; (d) elimination or reduction of factors that may maintain overt pain behaviors outside the treatment environment, including economic reinforcers, social attention and avoidance of responsibilities; and (e) time-contingent delivery of medication that progressively diminishes requirements for medication.

The operant approach is particularly valuable for changing medication use, whether the goal of treatment is to substitute non-opioid for opioid analgesics, and supply antidepressants, or to reduce all drug intake to nil. Analgesic use is often reinforced by reduced pain, even briefly, or by psychological effects including sedation. Fordyce [23] devised a sequential treatment strategy which calls for delivery of medications on a prescribed-as-needed (PRN) basis to establish the baseline, then on a fixed time basis as they are gradually withdrawn.

There are very real constraints on the extent to which the operant approach can be applied as systematically as required. Extensive use of response prevention can present ethical problems, and there are often social or societal "incentives" for remaining disabled. Additionally, social support can be construed rather as beneficial for health rather than reinforcing disability.

Sensory processes

The primary psychological interventions arising from the respondent formulation of pain have been relaxation therapies and biofeedback. Progressive muscle relaxation is the most common form of relaxation training, teaching tension and relaxation of major muscle groups throughout the body and ending with a focus on the latter. Biofeedback similarly involves muscle relaxation, learned through feedback of bodily responses as visual or auditory information. Electromyographic (EMG) feedback, aimed at reducing muscle tension, is the most common with chronic pain patients, primarily for headache [24], but also low back pain [10] and temporomandibular joint pain [25]. Relaxation training and biofeedback may be used alone or in combination. Common problems include failure to develop the skill, so that efforts at use may be counterproductive, and reliance on biofeedback equipment to cue muscle responses.

Cognitive interventions

The numerous psychological interventions available to health practitioners are often combined in CBT. Early forms of cognitive intervention included the use of hypnosis and imagery training. Hypnosis involves suggestions for decreasing discomfort or transforming pain into less noxious sensations. Imagery involves the purposeful use of visual images to strengthen distraction and/or to transform aspects of the painful experience. Evidence is weak on benefits in persistent pain, and where these are used it is mainly within the broader domain of CBT.

CBT programs are diverse in the strategies deployed and it is difficult describing precise features of the "ingredients" of practice. It also should be noted that the approach complements multidisciplinary care as certain professionals (e.g. physiotherapists, physicians) may be better trained to deliver particular features of CBT. The following, summarized by Hadjistavropoulos and Williams [26], are generally regarded to be core components:

1 Education about pain is vital to having the patient understand that persistent pain is not a warning to be cautious and exert all efforts to obtain pain relief and is achieved through

explaining pain mechanisms and the integral role of psychology and behavior in pain.

2 Exercise and fitness training is used to reverse presumed deconditioning due to reduced activity and to address fears about certain movements or physical demands. Active goal setting and independent exercise is encouraged.

3 Acquisition of skills for self-management of pain is encouraged through direct instruction, modeling of appropriate behavior and rehearsal and reinforcement, whether working on relaxation, activity pacing, interactions with friends and with healthcare staff, stress management or sleep problems. Behavioral change by personal contingency management enables patients to become more aware of unhelpful contingencies, and to encourage others to engage in similar selective reinforcement.

4 Goal setting, by the patient with assistance from staff, identifies short and long-term goals, skills deficits, and methods for achieving these goals. Activity scheduling and pacing start from a modest baseline and build by small increments the patient's capacity for activity, interspersed with programmed breaks or changes of activity. The aim is to achieve more, and more reliably, within the limits of pain, rather than to make heroic efforts to achieve goals despite pain, often unsuccessfully. Increasingly critical to the goal setting process is attention to motivational enhancement.

5 Cognitive therapy is the cornerstone of CBT, but the most variable in content and technique. It includes attention diversion components, relaxation, problem solving and cognitive restructuring strategies. It addresses patients' elicited concerns and emotional difficulties, teaches them to identify catastrophizing and other unhelpful habits of thinking, and provides them with a means to challenge and change their thoughts. This is not readily accomplished through didactic instruction, but typically requires substantial socratic dialogue with the patient and personal practice.

6 Generalization and maintenance are emphasized in CBT. Skills are practiced in different settings and barriers to change are anticipated and the patient prepared to address them. Essentially, patients are encouraged to anticipate setbacks and

plan for successful management. The simple model of adherence to program content as the key to maintenance is unsatisfactory [27].

In terms of delivery, CBT is often delivered to groups over a fixed time and number of sessions, with in-session and between-session rehearsal and application to individual goals. While patients have unique pain histories, they share sufficient problems in managing pain to share experiences in a group. This also serves to normalize the experience of isolated patients, validates their difficulties and efforts to manage them, and provides vicarious learning in pain management. Inpatient programs may be necessary for more severely disabled and distressed patients, but outpatient programs are also effective and cost less [28,29].

While the CBT approach has been widely disseminated and accepted, many issues urgently require clinical research. While clinicians believe that they match interventions to the requirements of particular patients, there is no evidence base for their decisions, since there are no unique relationships of intervention to outcome. Abbreviated or remote interventions, or those which dispense with clinical expertise, tend to produce very small effects, verging on clinical insignificance [17].

Emotional processes

Complementing the foregoing in attempting to control dysfunctional emotions are the exposure-based treatments derived from the fear avoidance model of pain [18]. With this approach, clinicians focus on assisting patients in constructing hierarchies for graded return to each activity limited by fear of pain or of damage [19]. Most recently, given evidence that the struggle to control and eliminate pain may be counterproductive and contribute to frustration and pain [30], clinicians have targeted emotional responses to pain by having the patient disengage from and accept pain and emotions concerning pain along with pursuing meaningful life activities despite pain [9].

Interpersonal distress and dysfunction

Family and/or marital therapy are increasingly well systematized in the treatment of chronic pain, yet still used in many different forms. Some therapists take the traditional family systems approach and focus on restoring balance in the family system. Alternatively, the family therapist may adapt the operant or CBT perspectives described above to change in the family. The CBT approach focuses upon how the family's beliefs concerning pain, disability and emotional behavior determine how they all deal with the challenges of chronic pain and encouraging direct and open communication about pain and related problems [31].

Conclusions

All psychological interventions described above are delivered with the recognition that patients are seeking help, or have been referred for assistance, because they are stuck in their attempts to manage their pain. Given the above evidence, it is apparent that psychological interventions should not be regarded as a treatment of last resort following failure of biologically based treatments [26], but rather should be standard in chronic pain treatment. When provided, psychological interventions make an important contribution to multidisciplinary treatment.

References

1 Hoffman BM, Papas RK, Chatkoff DK *et al.* (2007) Meta-analysis of psychological interventions for chronic low back pain. *Health Psychol* **26(1)**:1–9.

2 Linton S. (2000) A review of psychological risk factors in back and neck pain. *Spine* **25**:1148–56.

3 Dixon KE, Keefe FJ, Scipio CD *et al.* (2007) Psychological interventions for arthritis pain management in adults: a meta-analysis. *Health Psychol* **26**:–50.

4 Keefe FJ, Ahles TA, Sutton L *et al.* (2005) Partner-guided cancer pain management at the end of life: a preliminary study. *J Pain Symptom Manage* **29**:263–8.

5 Fordyce WE. (1976) *Behavioural methods for chronic pain and illness*. CV Mosby, St. Louis, MO.

6 Linton S. (1982) A critical review of behavioural treatments for chronic benign pain other than headache. *Br J Clin Psychol* **21**:321–37.

7 Turk DC, Rudy TE. (1989) A cognitive-behavioral perspective on chronic pain: beyond the scalpel and syringe. In Tollison CD, ed. *Handbook of Chronic Pain Management* Williams & Wilkins, Baltimore, MD. pp. 222–36.

8 Kerns RD, Payne A. (1996) Treating families of chronic pain patients. In Gatchel RJ, Turk DC, eds. *Psychological Approaches to Pain Management*. Guilford Press, New York. pp. 283–304.

9 Vowles KE, McCracken LM. (2008) Acceptance and values-based action in chronic pain: a study of treatment effectiveness and process. *J Consult Clin Psychol* **76**:397–407.

10 van Tulder MW, Ostelo R, Vlaeyen JW *et al.* (2000) Behavioral treatment for chronic low back pain: a systematic review within the framework of the Cochrane Back Review Group. *Spine* **25**:2688–99.

11 Craig KD, Versloot J, Goubert L *et al.* (2010) Perceiving others in pain: automatic and controlled mechanisms. *J Pain* **11(2)**:101–8.

12 Chambless DL, Ollendick TH. (2001) Empirically supported psychological interventions. *Ann Rev Psychol* **52**:685–716.

13 Sullivan MJ, Thorn B, Haythornthwaite JA *et al.* (2001) Theoretical perspectives on the relation between catastrophizing and pain. *Clin J Pain* **17**:52–64.

14 Turner J, Holtzman S, Mancl L. (2007) Mediators, moderators and predicts of therapeutic change in cognitive behavior therapy for chronic pain. *Pain* **127**:276–86.

15 Keefe FJ, Somers TJ, Kothadia S. (2009) Coping with pain. *Pain Clin Updates* **17**:1–5.

16 Guzmán J, Esmail R, Karjalainen K *et al.* (2001) Multidisciplinary rehabilitation for chronic low back pain: systematic review. *Br Med J* **322**:511–6.

17 Eccleston C, Williams AC de C, Morley S. (2009) Psychological therapies for the management of chronic pain (excluding headache) in adults. *Cochrane Database Syst Rev* **15(2)**:CD007407.

18 Vlaeyen JW, Linton SJ. (2000) Fear-avoidance and its consequences in chronic musculoskeletal pain: a state of the art. *Pain* **85**:317–32.

19 Vlaeyen JW, De Jong JR, Onghena P *et al.* (2002) Can pain-related fear be reduced? The application of cognitive-behavioural exposure *in vivo*. *Pain Res Manag* **7**:144–53.

20 Eccleston C, Crombez G. (2007). Worry and chronic pain: a misdirected problem solving model. *Pain* **132**:233–6.

21 Cano A, Williams AC deC. (2010) Social interaction in pain: reinforcing pain behaviors or building intimacy? *Pain* **149(1)**:9–11.

22 Sanders SH. (1996) Operant conditioning with chronic pain: back to basics. In: Gatchel RJ, Turk DC, eds. *Psychological Approaches to Pain Management*. Guilford Press, New York. pp. 112–30.

23 Fordyce WE. (1973) An operant conditioning method for managing chronic pain. *Postgrad Med* **53**:123–38.

24 Nicholson R, Penzien D, McCrory DC *et al.* (2004) Behavioural therapies for migraine headache. *Cochrane Database Syst Rev* **1**:CD004601.

25 Crider AB, Glaros AG. (1999) A meta-analysis of EMG biofeedback treatment of temporomandibular disorders. *J Orofac Pain* **13**:29–37.

26 Hadjistavropoulos HD, Williams AC de C. (2004) Psychological interventions and chronic pain. In: Hadjistavropoulos T, Craig KD, eds. *Pain: Psychological Perspectives*. Lawrence Erlbaum, Mahwah, NJ. pp. 271–302.

27 Curran C, Williams AC deC, Potts H. (2009) Cognitive-behavioral therapy for persistent pain: does adherence after treatment affect outcome? *Eur J Pain* **13**:178–88.

28 Gatchel RJ, Okifuji A. (2006) Evidence-based scientific data documenting the treatment and cost-effectiveness of comprehensive pain program for chronic nonmalignant pain. *J Pain* **7**:779–93.

29 Williams AC de C, Richardson PH, Nicholas MK *et al.* (1996) Inpatient vs. outpatient pain management: results of a randomised controlled trial. *Pain* **66**:13–22.

30 McCracken LM, Carson JW, Eccleston C *et al.* (2004) Acceptance and change in the context of chronic pain. *Pain* **109**:4–7.

31 Keefe FJ, Blumenthal J, Daucom D *et al.* (2004) Effects of spouse-assisted coping skills training and exercise training patients with osteoarthritic knee pain: a randomized controlled study. *Pain* **110**:530–49.

Chapter 25

Pain catastrophizing and fear of movement: detection and intervention

Michael J.L. Sullivan & Timothy H. Wideman

Department of Psychology, McGill University, Montreal, Canada

Introduction

Over the past two decades, considerable research has accumulated indicating that medical status variables cannot fully account for presenting symptoms of pain and disability in individuals with chronic pain conditions [1]. Biopsychosocial models have been put forward suggesting that a complete understanding of pain experience and pain-related outcomes will require consideration of physical, psychological and social factors [2]. Catastrophic thinking and fear of movement are two psychological variables that have been shown to be significant determinants of pain and disability associated with persistent pain conditions. This chapter briefly reviews what is currently known about the impact of pain catastrophizing and fear of movement on pain outcomes. The chapter describes assessment techniques and intervention approaches for individuals who present with high levels of pain catastrophizing and fear of movement.

Clinical Pain Management: A Practical Guide, 1st edition.
Edited by Mary E. Lynch, Kenneth D. Craig and
Philip W.H. Peng.
© 2011 Blackwell Publishing Ltd.

Pain catastrophizing (maladaptive coping)

Pain catastrophizing has emerged as one of the most robust and powerful predictors of pain-related outcomes [3]. Pain catastrophizing has been defined as an exaggerated negative response to actual or anticipated pain [3]. The term catastrophizing is used to describe a particular response to pain symptoms that includes elements of rumination (i.e. excessive focus on pain sensations), magnification (i.e. exaggerating the threat value of pain sensations) and helplessness (i.e. perceiving oneself as unable to cope with pain symptoms). Several investigations have revealed a relation between pain catastrophizing and pain and disability in patients with a variety of acute and persistent pain conditions [4].

Catastrophizing has been associated with increased pain and pain behavior, increased use of healthcare services, longer hospital stays, increased use of analgesic medication and higher rates of unemployment [3]. In samples of patients with chronic pain, catastrophizing has been associated with heightened disability, predicting the risk of chronicity and the severity of disability better than illness-related variables or pain itself [5]. Recent research suggests that individuals with high

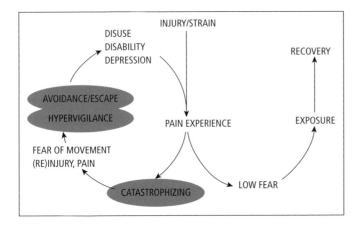

Figure 25.1 The Fear-Avoidance Model of Pain and Disability.

catastrophizing show poorer response to a variety of interventions including analgesics, surgery and rehabilitation [4]. A relation between catastrophizing and pain-related outcomes has been observed in children as young as 7 years [6].

Fear of movement associated with pain

Fear of pain has been defined as a "highly specific negative emotional reaction to pain eliciting stimuli involving a high degree of mobilization for escape/avoidance behavior" [7]. Fear of movement is a type of pain-related fear characterized by avoidance of activity associated with pain, or premature termination (i.e. escape) of activity causing pain [8]. Escape refers to behaviors that are enacted with the goal of terminating pain experience. Avoidance behavior refers to behavior that postpones the pain experience. Once learned, avoidance behaviors can be self-perpetuating. Self-perpetuation of avoidance behavior occurs when individuals develop the expectation that future activities will be associated with pain. Extreme avoidance of movement can contribute to significant disability. Although the role of fear of movement has been extensively studied in individuals with low back pain, recently investigators have examined pain-related fears in patients with other types of pain conditions such as arthritis and whiplash injury [9].

The negative impact of pain catastrophizing and fear of movement has been interpreted primarily within the context of Vlaeyen *et al.*'s Fear-Avoidance Model of Pain (Figure 25.1) [8]. According to the Fear-Avoidance Model, individuals differ in the degree to which they interpret their pain symptoms in a "catastrophic" or "alarmist" manner. The model predicts that catastrophic thinking following the onset of pain will contribute to heightened fear of movement. In turn, fear is expected to lead to avoidance of activity that might be associated with pain [8]. Prolonged inactivity is expected to contribute to depression and disability. The model is recursive such that increased pain symptoms, distress and disability become the input for further catastrophic or alarmist thinking [8].

Research to date has supported the view that catastrophizing and fear of movement are risk factors for problematic recovery following the onset of a pain condition [4]. It has been suggested that assessment of catastrophizing and fear of movement should be part of the routine evaluation of patients with pain conditions. There has also been a call for the development of interventions that are designed to specifically target catastrophizing and fear of movement [10].

Assessment of catastrophizing

Several assessment instruments have been developed to assess pain catastrophizing. Considerable research on catastrophizing has used the Coping Strategies Questionnaire (CSQ) [11]. The CSQ consists of seven coping subscales, including a 6-item catastrophizing subscale. Respondents are asked to rate the frequency with which they use the different strategies described by scale items. The catastrophizing subscale of the CSQ contains items reflecting pessimism and helplessness in relation to coping with pain. Self-report measures have also been developed for assessing catastrophizing in children and adolescents [6]. Interview methods have also been used; however, their application to clinical settings has been limited.

The Pain Catastrophizing Scale (PCS) [12] is currently the most widely used measure of pain catastrophizing. The PCS is a self-report questionnaire that assesses three dimensions of catastrophizing: rumination ("I can't stop thinking about how much it hurts"), magnification ("I worry that something serious may happen") and helplessness ("It's awful and I feel that it overwhelms me"). Electronic copies of the PCS can be downloaded in various languages from the website (http://sullivan-painresearch.mcgill.ca/pcs.php).

The PCS consists of 13 items describing different thoughts and feelings that individuals may experience when they are in pain [12]. On this measure, respondents are asked to rate the frequency with which they experience different catastrophic thoughts and feelings when they are in pain on a 5-point scale with the endpoints (0) not at all and (4) all the time. The reliability and validity of the PCS has been well established [13]. The PCS yields a total score and subscale scores for rumination, magnification and helplessness. Total scores above 20 are considered to fall within the risk range [14]. Individuals who obtain scores above 20 are more likely to follow a problematic course of recovery and poorer response to pain treatment or rehabilitation.

Treatments aimed at reducing catastrophizing

The robust relation between catastrophizing and pain has prompted a growing number of clinicians and researchers to identify catastrophizing as a central factor in the clinical management of disabling pain conditions [4]. Research suggests that a variety of intervention approaches can be used to reduce catastrophic thinking. For example, following multidisciplinary treatment for pain, significant reductions in catastrophizing are often noted [15]. Reductions in catastrophizing have also been observed following physiotherapy, suggesting that even interventions that would not be considered psychosocial in nature might still yield reductions in catastrophizing [16]. It is not clear, however, that such non-targeted approaches yield reductions in catastrophizing of sufficient magnitude to impact in a meaningful manner on clinical outcomes. Given the treatment-resistant nature of persistent pain conditions, it is likely that multipronged approaches, using techniques that aim to reduce the frequency of catastrophic thinking, the negative impact of catastrophic thinking as well as the correlates of catastrophic thinking, such as fear, depression and disability beliefs, will be required.

Recently, intervention programs have been developed that specifically target catastrophic thinking as a primary goal of treatment. Thorn *et al.* [17] have described a 10-week cognitive behavioral intervention designed to reduce catastrophic thinking in those with headache. In this treatment program, thought recording and cognitive restructuring techniques are used as a means of monitoring and modifying catastrophic thoughts. Clients use thought monitoring forms to become more aware of the thoughts they experience during episodes of pain exacerbation. In collaboration with the clinician, clients explore the negative consequences of their catastrophic or pessimistic thinking and are encouraged to consider less catastrophic or pessimistic appraisals of the problematic pain situation.

Sullivan *et al.* [18] have described a 10-week program (Progressive Goal Attainment Program [PGAP]) comprising goal-attainment techniques and activity mobilization strategies designed to target catastrophic thinking. The program consists of a maximum of 10 weekly contacts between a trained PGAP provider and a pain patient. The program never extends beyond 10 weeks because data suggest that if the techniques of PGAP are effective in promoting rehabilitation progress, their impact is observed within 10 weeks. A client workbook is provided to the client and serves as the platform for the intervention techniques that are used in the program. An information video is used as a standardized vehicle for the provision of education and reassurance information emphasizing the importance of activity resumption for promoting recovery. The information video orients the participants to the objectives of the program and describes the main procedures of the program.

PGAP incorporates a variety of techniques that have been shown to either reduce catastrophizing, or reduce the negative impact of catastrophizing. Disclosure techniques are used to reduce pain severity and emotional distress that might be maintaining high levels of catastrophizing. Activity mobilization techniques are used to decrease downtime in order to create a more enriched stimulus environment that will reduce the frequency and impact of catastrophic thoughts. Since fear of movement and disability beliefs are significant correlates of catastrophizing, fear reduction techniques and belief change techniques are incorporated to indirectly target catastrophic thinking. As in the intervention approach described by Thorn et al. [17], thought monitoring and cognitive restructuring are also used to directly target catastrophic thinking.

In one study of patients with chronic cervical pain, individuals who were participating in a functional restoration physical therapy program were compared with a sample of individuals who received PGAP in addition to the same physical therapy intervention [18]. The results showed that, at treatment termination, there were no significant differences in pain severity or pain-related fear. However, the individuals who received PGAP showed greater reductions in catastrophizing and were more likely to return to work. More recently, Sullivan & Adams [19] examined the added value of including PGAP in the rehabilitation of individuals with recent onset (<12 weeks) musculoskeletal pain conditions. At 1 year follow-up, individuals who received PGAP, compared with physiotherapy alone, required fewer additional treatment services, required less pain medication and were more likely to return to work. However, the two groups did not differ significantly on their self-reported pain severity. These results suggest that programs like PGAP might not prevent chronic pain, but might prevent disability associated with chronic pain.

Assessment of fear of movement

Several scales have been developed to assess pain-related fears including the Tampa Scale for Kinesiophobia (TSK) [20], the Fear-Avoidance Beliefs Questionnaire (FAB-Q) [21] and the Fear of Pain Questionnaire III (FPQ-III) [22]. The FAB-Q is most relevant for individuals who might have specific fears of work-related activities. The FPQ-III assesses the degree to which individuals are fearful of different pain-inducing situations (e.g. dental pain, surgery) but is not specific to activity or movement.

The TSK [20] is the most widely used measure of fear of movement. Respondents are asked to make ratings of their degree of agreement with each of the 17 statements. Four items of the TSK (items 4, 8, 12 and 16) are reversed such that higher scores represent less, as opposed to more, fear of movement. Respondents' ratings are summed to yield a total score where higher values reflect greater fear of movement. The TSK has been shown to be internally reliable and to be associated with various indices of disability [23]. Recently, attempts have been made to produce a shorter measure by deleting items of the TSK. Versions containing 11 and 14 items are available [24]. An electronic copy of the 17-item TSK can be obtained from the website (www.workcover.vic.gov.au/wps/wcm/resources/file/eb5c6742bb4ae48/tampa_scale_kinesiophobia.pdf).

The item content of the TSK is most relevant for individuals with pain from musculoskeletal injury, or from pain that is exacerbated by activity (e.g. arthritis). Patients with pain from headache, neuropathy, spinal injury or multiple sclerosis sometimes indicate that they have difficulty understanding how certain items pertain to their condition.

Treatments aimed at reducing fear of movement

Clinical interventions that have been shown to reduce levels of fear of movement include:

1 Education, reassurance and activity encouragement;

2 Graded exposure to feared activities;

3 Activity monitoring, progressive goal setting and graded activity; and

4 Cognitive behavioral therapy (CBT) techniques [9].

Each of these interventions can be effective when delivered independently in primary care settings or when combined within a multidisciplinary treatment program. Clinical trials that have evaluated the efficacy of the latter have shown that these programs are associated with meaningful improvement in measures of fear of movement, pain intensity, activity interference, psychosocial risk factors and work disability [18,25].

Interventions that use education, reassurance and activity encouragement aim to provide patients with information and advice about how to reduce their levels of fear-related disability [26]. Educational interventions typically inform patients about their pain condition, the expected trajectory of their recovery and the signs or symptoms that may indicate serious danger (i.e. red flags). Education aims to demedicalize and demystify patients' pain conditions and can be conceptualized as a precursor for encouraging the resumption of normal activities [27]. The key messages communicated through reassurance and activity encouragement are that pain is not a reliable signal of tissue damage, that the pain condition is not life threatening or permanently disabling, and that it is safe, and beneficial, to engage in physical activity. Patients with elevated levels of fear will often require support in shifting their focus from the severity of their injury to returning to normal activity. It may therefore be helpful for clinicians to consider activity encouragement and reassurance as therapeutic strategies that permeate the recovery process rather than as discrete interventions. The mediums through which these interventions are implemented can vary significantly

(e.g. information booklets, one-to-one sessions, group classes, online forums), which makes them relatively easy to integrate into primary care settings. Past research conducted with acute and subacute pain populations has shown that these interventions result in significant improvements in fear of movement, emotional functioning, pain intensity and self-reported disability [28].

Graded exposure to feared activities is a systematic behavioral intervention that helps patients overcome their fears of specific movements by progressively engaging them in previously avoided activities [8]. Clinicians help patients to identify and rank feared activities in a hierarchy, from least to most feared. Next, patients are asked to rate their fear of performing their least feared activity on a scale of 0 (no fear) to 10 (extreme fear), and to communicate the negative physical consequences they expect to occur upon engaging in this behavior. Patients are then encouraged to perform the behavior and asked to rate their level of fear following exposure. Research suggests that as patients gain exposure to each activity, their level of fear for this specific movement declines [9]. As fear dissipates, the next activity on the hierarchy is introduced and the procedure is repeated. This intervention is typically initiated in one-on-one clinical settings and complemented with, and ultimately progressed to, self-guided home exercises. While graded exposure is one of the most effective interventions for reducing the fear of specific movements, its effects do not seem to generalize to untargeted activities [29]. For this reason, this intervention is more likely to translate into improved disability levels when feared activities that hinder essential daily function are targeted (e.g. work-related activities).

It has been suggested that individuals' fears of movement, and their ensuing avoidance of activity are fueled by over-predictions of harm or pain exacerbation [8]. If individuals can be encouraged to engage in activities that they fear will bring about pain (or symptom exacerbation), they are provided with an opportunity to correct their over-predictions [9]. In other words, experience can allow individuals to alter their exaggerated predictions of threat or harm associated with potentially pain-inducing activities and, in turn, decrease the probability of avoidance behavior.

Activity monitoring, progressive goal setting and graded activity are therapeutic strategies that aim to provide patients with direction, structure and support to enable an increase in their levels of physical activity [18]. These interventions are initiated by establishing the patient's baseline activities level. Asking patients to record a week of daily activity logs can facilitate this step [18]. Once patients have identified and described their objectives, graded activity is used to progressively increase their activity participation. Based on the patient's baseline levels of activity, the clinician and patient establish daily activity quotas. At the next follow-up session, the clinician reviews the patient's success with achieving the activity quotas and increases or maintains them accordingly. Care must be taken to start with activity quotas that have a high probability of success. By completing quotas without significantly increasing pain levels, patients will be encouraged by positive feelings of achievement and motivated to engage in progressively higher quotas. When delivered over a 10-week period in primary care settings, these interventions have been associated with long-term improvements in fear of movement, pain intensity and activity limitations. When delivered in occupational health centers these interventions have also been shown to significantly reduce the number of work absenteeism days [30].

CBT techniques are a class of interventions that use a structured approach to modifying fear-related thoughts, feelings and activities [1]. Thought monitoring and thought restructuring are two CBT techniques that are commonly used in the treatment of fear of movement [1,17]. Patients with elevated levels of fear commonly react to pain with thoughts that increase the threat value of the painful experience, and with avoidant behavior that limits exposure to the pain-related activity [9]. The clinician works with the patient to alter his or her threat appraisals of pain-eliciting situations. Past research that has used CBT interventions to target fear of movement has shown that these treatments are associated with significant improvements in fear, activity interference and measures of work disability [1,9].

Conclusions

Research has pointed to psychological variables such as catastrophizing and fear of movement as significant determinants of pain and pain-related disability. Measurement instruments have been developed to assist clinicians in identifying pain patients at risk for problematic recovery or poor treatment response. There are also data to suggest that intervention approaches that have been shown to reduce catastrophizing and fear of movement yield improvement in a number of clinical outcomes.

References

1 Gatchel R, Peng YB, Peters ML *et al.* (2007) The biopsychosocial approach to chronic pain: scientific advances and future directions. *Psychol Bull* **133**:581–624.

2 Turk DC. (1996) Biopsychosocial perspective on chronic pain. In: Gatchel RJ, Turk DC, eds. *Psychological Approaches to Pain Management: A Practitioner's Handbook*. Guilford, New York. pp. 3–32.

3 Sullivan MJL, Thorn B, Haythornthwaite JA *et al.* (2001) Theoretical perspectives on the relation between catastrophizing and pain. *Clin J Pain* **17(1)**:52–64.

4 Quartana PJ, Campbell CM, Edwards RR. (2009) Pain catastrophizing: a critical review. *Expert Rev Neurother* **9(5)**:745–58.

5 Sullivan MJL, Lynch ME, Clark AJ. (2005) Dimensions of catastrophic thinking associated with pain experience and disability in patients with neuropathic pain conditions. *Pain* **113(3)**: 310–5.

6 Crombez G, Bijttebier P, Eccleston C *et al.* (2003) The child version of the pain catastrophizing scale (PCS-C): a preliminary validation. *Pain* **104(3)**:639–46.

7 McNeil DW, Au AR, Zvolensky MJ *et al.* (2001) Fear of pain in orofacial pain patients. *Pain* **89(2–3)**:245–52.

8 Vlaeyen JW, Linton SJ. (2000) Fear-avoidance and its consequences in chronic musculoskeletal pain: a state of the art. *Pain* **85(3)**:317–32.

9 Leeuw M, Goossens ME, Linton SJ *et al.* (2007) The fear-avoidance model of musculoskeletal pain: current state of scientific evidence. *J Behav Med* **30(1)**:77–94.

10 Sullivan MJ, Lynch ME, Clark AJ. (2005) Dimensions of catastrophic thinking associated with pain experience and disability in patients with neuropathic pain conditions. *Pain* **113(3)**: 310–5.

11 Rosenstiel A, Keefe F. (1983) The use of coping strategies in chronic low back pain patients: relationship to patient characteristics and current adjustment. *Pain* **17**:33–44.

12 Sullivan M, Bishop S, Pivik J. (1995) The Pain Catastrophizing Scale: development and validation. *Psychol Assess* **7**:524–32.

13 Van Damme S, Crombez G, Bijttebier P *et al.* (2002) A confirmatory factor analysis of the Pain Catastrophizing Scale: invariant factor structure across clinical and non-clinical populations. *Pain* **96**:319–24.

14 Sullivan MJL, Ward LC, Tripp D *et al.* (2005) Secondary prevention of work disability: community-based psychosocial intervention for musculoskeletal disorders. *J Occup Rehabil* **15(3)**:377–92.

15 Burns J, Kubilis A, Bruehl S *et al.* (2003) Do changes in cognitive factors influence outcome following multidisciplinary treatment of chronic pain? A crossed-lagged panel analysis. *J Consult Clin Psychol* **71**:81–91.

16 Smeets RJ, Vlaeyen JW, Kester AD *et al.* (2006) Reduction of pain catastrophizing mediates the outcome of both physical and cognitive-behavioral treatment in chronic low back pain. *J Pain* **7(4)**:261–71.

17 Thorn B, Boothy J, Sullivan M. (2002) Targeted treatment of catastrophizing for the management of chronic pain. *Cogn Behav Pract* **9**: 127–38.

18 Sullivan MJL, Adams H, Rhodenizer T *et al.* (2006) A psychosocial risk factor: targeted intervention for the prevention of chronic pain and disability following whiplash injury. *Phys Ther* **86(1)**:8–18.

19 Sullivan MJL, Adams H. (2010) Psychosocial techniques to augment the impact of physical therapy interventions for low back pain. *Physiother Can* **62(3)**:180–9.

20 Kori S, Miller R, Todd D. (1990) Kinesiophobia: a new view of chronic pain behavior. *Pain Manage* **(Jan)**:35–43.

21 Waddell G, Newton M, Henderson I *et al.* (1993) A Fear-Avoidance Beliefs Questionnaire (FABQ) and the role of fear-avoidance beliefs in chronic low back pain and disability. *Pain* **52**:157–68.

22 McNeil D, Au A, Zvolensky M *et al.* (2000) Fear of pain in orofacial pain patients. *Pain* **89**:245–52.

23 Roelofs J, Sluiter JK, Frings-Dresen MH *et al.* (2007) Fear of movement and (re)injury in chronic musculoskeletal pain: evidence for an invariant two-factor model of the Tampa Scale for Kinesiophobia across pain diagnoses and Dutch, Swedish, and Canadian samples. *Pain* **131(1–2)**:181–90.

24 Woby SR, Roach NK, Urmston M *et al.* (2005) Psychometric properties of the TSK-11: a shortened version of the Tampa Scale for Kinesiophobia. *Pain* **117(1–2)**:137–44.

25 Staal JB, Hlobil H, Twisk JW *et al.* (2004) Graded activity for low back pain in occupational health care: a randomized, controlled trial. *Ann Intern Med* **40(2)**:77–84.

26 Waddell G. (2004) *The Back Pain Revolution*, 2nd edn. Churchill Livingstone, London, UK.

27 de Jong JR, Vlaeyen JW, Onghena P *et al.* (2005) Fear of movement/(re)injury in chronic low back pain: education or exposure *in vivo* as mediator to fear reduction? *Clin J Pain* **21(1)**: 9–17; discussion 69–72.

28 Asenlöf P, Denison E, Lindberg P. (2005) Individually tailored treatment targeting activity, motor behavior, and cognition reduces pain-related disability: a randomized controlled trial in patients with musculoskeletal pain. *J Pain* **6(9)**:588–603.

29 Goubert L, Francken G, Crombez G *et al.* (2002) Exposure to physical movement in chronic back pain patients: no evidence for generalization across different movements. *Behav Res Ther* **40(4)**:415–29.

30 Staal JB, Hlobil H, Twisk JW *et al.* (2004) Graded activity for low back pain in occupational health care: a randomized, controlled trial. *Ann Intern Med* **140(2)**:77–84.

Part 8

Complementary Therapies

Chapter 26

Complementary and alternative medicines

Mark A. Ware

Departments of Anesthesia, Family Medicine, Pharmacology & Therapeutics, McGill University, Montreal, Canada

Introduction

Pain is the most common reason for patients to use complementary and alternative medicines (CAM) [1]. Estimates of the size of the CAM market in the USA are in the range $30–40 billion, a remarkable sum considering most of this money is spent out of pocket (not covered by any health insurance plan) and that the majority of CAM products and practices are unregulated. However, while these points may seem to constitute good reasons *not* to use CAM, as we discuss later, they may also be exactly the reasons why patients *do* turn to such therapies. The use of CAM by patients with pain is undeniably a complex issue and there are no simple answers.

The purpose of this chapter is to provide the pain clinician with tools in approaching the topic of CAM with patients in a clinical context. Some of the more well-studied CAM modalities are presented but the reader is referred for further detail to recent textbooks [2,3] where the evidence base for CAM in pain management has been well covered.

Clinical Pain Management: A Practical Guide, 1st edition.
Edited by Mary E. Lynch, Kenneth D. Craig and
Philip W.H. Peng.
© 2011 Blackwell Publishing Ltd.

Definition of CAM

CAM consists of many diverse and different practices and products, making it difficult to lump them into one definition. Since the earliest epidemiological studies of CAM use, the definition has been one of exclusion. In this manner, CAM is usually considered to include practices or products which are not routinely taught in medical school [4] or which fall outside of a conventional or culturally acceptable system of medicine (WHO). Under the World Health Organization (WHO) definition, traditional Chinese medicine (TCM) may be defined as an alternative therapy in North America, but as a mainstream approach in mainland China. For most pain practitioners, CAM treatments will usually include those that have not been given any formal consideration in pain education and for which there is little or no underlying scientific method or mechanism or evidence base. This means, of course, that with emerging evidence and mechanistic explanations, CAM therapies may become mainstream, so the concept of CAM itself is evolving constantly.

The US-based National Center for Complementary and Alternative Medicine (NCCAM) [5] has published a framework for organizing CAM into five main themes as shown in Table 26.1. It is clear that while this encompasses a very wide range of

Table 26.1 Classification of complementary and alternative medicines (CAM).

1 Medical systems that are built on complete systems of theory and practice (e.g. traditional Chinese medicine [TCM], Ayurvedic medicine, naturopathy)*
2 Mind–body interventions (e.g. meditation, yoga)
3 Biologically based therapies (e.g. minerals and vitamins and herbal remedies)
4 Manipulation and body-based methods (e.g. chiropractic, osteopathic treatments, massage therapy)
5 Energy therapies (e.g. treatments in which the energy field of the patient is allegedly modified such as Reiki, therapeutic touch and magnets)

* Note that individual components of medical systems may also be included under other headings (e.g. t'ai chi and qigong, which are integral parts of TCM, may be considered as mind–body interventions as well as body-based methods). To some extent the classification depends on the context in which the CAM practice is offered (e.g. yoga undertaken for physical fitness in a Western country may be considered more body-based than yoga for spiritual development under an Ayurvedic paradigm).

Table 26.2 Questions about CAM use.

Do you take any vitamins or supplements for your pain? Which ones?
Have you visited any alternative practitioners for your pain? Did it help?
Have you ever tried any unconventional therapies? With what effect?
Have you considered any such therapies? Why?
Have you ever tried any "weird and wonderful" remedies for your pain?

modalities, it provides a useful framework for classifying most CAM modalities encountered in pain practice.

Asking about CAM

Discussing CAM use with patients challenges our competencies as communicators and scholars because it is, by definition, an area in which we have little or no expertise. Rather, we must become partners in the decision-making process (and we may even learn from the interaction ourselves). Aspects of CAM appear as part of the International Association for the Study of Pain (IASP) core curriculum for professional education in pain [6], most likely because of the recognition that CAM use is widespread and the pain clinician needs to be able to manage the topic. Managing CAM use begins with the way in which the topic is first discussed in the clinical encounter.

CAM use is often brought up in a chronic pain consultation by the patients themselves. This may be in the context of a spontaneous question ("By the way, doctor, what do you think of craniosacral therapy for my low back pain?"). In response to this type of question, especially when asked almost incidentally at the end of an interview, it may be tempting to be very dismissive ("Nothing to it, it's hocus-pocus. Forget about it."). Alternatively, a patient may have found some information on a CAM topic in the newspaper or on the Internet and will produce the material to discuss ("Have you ever heard of this, doctor? What do you think?"). It is well known, however, that most patients do not discuss their use of CAM with their physician(s). To maximize the opportunities that discussions around CAM can offer, CAM use should be addressed directly.

Along with questions about medications, the pain practitioner should ask about use of unconventional therapies (those tried, those that worked and which did not) as well as those that the patient is considering. Such a question does not endorse all CAM practices, but should be seen as part of getting to know the patient, and their needs, better. As will be argued later, understanding why the patient is interested in CAM is as important as which CAM practices they actually use. Table 26.2 contains a list of examples of questions that may be asked to open up the discussion of CAM use, the reasons and the results.

Absence of evidence or evidence of absence

In this era of evidence-based medicine, it is reasonable to demand evidence as a requirement for further discussions of complementary medicine utilization. However, reliance on evidence alone will not lead to a meaningful dialogue between practitioners and patients because many CAM practices are not supported by evidence or, in some cases, by any form of biological plausibility. In such a case, a practitioner may be tempted to discredit the proposed therapy as unscientific, or worse, quackery. However, while both the scientific and research evidence may point to an absence of any meaningful mechanism of action, the fact remains that large numbers of the population use them. A prime example of this is homeopathy, widely used in Europe and North America where it is a big business, and indeed entire schools and hospitals have been dedicated to homeopathic treatments. Dismissing homeopathy with a wave of the hand may miss an opportunity for dialogue and education.

Why do patients use CAM?

Surveys of CAM use suggest that patients turn to CAM for several reasons, which have been classified as positive or negative (Table 26.3) [7]. Positive reasons include a perception that CAM is "natural" and therefore safe; a sense that CAM practitioners take a more "holistic" approach; and easier access to CAM practitioners. Negative reasons include a perceived failure of existing conventional therapies; a perception (sometimes justified) that conventional medicine has intolerable side effects or risks; dissatisfaction with the Western medical paradigm at large; or a distrust of big pharmaceutical companies' motives.

Once the clinician is aware of some of the underlying reasons why patients turn to CAM, as well as improved awareness of a patient's CAM use, the next issue becomes: why is this particular patient interested in this particular therapy? The reasons shown above may explain the deeper motives, and may be explored in more detail (if time permits), but it is perhaps more useful to enquire whether the patient is looking for treatment for a symptom or symptom complex that is not being adequately addressed by conventional medicine. It may be useful to respond to a question about a given

Table 26.3 Reasons for use of CAM.

Negative reasons	Positive reasons
Dissatisfaction with conventional healthcare; ineffective; toxicity/ adverse events; poor doctor–patient relationship; insufficient time with doctor; long waiting list; advent of "high tech, low touch" medicine	Perceived effectiveness and safety
Rejection of science and technology	Philosophical congruence: spiritual dimension; holism; "natural," active role of patient; understandable explanations
Rejection of the "establishment"	Control over treatment
Desperation	"High touch, low tech" Good therapeutic relationship; enough time available at visits; equal terms with therapist; emotional factors; empathy Non-invasive Accessible Pleasant experience Affluence

Source: After Ernst [7].

therapy with a statement such as: "What is it that you're hoping to achieve by exploring this particular therapy? Is there something that you would like this therapy to address that we haven't addressed in our care plan to date?"

A patient's choice to use CAM may also represent a desire to exercise control over their pain management. Most would agree that a patient's active participation in self-care is desirable. An empathic practitioner may therefore harness interest in CAM to good effect by inviting the patient to share what they have learned from their own research (Table 26.4). These questions should be asked in a nonjudgmental way.

Table 26.4 Engaging patient decision-making in using CAM.

What do they know about the therapy?
How much does it cost?
How long is treatment expected to be?
What outcome is the patient expecting?
What outcome does the CAM product or practice offer or claim?
Are there any side effects?
Who is the person offering the treatment? Do they have any qualifications?
What quality controls are there on the products involved?
Does the use of the CAM modality mean that the patient cannot use (or afford) their regular medication or treatment?

If done effectively, this line of questioning will create an alliance between the doctor and patient in exploring the CAM modality together. This serves two purposes: first, it encourages the patient to be an advocate and an active participant in making their own healthcare decisions, and, second, it educates the healthcare practitioner about a given modality and informs a discussion of the issues at stake. At the end of this chapter, a short list of credible websites is provided which may serve a useful role in this discussion. These sites can be bookmarked for easy access on a practitioner's desktop or portable device.

A question of quality

For many physicians, issues of safety and efficacy (see below) come second to concerns about the source and purity of CAM products or the qualifications of CAM practitioners. These are issues of quality. If a patient presents with a newspaper report of a novel therapy or something that a friend has told them about, a discussion around the qualifications of the practitioner or the source of the medication may reveal that in many situations surrounding CAM there are no controls over the credibility or training or qualifications of the practitioner, and globally there is very little control over the quality or standardization of products

such as vitamins and herbal medicines. In Canada in 2004, the Natural Health Products (NHP) Regulations were put into place in an attempt to provide some form of quality control over natural health products (e.g. orally administered vitamins, minerals, herbs and dietary supplements) [8]. This is a rational approach towards regulating manufacturers who may otherwise prepare, provide and promote preparations for self-care in the absence of any regulatory scrutiny. In the UK in 2000, the House of Lords recognized three categories of CAM with respect to regulation [9]:

• *Group 1:* those that have well-developed professional self-regulation (chiropractic, osteopathy and, increasingly, acupuncture and herbal medicine);

• *Group 2:* those that complement conventional medicine (aromatherapy, Alexander technique, bodywork therapies, massage, counseling, stress therapy, hypnotherapy, reflexology, meditation); and

• *Group 3:* those in which there is no convincing research-based evidence for efficacy and includes 3a, traditional systems of healthcare such as Ayurvedic and Chinese herbal medicine, as well as 3b, other alternative disciplines such as crystal therapy and dowsing.

In countries where a regulatory approach to a particular CAM modality exists (e.g. homeopathy in Germany, TCM in Australia, NHPs in Canada), it is therefore suggested that patients be directed to use only such products and services as have been approved by their local regulators. Practitioners should therefore familiarize themselves with local CAM regulations.

In certain jurisdictions, practitioners of CAM modalities such as acupuncture and chiropractic undergo intensive training and certification by local regulatory authorities. Thus, if a patient chooses to undertake chiropractic as part of the treatment for their back pain, they should be advised to seek licensed practitioners. In some regions, a register of accredited practitioners may be available. In this way, the pain practitioner may be reassured that at the very least the patient will be given the best that such practices have to offer.

Making sense in the information age

In seeking information on CAM, it is important to realize that with the advent of the information age, the patient has enormous access to discussion groups, information sites and networks concerning their own disorder as well as practices and practitioners who are seeking to publicize their own approaches. In many cases, the popular press has a role in perpetuating some of these approaches. Helping a patient to navigate their way through the maze of information that may be found on the Internet is a very valuable approach toward the discussion around CAM. Knowledge of a few credible websites may provide the practitioner with a resource that may be shared with the patient and explored and discussed with them in a few short minutes during a routine clinical visit. This may help both patient and practitioner understand more about the treatment, including its risks, benefits and lack or strength of evidence provided. Patients appreciate the time and effort taken by a practitioner to help them understand better the treatment. An open and honest discussion around such a treatment helps build a strong doctor–patient relationship.

Finding the evidence base

Over the past 40 years, a number of treatments that were once considered "alternative" therapies have become mainstream. Examples of this include forms of psychotherapy such as cognitive behavior therapy, aspects of counseling and exercise recommendations, dietary and nutritional advice, forms of massage therapy and trigger point release. On what basis were these therapies transferred into conventional care? One may also ask which therapies that we currently see as alternative may, in the course of time, become conventional? The response to these questions is the availability of evidence.

Finding evidence of efficacy for CAM is challenging, because the gold standard for determining efficacy of a treatment in today's age is the randomized controlled trial. Such trials are easier when

Table 26.5 CAM therapies for pain supported by good or encouraging evidence. Good or encouraging evidence suggests that at least one randomized controlled trial or meta-analysis has found evidence of efficacy of the CAM modality with a favorable safety profile.

CAM modality	Pain condition
Acupuncture	Dental pain, myofascial pain, osteoarthritis (knee)
Biofeedback	Migraine
Chiropractic	Back pain
Chondroitin	Osteoarthritis
Devil's claw (*Harpagophytum procumbens*)	Back pain
Diet	Rheumatoid arthritis
Exercise	Fibromyalgia, depression
Feverfew (*Tanacetum parthenium*)	Migraine prevention
Glucosamine	Osteoarthritis
Hypnotherapy	Abdominal pain, labor pain, perioperative pain, procedural pain
Massage	Back pain
Osteopathy	Various types of chronic pain
Relaxation techniques	Angina, migraine, depression
S-adenosyl methionine	Osteoarthritis
T'ai chi	Osteoarthritis
Willow (*Salix* spp.)	Back pain

Source: after Ernst [1].

pharmaceutical preparations such as tablets, tinctures or creams are the agents of study compared to complex practices such as t'ai chi, acupuncture or osteopathic adjustments. In these situations, a credible inactive control or placebo is extremely difficult (if not impossible) to design and implement. Clinical trials of complementary therapies are often criticized for the validity of the control group, and this renders many such studies subject to considerable biases. Despite these challenges, a great deal of effort has gone into trying to evaluate the safety and efficacy of some CAM modalities. Table 26.5 lists a range of CAM treatments for various chronic pain conditions for which the evidence base is fairly supportive. Space prohibits a detailed review of all these treatments, and the evidence base is constantly changing, but increasingly such trials are being carried out and published and are available through standard literature search engines (e.g. Medline).

It is worth reflecting on the fact that the vast majority of CAM studies and systematic reviews focus only on efficacy outcomes. The safety of CAM is subject to the same difficulties as conventional medicine: a lack of spontaneous reporting of adverse events. Since CAM use is often not discussed with physicians, potential drug–CAM interactions (especially with herbal remedies) may go unnoticed until they become severe. Practitioners are encouraged to report to suspected CAM adverse events using local reporting mechanisms.

In situations where there is no published evidence of efficacy or safety, then the practitioner must rely on the possible mechanism of action of a given CAM treatment. Homeopathy, a treatment in which the treating agent is diluted to the point at which, on physical principles, there is none of the original substance left in the solution, likely poses very little direct risk to the patient. However, cervical manipulation, which consists of rapid high intensity and low amplitude neck movements, poses potential risk of cervical spine injury and vertebral artery dissection. In both cases, evidence of harm and benefit may be weighed and the question then becomes: how credible is the evidence on both sides? Until valid data are available, the risk side of the equation for cervical manipulation should be weighted more heavily than for homoeopathy, on the basis of mechanisms alone, and the decision to proceed with such treatment based on such uncertainty.

Integrating CAM into pain medicine

As with any treatment, a decision to proceed with a CAM modality is ideally based on a careful and informed consideration of risks and benefits. It is hoped that this chapter will give the pain practitioner tools to be able to have this discussion with their patient. It is important to reinforce the need for the practitioner to remain open to the needs of the patient. A hasty response to a question about a complementary therapy is unlikely to change a patient's behavior, as they will be likely to go in pursuit of the treatment anyway, and the practitioner will appear ill-informed or simply biased against such treatments. A more proactive approach, such as that described in this chapter, based on asking specific questions about CAM, understanding the reasons behind CAM choices, recognizing a framework of CAM modalities, possessing a template for discussing CAM issues and having access to reliable sources of information on CAM specific questions, will undoubtedly enhance the doctor–patient relationship. Making the patient part of their own care team, empowering them to make decisions and encouraging them to give feedback on the success or benefits of the treatment will likely contribute to their care far more meaningfully than hastily dismissing CAM use as quackery. Increasing numbers of pain clinics are moving towards including evidence-based CAM in their scope of practice; the outcomes of such "integrative" pain clinics deserve careful study in the future.

References

1 Ernst E, Pittler MH, Wider B. (2007) *Complementary Therapies for Pain Management: An Evidence-Based Approach*. Mosby Elsevier.

2 Kligler B, Lee R. (2004) *Integrative Medicine: Principles for Practice*. McGraw-Hill.

3 Barnes PM, Powell-Griner E, McFann K *et al.* (2004) Complementary and alternative medicine use among adults: United States, 2002. *Adv Data* **343**:1–19.

4 Eisenberg DM, Kessler RC, Foster C *et al.* (1993) Unconventional medicine in the United States: prevalence, costs, and patterns of use. *N Engl J Med* **328(4)**:246–52.

5 National Center for Complementary and Alternative Medicine (NCCAM). (2007) What is CAM? Available from: http://nccam.nih.gov/health/whatiscam/. Accesssed August 23, 2007.

6 Anon. (2005) Complementary therapies. In: Charlton JE, ed. *Core Curriculum for Professional Education in Pain*, 3rd edn. IASP Press, Seattle. pp. 1–4.

7 Ernst E. Complementary medicine for pain. Wellcome Trust. Available from: http://www.wellcome.ac.uk/en/pain/microsite/medicine1.html. Accessed August 23, 2007.

8 Natural Health Products Directorate, Health Canada. Available from: http://www.hc-sc.gc.ca/dhp-mps/prodnatur/index_e.html. Accessed August 30, 2007.

9 House of Lords Select Committee on Science and Technology Sixth Report, 2000. Available from: http://www.parliament.the-stationery-office.co.uk/pa/ld199900/ldselect/ldsctech/123/12302.htm. Accessed January 12, 2010.

Recommended websites

National Centre for Complementary and Alternative Medicine (NCCAM): http://nccam.nih.gov/health/whatiscam

International Society for Complementary Medicine Research (ISCMR): www.iscmr.org/index.html

Natural Standard: For each therapy covered by Natural Standard, a research team systematically gathers scientific data and expert opinions. Validated rating scales are used to evaluate the quality of available evidence. Information is incorporated into comprehensive monographs which are designed to facilitate clinical decision-making. All monographs undergo blinded editorial and peer review prior to inclusion in Natural Standard databases: www.naturalstandard.com

Part 9

Specific Clinical States

Chapter 27

Chronic low back pain

Eugene J. Carragee & Don Young Park

Department of Orthopedic Surgery, Stanford University School of Medicine, Redwood City, USA

Introduction

Low back pain (LBP), either episodic or recurrent, is an extremely common symptom but only a very small proportion of persons having LBP see a clinician for any episode. In societies where very heavy labor is a necessary component of subsistence living, LBP episodes resulting in an inability to perform heavy labor may threaten basic needs. However, in recent years it has been in industrialized societies that chronic LBP illness has become a major clinical and financial problem. To a great extent, LBP illness is an enigmatic clinical entity. The etiology of LBP is sometimes clear, such as infections, tumors or major trauma, but more often the local pathology is obscure and there often appears to be complex psychological, social or neurophysiological issues predominating the clinical picture.

Clinical evaluation

Most persons with LBP do not seek medical care. The majority of LBP episodes are benign and self-

Clinical Pain Management: A Practical Guide, 1st edition. Edited by Mary E. Lynch, Kenneth D. Craig and Philip W.H. Peng.
© 2011 Blackwell Publishing Ltd.

limited, although minor persistent pain or recurrences are common. In a prospective evaluation of 200 working adults, asymptomatic for LBP at baseline, followed over 5 years, nearly all subjects had at least one LBP episode during the study period [1]. In fact, there were 625 LBP episodes lasting greater than 48 hours reported. Of these only 33 episodes (5%) were evaluated by a clinician. As in usual practice, the overwhelming majority of cases had no diagnosis made and no specific treatment prescribed.

When an initial diagnostic assessment is performed in the acute period (days to several weeks of symptoms), the focus is usually on identifying or "ruling out" serious illness rather than definitively making a pathoanatomic diagnosis. This primary diagnostic evaluation usually involves a screening for "red flags" of serious disease by history and detecting systemic disease, spinal deformity and neurologic signs by examination (Table 27.1). In a large primary care setting (including primary care physical therapists), less than 1% of the 1200 patients newly referred for LBP evaluations had serious pathology [2]. Obviously, in other practices with more frequent and serious underlying diseases, this may be somewhat higher (3–4%).

It is important to clearly differentiate primary back and buttock pain from primary radicular pain (indicated by predominant leg pain, sensory

Table 27.1 Red and yellow flags in the evaluation of low back pain.

Red flags	Yellow flags
Major trauma	Negative attitudes that
New onset age >55 years	back pain is harmful or
Constitutional symptoms	potentially severely
(fever, chills, weight loss)	disabling
Recent infection, IV drug	Fear-avoidance behavior
use, immune	and reduced activity levels
suppression	An expectation that
Severe pain with rest,	passive, rather than active,
night pain	treatment will be
Neurologic weakness or	beneficial
cauda equina symptoms/	A tendency to depression,
signs (bowel, bladder	low morale and social
symptoms, saddle	withdrawal
sensory loss)	Social, financial or
	compensation problems

changes, weakness or bowel and bladder disturbance) because the treatment will be very different. There is rarely any surgical or invasive intervention indicated for back pain syndromes early in the clinical course. Conversely, patients with primary neurological compression syndromes (e.g. radiculopathy from disc herniation or stenosis, neurogenic claudication symptoms and cauda equina symptoms) should be more closely evaluated and effective interventions might be indicated early on or even urgently. The treatment of neurological compression syndromes is beyond the scope of this chapter.

In the patient who does not recover good function in 4–8 weeks, a secondary diagnostic survey is indicated. This follow-on evaluation should identify both serious psychosocial and neurophysiological barriers to recovery ("yellow flags") and also definitely "rule out" those serious pathologic conditions considered initially (Table 27.1). Laboratory testing, erythrocyte sedimentation rate (ESR) or C-reactive protein (CRP) and imaging (most efficiently with a rapid sequence sagittal magnetic resonance scan of the lumbar spine) are extremely sensitive for inflammatory disease, infection, malignancy and insufficiency fracture [3]. These

tests are so sensitive that these serious conditions are usually identified even in the early stages, and very few serious pathologic findings will be missed.

Most commonly, however, only benign degenerative changes are found on evaluation. Because the next phase of treatment is usually non-specific (analgesics, anti-inflammatory medication, conditioning, supportive measures and the expectant passage of time), an anatomic diagnosis of high precision is usually not pursued. It must be emphasized that a failure to report significant recovery by this time is unusual. The clinician must be concerned there are non-spinal issues (e.g. the illnesss is linked to a compensation dispute, is part of a widespread chronic pain illness or is complicated by major depression) that are contributing or predominating this patient's failure to return to usual activities.

In patients who report they are still having troubles that are highly bothersome despite 3–6 months of illness, further anatomic evaluation may be considered. This tertiary diagnostic evaluation may be undertaken if the primary and secondary evaluations have revealed neither serious structural pathology nor significant confounding psychosocial or neurophysiological factors. This examination may include flexion and extension radiographs looking for instability, computed tomography (CT) scan looking for occult facet or pars fractures, pelvic or vascular examination looking for visceral pathology (Table 27.2).

Diagnostic injections (discography, anesthetic facet or sacroiliac joint blockades) are highly controversial. There are no good validation studies to confirm the diagnostic accuracy of these studies nor is there evidence that these procedures improve outcomes [4]. There is consensus in the American Pain Society Guidelines, American College of Occupational and Environmental Medicine Guidelines, Veteran Administration Guideline and the European COST Guidelines that these diagnostics injections have weak or absent supporting evidence or are frankly not recommended. There is some evidence that the use of discography may result in worse outcomes in patients with psychological distress or compensation issues. Clinicians

Table 27.2 Common pathologic findings and implications in patients with persistent low back pain and disability (no radicular symptoms).

Findings	Likelihood of causing symptoms	Course of action
Malignant primary or metastatic tumor	High	Specific to tumor, neurologic risk and spinal stability
Pyogenic or granulomatous osteomyelitis/discitis	High	Specific to infection, neurologic risk and spinal stability
Acute compression fracture	High	Specific to deformity, neurologic risk and spinal stability
Unstable isthmic or degenerative spondylolisthesis	High	Reassurance if neurologically normal and slip is small. Surgical evaluation if highly unstable, neurologic risk
Disc herniation without sciatica	Unclear. Suspect related if massive extruded herniation	Reassurance if small. Surgical evaluation if massive and causing severe stenosis
Scoliosis (>40°) or with rotatory listhesis	Moderate	Specific to deformity, neurologic risk and spinal stability
Reactive endplate changes (massive)	Moderate, associated with instability	Specific local treatment may be indicated (e.g. fusion)
Stable isthmic or degenerative spondylolisthesis	Moderate	Specific local treatment may be indicated (e.g. fusion)
Scoliosis (<15–40°) Schmorl's nodes (isolated) Minor kyphosis	Low	Reassurance, general measures
Scoliosis (<15%)	Extremely low	Reassurance, general measures
Disc degeneration	Extremely low	Reassurance, general measures
Anular fissure	Extremely low	Reassurance, general measures
Facet arthrosis without large cyst or deformity	Extremely low	Reassurance, general measures

utilizing these tests should discuss their risks and limitations frankly with patients.

Trivial findings and the "pseudo-diagnosis"

Too often, as a matter of convenience or poor understanding of common degenerative pathology, patients are given anatomic diagnoses with little supporting evidence (e.g. "discogenic pain" or "facet syndrome"). These diagnoses are often made on the basis of minor facet or disc abnormalities or unvalidated diagnostic injections, but are almost never corroborated (Table 27.2) [4]. These findings are very frequently seen in asymptomatic individuals. Only a small minority of persons with these findings will present with serious LBP.

Attributing a patient's illness to the presence of those anatomic diagnoses with little supporting evidence diverts the attention of the patient and family from other possible causes or contributors of persistent LBP illness. This is particularly true in the patient with multiple chronic pain problems, psychological distress, compensation disputes and substance abuse disorders which frequently complicate the treatment of this condition and are associated with a prolonged clinical course.

Natural history

The natural history of LBP is well described in the literature. Although the lifetime adult prevalence of LBP is estimated to be 80% or greater, the majority of patients eventually have significant recovery. In those patients, however, recurrences are common [3,5,6]. The point prevalence of LBP with some impairment is estimated at 15–30%. Most of these patients will typically have pain lasting less than 6 weeks. However, 10–15% of patients annually report chronic LBP as the duration of the back pain persists longer than 3 months [3]. Not all patients with persistent LBP have serious impairment. Carragee *et al.* [7] reported on a large cohort of subjects with varying degrees of back pain and found that 10% had persistent LBP but denied functional loss, seeking medical care or activity modification. Conversely, few persons reporting no history of LBP on annual surveys will in fact continue without reported back pain when monthly surveys are performed [8]. Thus, it appears many episodes of LBP are poorly recalled and few people go more than 1 year without one or more episodes.

Progression to chronic low back pain

Risk factors for the development of chronic LBP may be categorized into morphologic, demographic, psychosocial and genetic factors. Magnetic resonance imaging (MRI) studies of asymptomatic adults demonstrate herniated discs in up to 70% of subjects, degenerative discs in 50% and annular fissures in 20% [6,9,10]. Multiple MRI studies have failed to demonstrate causality or even high correlations of these common structural abnormalities with chronic LBP [1,9–15]. Only weak associations with LBP progression were demonstrated with the presence of a high intensity zone (HIZ) within the disc, moderate or severe vertebral endplate changes, severe degenerative disc disease and canal stenosis.

Studies of asymptomatic subjects with baseline MRI demonstrated that repeat MRI with a new LBP episode did not commonly discover new or progressive structural changes [10,11,15]. Carragee *et al.* [11] found that 86% of subjects with repeat MRI at mean 6 weeks after a new LBP episode did not demonstrate any new findings other than those associated with aging or a slowly evolving proc-

esses. Furthermore, minor trauma has not been significantly correlated with progression of LBP nor has minor trauma been found to be the cause of clinically significant structural changes on MRI [1].

Of the demographic risk factors predicting progression to chronic LBP, age over 30 years old is consistently associated with development of debilitating chronic LBP [16]. Typically, the incidence of disabling back pain diminishes after age 50. Comparative population studies of low and high income countries demonstrated that populations in affluent countries are 2–4 times more likely to have the diagnosis of LBP, despite the high proportion of low-income populations performing heavy physical labor [17]. In addition, the prevalence of LBP is higher in urban populations than rural populations and those working in enclosed workshops. Employment in jobs in certain areas, such as work in enclosed workshops, manual and psychologically stressful work, is a significant risk factor for reporting occupational disability due to persistent back pain [10,17].

Much research has been dedicated to the interplay of psychological risk factors with progression of chronic LBP. Coexisting depression and anxiety has a significant role in the development of chronic LBP [1,10,18]. Jarvik *et al.* [14] demonstrated that depression was a stronger predictor for chronic LBP, as depressed patients were 2.3 times more likely to have persistent LBP. A review of the scientific literature found strong evidence for psychological distress and depressive mood as predictors for the transition from acute to chronic LBP [18].

Multiple studies pointed to other social or neurophysiological factors, such as chronic non-lumbar pain issues, smoking history and worker's compensation cases, as primary predictors of progression to chronic LBP disability [1,10,18]. These factors were much stronger predictors of LBP persistence than common degenerative structural findings [1]. Minor traumatic events that incited chronic LBP were highly correlated persistence of LBP only when associated with compensation claims [1]. Boos *et al.* [10] found that psychosocial aspects of work, such as physical job characteristics, adverse work influence on personal life and the quality of social support at the workplace, played a more important role in the duration of LBP than MRI identified disc abnormalities.

Multiple genetic factors may contribute to the development of chronic LBP in certain susceptible individuals by affecting the structure of the intervertebral disc, influencing the inflammatory response and abnormally modulating pain perception [19,20]. Genes responsible for the structural integrity of the intervertebral disc may play a part by affecting the rate of disc degeneration. While genetic associations with disc degeneration have been described, association with chronic LBP, per se, has been less clear or absent.

Genetic variations in cytokine genes, specifically the interleukin-1 (IL-1) gene locus may have a role in development of LBP by creating a pro-inflammatory milieu that sensitizes nociceptors innervating the discs and surrounding spinal tissue. Polymorphisms of IL-1α, IL-1β and IL-1 receptor antagonist have been shown to affect bone mineral density and promote degenerative disc disease [21]. Inflammatory mediators such as IL-1, IL-6 and tumor necrosis factor α (TNFα) are key factors in propagating the inflammatory response that may become enhanced and difficult to control with certain genetic polymorphisms.

Treatment of chronic LBP with only common degenerative changes

Treatment of the major structural pathology (e.g. infection, tumor) is disease-specific. However, common degenerative findings themselves seldom account for the totality of the illness observed. It is highly likely that significant psychological, social or neurophysiological factors contribute to the problem and treatment should be directed at the whole person.

Most people with LBP do not seek medical care. Many persons will self-treat with over-the-counter medications and activity modification [1,3,6]. In patients with persistent LBP with only common degenerative findings, reassurances that a serious underlying disease is not present and that the spine is not "fragile" or unstable are critical interventions that are often neglected. The best evidence for treatment indicates a multimodal regimen that includes a psychological support, regular exercise program, weight loss and medications, can be beneficial [3,6]. Cognitive behavioral approaches have been proven more effective than primary pain-directed approaches [3]. Injections, percutaneous interventions and surgery are best indicated for patients with primary radiculopathy, not those with predominant chronic LBP alone.

Pharmacotherapy

There is good evidence that non-steroidal anti-inflammatory drugs (NSAIDs) are effective for chronic LBP but the effect size is very small, not necessarily superior to acetaminophen and it is not proven that one NSAID is superior to others [3,6].

Although non-benzodiazepine muscle relaxants appear useful in patients with acute non-specific back pain, the evidence supporting muscle relaxants for chronic LBP is less convincing [22]. Similarly, opioids may be a reasonable treatment option for acute back injuries, but the evidence supporting their use for chronic LBP is poor. In a meta-analysis examining the role of opioid treatment for chronic LBP, the authors concluded that opioids provided only a "non-significant" reduction in pain scores at the price of very significant risks [23]. In addition, concurrent substance misuse disorders were found in up to 43% of patients receiving opioid treatment for chronic back pain and aberrant medication-taking behavior was reported to range 5–25%. Finally, no analgesic benefit has been found for long-term opioid treatment (>16 weeks).

Tricyclic antidepressants, but not selective serotonin reuptake inhibitors, have been reported to be more effective than placebo for chronic non-specific LBP [3,6,24].

Alternative therapies

Chiropractic and other alternative treatment modalities are frequently used and in some LBP patient subgroups this may exceed 50% utilization rates [6,25,26]. Chou & Huffman [26], in their guidelines by the American College of Physicians and American Pain Society, found fair to good evidence supporting myriad alternative treatments for chronic LBP including acupuncture, yoga, massage and spinal manipulation.

Percutaneous injections, nerve ablation and heating techniques

Unlike for radicular pain processes, percutaneous interventions for LBP alone are poorly supported by available evidence. In patients with suspected facet joint or sacroiliac joint pain, there is very little evidence to support corticosteroid injections, and very weak evidence for radiofrequency denervation [3,4,27].

For suspected "discogenic pain" a variety of intra-discal measures have been suggested but none have proven efficacy. The best evidence available is regarding intradiscal electrothermal therapy (IDET) and this is conflicting. One randomized controlled trial (RCT) showed no benefit. Another RCT conducted in a highly selected patient population (without compensation claims, psychological distress or other comorbidities) showed no benefit in most patients but a small subgroup (20%). A third RCT was discontinued before the study was completed because of the early successes in the placebo group, ensuring a positive effect in the treatment group was unlikely [27].

Surgery

Surgical interventions for LBP secondary to major pathologies such as infections, tumors and fractures are often effective in protecting neurologic structures, preventing deformity and relieving pain. In patients with persistent radiculopathy from common degenerative conditions, surgery can reduce pain and improve function [3,6].

In patients with chronic LBP illness who present with common degenerative changes seen on imaging, surgical interventions (fusion or disc arthroplasty) are less effective. It is not clear that surgical interventions in this group provide a better outcome over a comprehensive rehabilitation program with cognitive behavioral therapy. Only 15–40% of patients can expect a highly functional outcome after surgery when patients are highly selected, excluding those with psychological problems, compensation issues or other comorbidities [3,6]. In patients with abnormal psychological testing, fusion is extremely unlikely to result in meaningful functional improvement.

Conclusions

Chronic LBP represents a large spectrum of disorders, ranging from minimal to severe disability. In the absence of serious pathologic findings (e.g. fracture, tumor, instability), serious reported disability is usually associated with psychological, social or neurophysiological comorbidities. The presence of multiple chronic pain problems, psychological distress, compensation disputes and substance abuse disorders frequently complicate the treatment of this condition and are associated with a prolonged clinical course. Specific spinal treatments are most effective when clear pathological causes are found. Treatment efforts directed at the whole person with a cognitive behavioral approach are most effective in patients in whom only common degenerative changes are found and comorbid psychosocial or pain processes are found.

References

1 Carragee E, Alamin T, Cheng I *et al.* (2006) Does minor trauma cause serious low back illness? *Spine* **31(25)**:2942–9.

2 Henschke N, Maher CG, Refshauge KM *et al.* (2009) Prevalence of and screening for serious spinal pathology in patients presenting to primary care settings with acute low back pain. *Arthritis Rheum* **60(10)**:3072–80.

3 Carragee EJ. (2005) Clinical practice: persistent low back pain. *N Engl J Med* **352(18)**:1891–8.

4 Chou R, Loeser JD, Owens DK *et al.* (2009) Interventional therapies, surgery, and interdisciplinary rehabilitation for low back pain: an evidence-based clinical practice guideline from

the American Pain Society. *Spine* **34(10)**: 1066–77.

5 Andersson GB. (1998) Epidemiology of low back pain. *Acta Orthop Scand Suppl* **281**:28–31.

6 Cohen SP, Argoff CE, Carragee EJ. (2008) Management of low back pain. *Br Med J* **337**:a2718.

7 Carragee EJ, Alamin TF, Miller J *et al.* (2002) Provocative discography in volunteer subjects with mild persistent low back pain. *Spine J* **2**:25–34.

8 Carragee EJ, Cohen SP. (2008) Life-time asymptomatic for back pain: a study of the validity of this back pain subgroup in soldiers. *Spine* **34(9)**:978–83.

9 Jarvik JG, Deyo RA. (2002) Diagnostic evaluation of low back pain with emphasis on imaging. *Ann Intern Med* **137(7)**:586–97.

10 Boos N, Semmer N, Elfering A *et al.* (2000) Natural history of individuals with asymptomatic disc abnormalities in magnetic resonance imaging: predictors of low back pain-related medical consultation and work incapacity. *Spine (Phila Pa 1976)* **25(12)**: 1484–92.

11 Borenstein DG, O'Mara JW Jr, Boden SD *et al.* (2001) The value of magnetic resonance imaging of the lumbar spine to predict low-back pain in asymptomatic subjects: a seven-year follow-up study. *J Bone Joint Surg Am* **83-A**:1306–11.

12 Carragee E, Alamin T, Cheng I *et al.* (2006) Are first-time episodes of serious LBP associated with new MRI findings? *Spine J* **6(6)**:624–35.

13 Carragee EJ, Alamin TF, Miller JL *et al.* (2005) Discographic, MRI and psychosocial determinants of low back pain disability and remission: a prospective study in subjects with benign persistent back pain. *Spine J* **5(1)**:24–35.

14 Jarvik JG, Hollingworth W, Heagerty PJ *et al.* (2005) Three-year incidence of low back pain in an initially asymptomatic cohort: clinical and imaging risk factors. *Spine (Phila Pa 1976)* **30(13)**:1541–8.

15 Carragee EJ, Barcohana B, Alamin T *et al.* (2004) Prospective controlled study of the development of lower back pain in previously asymptomatic subjects undergoing experimental discography. *Spine (Phila Pa 1976)* **29(10)**: 1112–7.

16 Deyo RA, Weinstein JN. (2001) Low back pain. *N Engl J Med* **344(5)**:363–70.

17 Volinn E. (1997) The epidemiology of low back pain in the rest of the world: a review of surveys in low- and middle-income countries. *Spine (Phila Pa 1976)* **22(15)**:1747–54.

18 Pincus T, Vogel S, Burton AK *et al.* (2006) Fear avoidance and prognosis in back pain: a systematic review and synthesis of current evidence. *Arthritis Rheum* **54(12)**:3999–4010.

19 Battié MC, Videman T, Parent E. (2004) Lumbar disc degeneration: epidemiology and genetic influences. *Spine (Phila Pa 1976)* **29(23)**: 2679–90.

20 Tegeder I, Lötsch J. (2009) Current evidence for a modulation of low back pain by human genetic variants. *J Cell Mol Med* **13**:1605–19.

21 Takahashi M, Haro H, Wakabayashi Y *et al.* (2001) The association of degeneration of the intervertebral disc with 5a/6a polymorphism in the promoter of the human matrix metalloproteinase-3 gene. *J Bone Joint Surg Br* **83(4)**:491–5.

22 Van Tulder MW, Touray T, Furlan AD *et al.*; *Cochrane Back Review Group.* (2003) Muscle relaxants for nonspecific low back pain: a systematic review within the framework of the cochrane collaboration. *Spine (Phila Pa 1976)* **1**:1978–92.

23 Martell BA, O'Connor PG, Kerns RD *et al.* (2007) Systematic review. Opioid treatment for chronic back pain: prevalence, efficacy, and association with addiction. *Ann Intern Med* **146**:116–27.

24 Staiger TO, Gaster B, Sullivan MD *et al.* (2003) Systematic review of antidepressants in the treatment of chronic low back pain. *Spine* **28**:2540–5.

25 Cherniack EP, Ceron-Fuentes J, Florez H *et al.* (2008) Influence of race and ethnicity on alternative medicine as a self-treatment preference for common medical conditions in a population of multi-ethnic urban elderly. *Complement Ther Clin Pract* **14**:116–23.

26 Chou R, Huffman LH. (2007) Nonpharmacologic therapies for acute and chronic low back pain: a review of the evidence for an American Pain Society/American College of Physicians clinical practice guideline. *Ann Intern Med* **147**: 492–504.

27 Urrútia G, Kovacs F, Nishishinya MB *et al.* (2007) Percutaneous thermocoagulation intradiscal techniques for discogenic low back pain. *Spine (Phila Pa 1976)* **32(10)**:1146–54.

Chapter 28

Fibromyalgia syndrome and myofascial pain syndromes

Winfried Häuser[1], Marcus Schiltenwolf[2] & Peter Henningsen[3]

[1] Department Internal Medicine I and Interdisciplinary Center of Pain Medicine, Klinikum Saarbrücken, Germany
[2] Universität Heidelberg, Stiftung Orthopädische Universitätsklinik, Heidelberg, Germany
[3] Department of Psychosomatic Medicine and Psychotherapy, Technische Universität München, Germany

Introduction

Musculoskeletal pain is the most prevalent type of pain occurring in the general population and in clinical samples. Musculoskeletal pain can be classified as local (one pain site), regional (several pain sites in one body region) or widespread. Widespread pain can be described as either as pain occurring axially or in all four extremities, or pain present on both sides of the body, above and below the waist.

Only a minority of musculoskeletal pain syndromes are caused by specific organ damage. The most frequent non-specific local and regional chronic musculoskeletal pain condition is myofascial pain syndrome (MPS), and the most frequent widespread pain condition is fibromyalgia syndrome (FMS). For patients not meeting the diagnostic criteria for FMS completely it is suggested the term chronic widespread pain (CWP) be used.

The presented recommendations on the management of FMS are derived from the interdisciplinary

German guideline on the classification, pathophysiology and management of FMS [1], the guideline on the management of FMS of the US American Pain Society [2] and a Canadian interdisciplinary consensus document [3]. The recommendations on the management of MPS are based on two narrative reviews [4,5] and on the Canadian Concil of Chiropractic Guidelines [6].

Definition and classification

According to the criteria of the American College of Rheumatology (ACR), FMS is defined as chronic (>3 months) widespread pain (including pain on both sides of the body, above and below the waist, and axial pain) and tenderness on manual palpation in at least 11 out of 18 defined tender points. Other key symptoms of FMS are physical and mental fatigue and non-restorative sleep. Depending on the criteria used and the setting of the studies, 30–80% of comorbid mental disorders (affective and anxiety disorders, post-traumatic stress disorder) and 20–80% of other functional somatic syndromes (e.g. irritable bowel syndrome, functional dyspepsia, tension headache, temporomandibular disorder) can be diagnosed. Because the ACR criteria do not require the exclusion of somatic diseases sufficiently explaining CWP in

Clinical Pain Management: A Practical Guide, 1st edition.
Edited by Mary E. Lynch, Kenneth D. Craig and Philip W.H. Peng.
© 2011 Blackwell Publishing Ltd.

inflammatory rheumatoid disorders (e.g. rheumatoid arthritis, Sjögren's syndrome, systemic lupus erythematosus) "fibromyalgia" can be diagnosed in 20–60% of patients with inflammatory rheumatoid disorders [7].

FMS is not a distinct nosological entity like a myocardial infarction. Symptoms of FMS are more like other continuous medical variables such as blood pressure or coronary sclerosis for which clinically relevant limits have been defined to differentiate normal from borderline and pathological conditions. Within this context FMS can be conceptualized as a cluster at the end of a continuum of distress caused by somatic (mainly pain and physical fatigue) and psychological (mainly sleeping and cognitive problems) symptoms. The tender point criterion leads to a preponderance of women. FMS is not a homogenous disorder, but a complex of various symptoms; patients differ in disability, coping, associated psychosocial conflicts and mental comorbidities.

The term "fibromyalgia syndrome" is preferable to "fibromyalgia," because the definition of FMS according to the ACR criteria is based on a combination of symptoms (CWP) and clinical findings (tenderness).

Myofascial pain syndrome (MPS) is defined as the sum of symptoms associated with an active myofascial trigger point (MTrP) (Table 28.1). An active MTrP causes spontaneous pain at rest with an increase in pain on contraction or stretching of the muscle involved. A latent MTrP is a focal area of tenderness and tightness in the muscle that does not result in spontaneous pain. Active MTrPs may have a role in patients with FMS, tension headache, neck and low back pain, temporomandibular disorders, extremity pain (shoulder, hip, limp), abominal and thoracic and pelvic/urogenital pain syndromes.

Prevalence

The prevalence of CWP and FMS in the general adult population range 10–26% and 0.7–3.3%, respectively. The sex ratio of women to men in CWP is 1–1.5 : 1, in FMS 2–21 : 1 [8]. Most patients with FMS are 40–60 years old, but CWP and FMS can also be diagnosed in children and adolescents.

There are no data on the prevalence and sex ratio of MPS in representative samples of the general population available. In clinical samples MPS prevails in women and those of middle age.

There are few data available on the comorbidity of FMS and MPS. Of patients diagnosed with MPS 18–40% also met the ACR criteria of FMS and in up to 75% of patients with FMS an MPS could be diagnosed.

Course and prognosis

A review of longitudinal studies on the natural course of FMS demonstrated that the symptoms of FMS persist in the long term in nearly all patients. Some patients adapt to the symptoms and the associated restrictions and report a better long-term satisfaction with their health status. FMS is not associated with a reduced life expectancy.

There are no longitudinal studies available on MPS. From clinical experience some MPS might remit spontaneously or resolve with appropriate correction of predisposing factors and therapy. MPS that has been present for longer than 6 months or has followed a chronic relapsing course tends to continue in this fashion. Local MPS can spread to a regional chronic pain syndrome or to CWP and/or FMS.

Table 28.1 The characteristics of a myofascial trigger point [4,5].

Focal point of tenderness to palpation in the muscle involved
Reproduction of pain complaint by trigger point palpation (about 3 kg pressure)
Palpation reveals an induration of the adjacent muscle ("taut band")
Restricted range of the muscle involved
Often pseudo-weakness of the muscle involved without atrophy
Often referred pain on continued pressure over trigger point

Diagnosis of fibromyalgia syndrome

History taking

A pain diagram helps to identify patients with CWP. Some patients report "pain all over." The site of maximum pain changes frequently in most patients. Most patients report a high affective component of pain (agonizing, terrible). Pain is usually aggravated by hard or repetitive physical exercise, psychological stress, wet and cold and can be ameliorated by heat and rest. Other key symptoms (fatigue, sleep disturbances) should be actively explored. Patients should be screened for symptoms of other functional somatic syndroms and mental disorders as well as current psychosocial stressors. Moreover, restrictions of daily activities should be explored. Finally, all types of medication used by the patient should be assessed because arthralgia, myalgia and fatigue can also be side effects of medication. Misuse of medication should be actively explored.

Physical examination

There is an ongoing debate on the utility of the tender point examination for the clinical diagnosis of FMS. The original ACR criteria had been primarily developed for the classification of FMS to identify a group of patients with similar clinical features for future systematic studies. Their practicability and validity for clinical diagnosis had never been tested outside a rheumatological setting. Nevertheless, a history of CWP > 3 months and the finding of tenderness of at least 11 of 18 tender points with manual palpation using approximately 4 kg pressure have become the gold standard of FMS diagnosis in clinical studies. The use of tender point examination for clinical diagnosis has been criticized for the following reasons. A cutoff of 11 positive tender points is arbitrary. The tender point count has been shown to be influenced by the interaction between patient and examiner and is highly correlated with distress. Despite efforts to standardize the procedure such as the manual tender point survey it has not been shown to be reproducible across different clinical settings. It is a poor marker of change in clinical studies. Most non-rheumatologists are reluctant to use the tender point examination because of the time spent and of lacking training in tender point examination during residency. Recently the ACR have published preliminary diagnostic criteria for fibromyalgia that do not use tenderpoint examination and rely on the widespread pain index (WPI) and symptom severity scale (SS). The WPI is essentially a count of the number of sites of pain and the SS consists of 0–3 point scale of severity of symptoms of fatigue, waking unrefreshed, and cognitive symptoms [9].

Irrespective of whether a tender point examination is performed, a complete physical examination including orthopedic and neurological examination is recommended to reveal signs of internal, bone and joint or neurological disorders mimicking the key symptoms of FMS.

Questionnaires

The use of standardized somatic symptom scales and questionnaires such as the Brief Pain Inventory [10], the Fibromyalgia Impact Questionnaire [11] or the Patient Health Questionnaire [12] can be considered.

Blood tests and diagnostic imaging

The following routine blood tests are recommended for the initial evaluation of patients with CWP (potential differential diagnoses are indicated in parentheses):

1 Blood sedimentation rate, C-reactive protein, red and white cell blood count (polymyalgia rheumatica, rheumatoid arthritis);

2 Creatinin kinase (muscle disease);

3 Calcium (hypercalcemia);

4 Thyroid-stimulating hormone (hypothyroidism);

5 Depending on history and examination further blood tests may be necessary if other differential diagnoses are suspected.

Without cinical signs, routine testing for antibodies associated with inflammatory rheumatoid diseases is not recommended. If no other diseases are suspected on clinical grounds, which require imaging studies for diagnosis such as joint diseases,

X-rays or other diagnostic imaging studies are not recommended.

Final diagnosis

Three defined diagnostic schemes are available:

• *ACR 1990 classification criteria:* CWP and tenderness on palpation of at least 11 of 18 tender points [13].

• *Survey criteria:* FMS is diagnosed by a questionnaire, the Regional Pain Scale (RPS), if the patient indicates pain in at least 11 of 19 pain sites and reports a fatigue score ≥6 on an 11-point visual analog scale [14].

• *ACR diagnostic 2010 criteria:* WPI >7 and SS >5 or WPI 3–6 AND SS >9 and exclusion of a somatic disease sufficiently explaining the pain [9].

• *Interdisciplinary German guideline symptom-based criteria:* all of the following four symptoms > 3 months must be present: (1) widespread pain; (2) physical and/or mental fatigue or non-restorative sleep and/or sleep disturbances; (3) sensations of stiffness and/or swelling in the hands and/or the feet and/or the face; and (4) exclusion of somatic diseases sufficiently explaining CWP. Inactive somatic diseases such as inflammatory rheumatoid disorder in remission or low disease activity or any mental disorder does not exclude the diagnosis of FMS [1].

Patients not meeting these criteria completely should be diagnosed with CWP.

Diagnosis of myofascial pain syndrome

History taking

Patients with MPS report a deep aching sensation, often with a feeling of stiffness in the involved area. Pain is aggravated by the use of involved muscles, psychological stress, cold and postural imbalance. Radiation from a trigger point can be described in terms of paresthesiae. MTrP activity may lead to the development of various autonomic changes such as lacrimation, regional excessive coldness or vertigo. Motor dysfunction includes restricted range, local weakness, reduced coordination and spasms in other muscles. In long-lasting myofascial pain general weakness, reduced work tolerance, fatigue and sleep disturbances are reported.

Physical examination

The usual recommendations for identifying a trigger point specify that gentle palpation should be performed across the direction of the muscle fibers in order to identify a longitudinal region of nodularity (i.e. the taut band). When the palpating finger is snapped around the taut band, a local contraction of the muscle may be obeserved in superficial muscles or felt by the examiner in deep muscles (i.e. the twitch response). Firm pressure over the taut band is painful and reproduces the patient's pain complaint. Continous pressure > 5 seconds may reproduce the pattern of referred pain. Neighboring joints should be examined by assessing range of movement and articular pain.

The data on the diagnostic reliability of these findings between experienced and non-experienced observers in studies are mixed. A poor discrimination of patients diagnosed with FMS and MPS was found by manual palpation [15].

Blood tests and diagnostic imaging

Blood tests and diagnostic imaging are not necessary for the diagnosis or exclusion of a MPS. In case of lacking rapid response to treatment, the exclusion of a borderline hypothyroidism or nutritional inadequacies can be considered.

Final diagnosis

There are no well-validated diagnostic criteria for the identification of an MTrP. The four most commonly applied criteria in clinical studies were: "tender spot in a taut band" of skeletal muscle, "patient pain recognition," "predicted pain referral pattern" and "local twitch response."

Basic mechanisms

Risk factors

Risk factors for CWP/FMS identified by longitudinal population-based studies are as follows [7]:

- *Biological:* family aggregation;
- *Psychological:* occupational psychological stressors, depressed mood, tendency to report somatic symptoms;
- *Social:* low class index, occupational mechanical burdens.

An adequate physical activity level and coping strategies adjustments to limited physical abilities and distraction from symptoms are associated with a good long-term prognosis.

The following factors are commonly cited but not proved by cross-sectional or longitudinal studies to predispose to MTrP: deconditioning, poor posture, repetitive mechanical stress, physical trauma, mechanical imbalance, muscle wasting or ischemia, visceral referred pain, joint disorders, vitamin deficiencies, non-restorative sleep, clima (damp, draughts, excessive cold or heat) and psychological stressors [4,5].

Pathophysiology

Several potential pathophysiological mechanisms in FMS have been described, but their causal relationship is unclear because of the cross-sectional nature of all these studies. Potential mechanisms include central nervous system pain processing abnormalities, hyporeactivity of the hypothalamus-pituitary-adrenal (HPA) axis, and disturbances in the dopaminergic and serotonergic systems; however, alterations of cytokines were proved to be epiphenomenal. At present, consistent or specific structural or biochemical abnormalities in the muscles or tender points of FMS patients have not been demonstrated. The biopsychosocial model of FMS postulates that there is heterogeneity in the genetic and psychological predispositions as well as in the vegetative, endocrine and central nervous system reactions. Different etiological factors and pathophysiological mechanisms lead to a common pathway of symptomatology currently classified as FMS [7].

The key pathophysiological abnormalities associated with MTrPs appear to be principally located at the center of a muscle in its motor endplate zone. Histological, biochemical and electromyographic abnormalities in trigger points have been

reported but these findings were not specific or require reproduction by other studies [16]. Active MTrPs may serve as one of the sources of noxious input leading to the sensitization of spinal and supraspinal pain pathways in FMS [17].

Impact of basic understanding on clinical management

Effective pharmacotherapy of FMS includes medications that inhibit pronociceptive input and augment modulatory signaling. Antidepressants are presumed to act on noradrenergic and serotonergic neurons that are implicated in the mediation of endogenous pain inhibitory mechanisms. Structural analogs of the neurotransmitter gamma-aminobutyric acid (GABA) are presumed to diminish the release of several neurotransmitters, including glutamate and substance P. Psychotherapy aims to reduce dysfunctional coping such as catastrophizing and fear-avoidance beliefs as well to resolve emotional or interpersonal conflicts and to improve attachment patterns. Aerobic exercise helps to restore physical working capacity and to promote self-efficacy.

In FMS and MPS physical therapies such as balneotherapy (bathing in warm or cold water or mud) and spatherapy (bathing in thermal or mineral water) may reduce muscle tension and increase the pain threshold in the nerve endings. Heat and hydrostatic pressure of water and these stimuli could decrease the pain sensation.

Needling and ischemic pressure in MPS might work through sensory stimulation as well as through mechanical disruptions.

Treatment of fibromyalgia syndrome

General principles of management of fibromyalgia syndrome

Self-management

At present FMS cannot be cured by any therapy. Even patients defined as responders in studies still report substantially elevated symptom scores and disability at the end of treatment. The aims of therapy therefore are the preservation or improvement of daily functioning and management of symptoms and disabilities. Management of symptoms includes both the acceptance of symptoms and of some limitations (e.g. hard physical work) as well as continous self-management (e.g. moderate aerobic exercise).

Collaborative therapy

The patient should be fully informed about the potential benefits and harms of any therapy. The choice of treatment options should be based on the impact of the key symptoms, patients' comorbidities, individual relevance of potential side effects and preferences and the availability of local resources. The harms and benefits of any therapy should be evaluated regularly by patient and physician.

Interventions strongly supported by evidence

Evidence regarding the most frequently used treatments of FMS is summarized in Table 28.2. Of the pharmacological treatments, only duloxetine, milnacipran and pregabalin were recently approved by the US Food and Drug Administration for the use in FMS in the USA, but not by the European Medicines Agency for use in Europe.

It is important to note that there are different effects of pharmacological and non-pharmacological treatments on the key symptoms of FMS. Systematic reviews with meta-analysis found significant and substantial (standardized mean difference > 0.2) effects on fatigue using aerobic exercise, amitriptyline, balneotherapy and multicomponent therapy; and on sleep using amitriptyline, duloxetine and pregabalin. Most studies on pharmacotherapy were limited to periods of 6 months or less. Positive effects were found for aerobic exercise on mood and aerobic exercise and multicomponent therapy on physical fitness at follow-ups. The evidence is limited to adult patients without severe physical (including rheumatic disorder) and mental disorder, except duloxetine was found to be effective for patients with comorbid major depression [18–24].

Table 28.2 Evidence of treatments for adult fibromyalgia syndrome.

Interventions strongly supported by evidence (systematic reviews including at least four RCTs with consistent results)	Aerobic exercise Amitriptyline Balneotherapy and spatherapy* Cognitive and cognitive behavioral therapy Cyclobenzaprine Duloxetine Hypnotherapy/guided imagery Milnacipran Multicomponent treatment programs Pregabalin
Interventions supported by evidence (at least two RCTs with consistent results)	Fluoxetine Homeopathy Paroxetine Sodium oxybate Tramadol with and without acetaminophen Vegetarian diet
Commonly used interventions currently unproven (only RCTs with low quality, RCTs with conflicting results or no RCT available)	Acetaminophen Acupuncture Lidocaine infusions Lymph drainage Massage Metamizol Muscle relaxants other than cyclobenzaprine Osteopathy Qigong Psychodynamic therapy Tender point injections Written emotional disclosure
Interventions strongly refuted by evidence (systematic reviews with at least two RCTs with negative results)	Anxiolytics Biofeedback as single intervention Citalopram Corticosteroids Neuroleptics Non-steroidal agents Patient education as single intervention Relaxation therapy as single intervention

RCT, randomized controlled trial.
* Balneotherapy (bathing in warm water or mud); spatherapy (bathing in thermal or mineral water).

There is moderate evidence that the most frequently used drug class in FMS, non-steroidal anti-inflammatory agents, are not effective. Furthermore, a systematic review found randomized controlled trials with negative results for anxiolytics, corticosteroids and neuroleptics. There is limited evidence for the efficacy of tramadol with and without acetaminophen. No controlled studies have been performed with other opioids [25]. Verum as well as placebo acupuncture have large effects for pain reduction. The small effect of verum compared with placebo acupuncture cannot clearly be distinguished from bias [26]. The evidence for the efficacy of other complementary therapies such as homeopathy is limited and inconsistent [27].

Because of the negative impact of comorbid mental disorders on FMS, anxiety and depressive disorders should be treated (Chapters 24 and 41).

Any pharmacological therapy as well as aerobic exercise should be started at a low level and increased slowly. The final recommended level of aerobic exercise (e.g. aquatic jogging, walking, cycling) is 2–3 times a week for 30 minutes at a moderate intensity (60–75% of the age-adjusted maximum heart rate [210 per min]) [18].

A stepwise treatment approach to fibromyalgia syndrome

A graded treatment approach is recommended (Figure 28.1). The following issues should be kept in mind: FMS cannot be cured and does not lead to reduced life expectancy. The order of the recommended treatment approaches can be changed according to patients' preferences and local availabilities. A combination of pharmacological and non-pharmacological therapies is appropriate. It is unknown whether a combination of pharmacological agents with different effects on the key symptoms of FMS will improve the outcome.

Treatment of myofascial pain syndrome

A systematic qualitative review demonstrated that "wet" and "dry" needling of MTrPs reduce pain

and that botulinum toxin does not offer any advantage over saline or local anesthetic [6]. A systematic qualitative review concluded that botulinum toxin A is not effective in pain relief for MPS [28]. Verum as well as placebo acupuncture are effective for short-term pain relief in temporomandibular disorder (TMD). Verum and placebo acupuncture are effective for short-term pain relief in TMD [29]. Low dose benzodiazepines proved superior to placebo in the majority of studies in TMD, but are not suitable for lengthy treatment because of the risk of dependence [30]. For other evidence-based treatments see Table 28.3.

Because of inadequate data on the long-term course of FMS and on long-term effects of therapies in MPS an algorithm of therapy is challenging; however, Figure 28.1 presents a suggested working algorithm for fibromyalgia based on current evidence.

Conclusions

In summary, FMS and MPS are the most common musculoskeletal pain conditions and are associated

Table 28.3 Evidence of treatments for myofascial pain syndromes.

Interventions strongly supported by evidence (systematic reviews including at least four RCTs with consistent results)	Needling with and without injection (saline, local anesthetic) Laser therapy Manual therapies (manipulation, ischemic pressure)
Interventions supported by evidence (at least two RCTs with consistent results)	Magnet therapy Frequency modulated neural stimulation (FREMS) High-voltage galvanic stimulation (HGVS) Interferential current
Commonly used interventions currently unproven (only one RCT with low quality, RCTs with conflicting results or no RCT available)	Local injections with botulinum toxin Pharmacological treatment Ultrasound

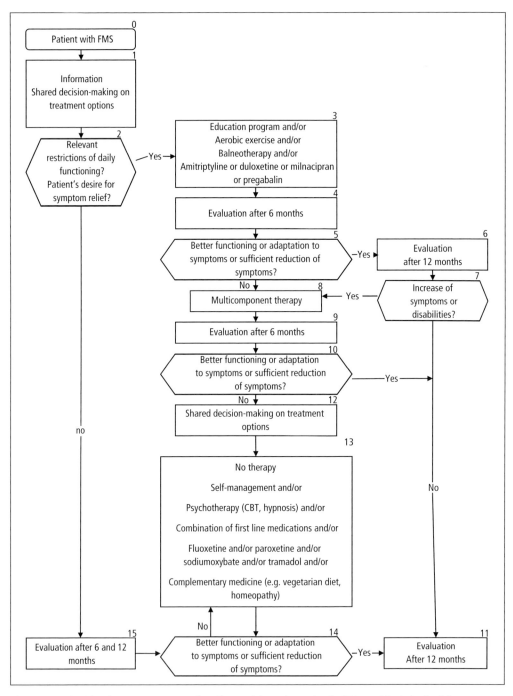

Figure 28.1 Algorithm for treatment approach to fibromyalgia syndrome (FMS). CBT, cognitive behavioral therapy.

with significant suffering and associated disability. Consequently, it is very important to assist patients with these conditions. As with other conditions causing chronic pain, a biopsychosocial approach is required. There is strong evidence for the efficacy of aerobic exercise, balneotherapy, multidisciplinary therapy (exercise and psychological therapy) and specific pharmacological agents (amitriptyline, duloxetine, milnacipran, pregabalin) in reducing some of the key symptoms of FMS. There is also strong evidence for short-term pain relief in MPS by needling and laser therapy; however, further research is required in order to determine the role for these treatments in the long term.

References

1 Häuser W, Eich W, Herrmann M et al. (2009) Fibromyalgia syndrome: classification, diagnosis, and treatment. Dtsch Arztebl Int **106**: 383–91.

2 Burckhardt CS, Goldenberg D, Crofford L et al. (2005) Guideline for the Management of Fibromyalgia Syndrome: Pain in Adults and Children. APS Clinical Practice Guideline Series No. 4. American Pain Society, Glenview, IL.

3 Jain AK, Carruthers BM, van de Sande MI et al. (2004) Fibromyalgia syndrome: Canadian clinical working case definition, diagnostic and treatment protocols – a consensus document. J Musculoskeletal Pain **11**:3–107.

4 Bennett R. (2007) Myofascial pain syndromes and their evaluation. Best Pract Res Clin Rheumatol **21**:427–45.

5 Cummings M, Baldry P. (2007) Regional myofascial pain: diagnosis and management. Best Pract Res Clin Rheumatol **21**:367–87.

6 Vernon H, Schneider M. (2009) Chiropractic management of myofascial trigger points and myofascial pain syndromes: a systematic review of the literature. J Manipul Physiol Ther **32**:14–25.

7 Sommer C, Häuser W, Gerhold K et al. (2008) Etiology and pathophysiology of fibromyalgia syndrome and chronic widespread pain. Schmerz **22**:267–82. [In German]

8 Gran JT. (2003) The epidemiology of chronic generalized musculoskeletal pain. Best Pract Res Clin Rheumatol **17**:547–61.

9 Wolfe F, Clauw DJ, Fitzcharles MA et al. (2010) The American College of Rheumatology Preliminary Diagnostic Criteria for Fibromyalgia and Measurement of Symptom Severity. Arthritis Care Res **62(5)**:600–10.

10 Cleeland CS, Ryan KM. (1994) Pain assessment: global use of the Brief Pain Inventory. Ann Acad Med Singapore **23**:129–38.

11 Bennett RM, Friend R, Jones KD et al. (2009) The Revised Fibromyalgia Impact Questionnaire (FIQR): validation and psychometric properties. Arthritis Res Ther **11**:R120.

12 Kroenke K, Spitzer RL, Williams JB et al. (2009) An ultra-brief screening scale for anxiety and depression: the PHQ-4. Psychosomatics **50**: 613–21.

13 Wolfe F, Smythe HA, Yunus MB et al. (1990) The American College of Rheumatology criteria for the classification of fibromyalgia: report of the multicenter criteria committee. Arthritis Rheum **33**:160–72.

14 Wolfe F. (2003) Pain extent and diagnosis: development and validation of the regional pain scale in 12 995 patients. J Rheumatol **30**:369–78.

15 Lucas N, Macaskill P, Irwig L et al. (2009) Reliability of physical examination for diagnosis of myofascial trigger points: a systematic review of the literature. Clin J Pain **25**:80–9.

16 Basford JR, An KN. (2009) New techniques for the quantification of fibromyalgia and myofascial pain. Curr Pain Headache Rep **13**: 376–813.

17 Ge HY, Nie H, Madeleine P et al. (2009) Contribution of the local and referred pain from active myofascial trigger points in fibromyalgia syndrome. Pain **147**:233–40.

18 Busch AJ, Schachter CL, Overend TJ et al. (2008) Exercise for fibromyalgia: a systematic review. J Rheumatol **35**:1130–44.

19 Häuser W, Bernardy K, Üceyler N et al. (2009) Treatment of fibromyalgia syndrome with antidepressants: a meta-analysis. JAMA **301**: 98–209.

20 Häuser W, Bernardy K, Üceyler N *et al.* (2009) Treatment of fibromyalgia syndrome with gabapentin and pregabalin: a meta-analysis of randomized controlled trials. *Pain* **145**: 169–81.

21 Häuser W, Petzke F, Sommer C. (2010) Systematic review: comparative efficacy and harms of duloxetine, milnacipran and pregabalin in fibromyalgia syndrome. *J Pain* **11(6)**: 505–21.

22 Häuser W, Bernardy K, Offenbächer M *et al.* (2009) Efficacy of multicomponent treatment in fibromyalgia syndrome: a meta-analysis of randomized controlled clinical trials. *Arthritis Rheum* **61**:216–24.

23 Thieme K, Gracely RH. (2009) Are psychological treatments effective for fibromyalgia pain? *Curr Rheumatol Rep* **11**:443–50.

24 Langhorst J, Klose P, Musial F *et al.* (2009) Efficacy of hydrotherapy in fibromyalgia syndrome: a meta-analysis of randomized controlled clinical trials. *Rheumatology* **48**:1155–9.

25 Sommer C, Häuser W, Berliner M *et al.* (2008) Pharmacological treatment of fibromyalgia syndrome. *Schmerz* **22**:313–23. [In German]

26 Langhorst J, Klose P, Musial F *et al.* (2010) Efficacy of acupuncture in fibromyalgia syndrome: a systematic review with a meta-analysis of controlled clinical trials. *Rheumatology (Oxford)* **49(4)**:778–88.

27 Baranowsky J, Klose P, Musial F *et al.* (2009) Qualitative systemic review of randomized controlled trials on complementary and alternative medicine treatments in fibromyalgia. *Rheumatol Int* **30(1)**:1–21.

28 Ho KY, Tan KH. (2007) Botulinum toxin A for myofascial trigger point injection: a qualitative systematic review. *Eur J Pain* **11**:519–27.

29 La Touche R, Angulo-Díaz-Parreño S, de-la-Hoz JL *et al.* (2010) Effectiveness of acupuncture in the treatment of temporomandibular disorders of muscular origin: a systematic review of the last decade. *J Altern Complement Med* **16(1)**:107–12.

30 Hersh EV, Balasubramaniam R, Pinto A.(2008) Pharmacologic management of temporomandibular disorders. *Oral Maxillofac Surg Clin North Am* **20**:197–210.

Chapter 29

Clinical pain management in the rheumatic diseases

Mary-Ann Fitzcharles

Montreal General Hospital Pain Center, Montreal General Hospital, McGill University, Montreal, Canada; Division of Rheumatology, McGill University, Montreal, Canada

Introduction

Rheumatic diseases include inflammatory arthritis (IA) of which rheumatoid arthritis (RA) is the most common degenerative arthritis, which includes peripheral and spinal osteoarthritis (OA), and the spectrum of soft tissue rheumatic complaints of tendonitis and bursitis [1]. Fibromyalgia, previously considered to be a soft tissue process, should no longer be classified as a rheumatic condition, as evidence points to dysregulation of pain-processing mechanisms and a neurologically based pathogenesis. The most common presenting symptom of each of these conditions is pain, with indications that rheumatic pain complaints are threefold greater today than 40 years ago. A further increase in musculoskeletal pain can be anticipated in the future because of the aging of the population and more OA of peripheral and spinal joints [2].

Rheumatic pain, the most prevalent pain syndrome worldwide, is the leading cause of disability in the USA, and will be experienced by almost all persons at some time during their lifetime [1]. Some form of arthritis currently affects at least 50% of individuals over the age of 65 years, with doctor-diagnosed arthritis present in more than 21% of

Clinical Pain Management: A Practical Guide, 1st edition.
Edited by Mary E. Lynch, Kenneth D. Craig and Philip W.H. Peng.
© 2011 Blackwell Publishing Ltd.

adults at any one time. Back pain is probably the most ubiquitous arthritic pain syndrome with a positive response in over 80% of individuals for lifetime pain.

As there is no imminent cure for either IA or OA, the pain associated with these conditions will continue to require attention. As with other painful conditions, rheumatic pain has important negative consequences to overall health with impaired quality of life and poor functional outcome. Therefore healthcare professionals should be sensitive to the complaint of pain in patients with arthritis and soft tissue rheumatism, and should assess and treat pain in parallel with management of the underlying disease.

Basic mechanisms in rheumatic pain

Rheumatic pain has previously been categorized as predominantly nociceptive. This concept is based on the premise that a primary inflammatory process initiates the pain message, which is conducted via first order sensory neurons through relays in the dorsal horn to the somatosensory cortex. However, recent study has demonstrated the presence of associated neurogenic mechanisms in rheumatic pain [3].

In the context of a purely nociceptive pathogenesis, treatments were previously focused on use of non-steroidal anti-inflammatory drugs (NSAIDs) and simple analgesics. Now that neurogenic mechanisms are also invoked, the scope of treatment options will broaden to include stronger analgesics and possibly adjuvant agents such as anticonvulsants, antidepressants and others.

Anatomic considerations

With the exception of healthy cartilage, all joint structures are richly innervated with sensory neurons, which can mediate the pain response [3]. Under normal circumstances, the structures of the joint are not sensitive to strong pressure or even vigorous movement. In contrast, diseased joints that have been primed by inflammatory molecules, develop sensitivity to seemingly benign movements, and have a low threshold of activation to noxious stimuli.

Pathogenic mechanisms in IA and OA show considerable similarities with both demonstrating variable degrees of inflammation and structural tissue damage. IA has a more pronounced inflammatory phase than OA, with synovial infiltration of immune cells, leading to invasion of ligaments, cartilage and bone. Structural changes occur in both with time, with radiographic erosions present in IA, and subchondral sclerosis and osteophyte formation in OA. Changes in juxta-articular bone, bone marrow edema and bone marrow vascular stasis all play a part in pain generation [4].

The active inflammatory setting

The major stimulus initiating pain in an active inflammatory process is the outpouring of inflammatory molecules at the local tissue site [3]. This occurs to a lesser degree in OA. This neuroactive and inflammatory milieu lowers the firing threshold of high threshold nociceptors to mechanical, thermal or chemical stimuli, and a cycle of pain is set in motion. The success of the numerous NSAIDs can be attributed to the importance of inflammatory mechanisms in rheumatic pain.

The chronic rheumatic process

In contrast, chronic pain resulting from tissue destruction and mechanical changes to cartilage, bone and soft tissues is mostly sustained by activation of neurogenic mechanisms. Peripheral and central sensitization contribute to the chronicity of pain. Afferent neuronal pathways are in turn influenced by descending neuron projections, synapsing in the laminae of the dorsal horns, with messages mediated by molecules such as serotonin, norepinephrine, endogenous opioids and cannabinoids. For these reasons, the management of chronic pain is more challenging and often less successful than that of acute pain.

Clinical practice

A specific diagnosis is the first step to effective management [5]. Locating the site of pain to either joint or soft tissue is followed by identification of joint pathology as either inflammatory or degenerative. IA encompasses a wide spectrum of connective tissue diseases occurring mainly in the middle years of life. Although RA is the most readily recognized IA, other conditions of equal importance are seronegative arthritis, with a negative rheumatoid factor, including psoriatic arthritis, inflammatory spondyloarthritis and reactive arthritis. Crystal-induced inflammation due to gout or pseudogout, another cause of acute joint inflammation, is seen in the older population and presents with acute pain and swelling localized to one or a few joint or tendon sites (Table 29.1). OA

Table 29.1 Classification of rheumatic painful conditions.

Inflammatory arthritis	Rheumatoid arthritis
	Seronegative arthritis:
	Psoriatic arthritis, inflammatory spondyloarthritis, reactive arthritis, other connective tissue diseases
	Crystal-related arthritis:
	Gout, pseudogout
	Infectious arthritis
Osteoarthritis	Peripheral osteoarthritis:
	Small joints hands
	Large joints (mostly weight-bearing)
	Spinal osteoarthritis
Soft tissue rheumatism	Tendonitis, bursitis

of peripheral joints as well as spine is termed a degenerative arthritis.

The first goal of treatment for IA must be to control the disease process, reduce the inflammatory activity and prevent chronic joint damage. This is usually achieved to a moderate degree with the use of disease-modifying agents (DMARDs) such as methotrexate, hydroxychloroquine and others, as well as the more recent use of biologic molecular directed agents. Failure to address the global disease will result in continued symptoms, even with the best attention to pain. In contrast, there is no DMARD available for treatment of OA, which is therefore treated symptomatically [6]. In the setting of continued pain there is often associated sleep disturbance, fatigue and mood disorder. Each of these factors must be addressed.

Musculoskeletal pain is described as dull and aching, interfering with daily function and sleep, but seldom extreme, except for severe inflammation of infection or crystal arthritis. Inflammatory pain generally improves with gentle exercise and is aggravated by immobility. Morning stiffness lasting for over an hour is common. OA pain can be associated with stiffness, but usually lasting minutes rather than hours. Rheumatic pain can vary considerably from day to day, and can also be influenced by weather changes as well as mood. Weather-related changes are more prevalent in women than in men, are not well understood and apply to temperature, barometric pressure and precipitation changes [7].

Treatment

Pain management must be tailored to the individual patient, taking into account age, comorbidity, specific rheumatic process and personal beliefs of the patient. Pain control for one individual may be facilitated by reduction of anxiety, whereas for another it may be simply the advice to use an assistive device such as a cane or a supportive pillow. Not every pain requires treatment with a pill [4].

Realistic treatment goals should be clearly identified with the objective to reduce the pain as well as improve function. Successful treatment usually combines both non-pharmacologic and pharma-

cologic interventions [4]. Accompanying pain of sleep disturbance, mood disorder and fatigue need also to be addressed. The efficacy of any treatment should be carefully balanced with treatment-related side effects, and the need for continued treatment must be carefully evaluated. Treatment of pain should also occur in parallel with the best management of the underlying rheumatologic process.

Exercise

Exercise provides important benefits and rarely causes harm [8]. Benefits include stimulation of reparative processes in cartilage, maintenance of muscle tone and activation of the natural descending inhibitory pain pathway. Exercise should be part of a normal healthy lifestyle routine, appropriate for the patient's age and physical condition, and enjoyable to encourage adherence. T'ai chi or a water exercise program are acceptable forms of exercise for many patients. Some people may prefer the slightly more active program of yoga, or a low impact exercise program. Exercise combined with weight reduction improves symptoms of arthritic pain in the lower limbs, with one unit of body weight translated into a 4-unit load through the knee joints with every step taken.

Practitioner administered treatments

Treatments by healthcare practitioners should be focused towards education and have a short duration. Patients should learn techniques to modulate pain, rather than develop a dependence on the healthcare provider, which promotes passive behaviors [9]. Advice regarding muscle strengthening and joint protection by a physiotherapist or occupational therapist is ideal, but is still unfortunately unrealistic for many. Treatments such as relaxation, meditation, hypnosis, massage, chiropractic and others, have mostly been categorized as complementary therapies [4,10]. Activation of descending inhibitory pathways is believed to be the mechanism of action for pain relief for many of these treatments, but further study is needed.

Herbal and diet

Complementary treatments in many forms have been used for years, often on the basis of hearsay and tradition rather than scientific rigor, but should not be immediately discarded for want of evidence. Patients with rheumatic pain use herbal products and dietary interventions extensively. There is increasing evidence that some agents modulate pain or have anti-inflammatory effects such as evening primrose oil, devil's claw (*Harpagophytum*), capsaisin and avocado/soya [11]. Several lines of evidence show that dietary omega-3 polyunsaturated fatty acids (e.g. alfa-linolenic acid) possess anti-inflammatory properties. Whether glucosamine has true chondroprotective properties in OA is debatable but, with a good safety record, can be tried for a period of 3 months in a dosage of 1500 mg/day with attention to change in OA symptoms. The healthcare professional should acknowledge that disclosure by the patient of use of complementary products speaks to a trusting doctor–patient relationship.

Topical treatments

Topical applications provide an attractive alternative to oral treatments for patients with musculoskeletal conditions. Good tissue levels of drug are achieved, especially when the painful area is close to the skin, such as in tendonitis in the elbow or wrist region, OA of the finger joints and OA of the knee. Although some systemic absorption does occur, plasma levels of drug are extremely low, contributing to tolerability of treatment and low level of side effects [12]. Topical agents that have been studied include NSAIDs, capsaicin, local anesthetics and others (Chapter 17) [12].

Injections into joints and soft tissues

Corticosteroid injections into joints, bursae and perilagamentous structures remain a useful therapeutic measure. Risks are low, infection is rare and treatment is cheap. Corticosteroids are useful in localized OA, tendonitis and inflammatory conditions such as crystal arthritis (gout or chondrocalcinosis), single active joint in IA or a painful sacroiliac joint in spondyloarthritis. The general rule of thumb, without an evidence base, is to administer no more than three injections per joint per year, with the objective for at least 3 months of pain relief. Intra-articular hyaluronic acid may have a role in the treatment of knee OA [13]. Even although hyaluronic acid is cleared from the joint in 24 hours, the postulated mechanism of action is a change in chondrocyte cell function and cartilage metabolism. The clinical efficacy is moderate, with a treatment regimen of three injections into a joint at weekly intervals. This may be repeated after 6 months, but cost remains an issue. The use of intrarticular opioids in arthroscopic knee surgery and chronic inflammation has also provided benefits (Chapter 17).

Systemic pharmacologic treatments

Analgesics and anti-inflammatory agents

NSAIDs are efficacious in mild to moderate rheumatic pain. In view of toxicity related to gastrointestinal, renal and cardiac effects, it is currently recommended that NSAIDs be used in the lowest doses and for the shortest period of time possible. [14]. In view of concerns regarding side effects of the NSAIDs, acetaminophen may be considered for milder pain (see also Chapter 18).

A recent systematic review identified that opioids were more effective than placebo for pain and functional outcomes in patients with nociceptive pain related to OA, RA and back pain in the short term; however, one-third of patients discontinued therapy as a result of side effects (average 5 weeks , range 1–16 weeks) [15]. A subsequent review of long-term trials in chronic non-cancer pain identified weak evidence that patients who are able to continue the opioids experience clinically significant pain relief with no conclusion regarding whether level of function improves but serious adverse events including iatrogenic opioid addiction were rare [16]. Thus, it is reasonable to consider a trial of opioid in appropriately selected patients with moderate to severe pain as long as patients are made aware of potential for adverse events and appropriate follow-up for risk–benefit and monitoring takes place (Chapter 16).

Corticosteroids

Corticosteroids can be a useful adjunct to pain management in the rheumatic diseases in a few particular settings. Either an intramuscular injection of a depot preparation of methylprednisolone or a short sharp course of oral corticosteroid for a few days to a few weeks can be used to settle a flare of IA or to treat an acute attack of crystal arthritis. In view of toxicity associated with prolonged use, the treatment strategy should be similar to that for NSAIDs, use of the lowest dose for the shortest period of time possible. Low dose oral corticosteroids, equivalent to less than 10 mg/day prednisolone, may be used concomitantly with a DMARD in IA and usually give excellent symptom relief. However, the risk–benefit ratio of long-term corticosteroid use needs to be evaluated for each patient. The notable exception is polymyalgia rheumatica, where low-dose corticosteroid is the treatment of choice.

Adjuvant drugs

Use of antidepressants as pain modulators has been reported in small trials of patients with arthritic disease, with improvements noted in about half of patients treated. The anticonvulsant gabapentin, acting on voltage-gated and ligand-gated ion channels and other receptors, has reduced pain behaviors in acute arthritis in the rat. Limited studies in osteoarthritis of the hip suggest a possible benefit.

Cannabinoids

There are a number of factors relevant to the rheumatic diseases that pertain to the cannabinoid system. The cannabinoid receptors, of which there are two known to date, are distributed not only throughout the nervous system, but also in the periphery at sites that include the skin, joint tissue and cartilage. The CB1 receptor is mostly associated with neural tissue, whereas the CB2 receptor is found on immunologic cells as well as chondrocytes and osteoclasts. Inflammatory pain in the rat model has been attenuated by activation of CB1

Table 29.2 Barriers to pain management.

Patient concerns	Side effects of medications
	Dislike of too many pills
	Treatments may not be effective when needed
	Masking disease process
	Fear of addiction
Physician	Additional time required
	Discomfort with treatments
	Lack of education
	Regulatory bodies

and CB2 receptors. Well-controlled studies examining cannabinoids in treatment of rheumatic pain are lacking; however, analgesic effects demonstrated in other types of non-cancer pain [17] along with preclinical evidence demonstrating anti-inflammatory effects suggest that it may be reasonable to consider cannabinoids in rheumatic disease (Chapter 18).

Obstacles to optimal pain management

Barriers to optimal pain management exist for patients with rheumatic pain from both the patient's as well as the healthcare professional's perspective (Table 29.2) [4]. Patients often believe that pain is a normal part of the rheumatic disease, and that pain management will mask the disease process. There is fear and distrust of medications because of side effects, concerns about loss of efficacy of pain treatments and risks of addiction. Compliance is poor with many studies reporting only 50% adherence to treatments. Physicians have also been remiss in neglecting optimal pain management, as this adds an extra dimension to patient care which is time-consuming, associated with concerns about regulatory scrutiny and has in the past been assigned as having secondary importance to management of the primary rheumatic disease [4].

Conclusions

Current treatment for rheumatic pain must address both disease-modifying and pain management approaches. This will include the use of appropriate DMARDs along with approaches for general pain management. Treatment should include healthful living such as healthy diet, exercise and weight control as well as quitting smoking. It is also appropriate to add additional analgesic agents, physical and psychological and specific complementary therapies to target the pain following the same principles reviewed in this and other chapters in this volume. Given that the pain leads to significant disability and compromise in quality of life, it is time for clinicians to give priority to the management of pain in rheumatic disease as well as targeting the disease process in order to reduce the inflammatory activity and prevent chronic joint damage.

References

1 Fitzcharles MA, Shir Y. (2008) New concepts in rheumatic pain. *Rheum Dis Clin North Am* **34(2)**:267–83.

2 Hootman JM, Helmick CG. (2006) Projections of US prevalence of arthritis and associated activity limitations. *Arthritis Rheum* **54(1)**: 226–9.

3 Kidd BL. (2006) Osteoarthritis and joint pain. *Pain* **123(1–2)**:6–9.

4 Fitzcharles MA, Almahrezi A, Shir Y. (2005) Pain: understanding and challenges for the rheumatologist. *Arthritis Rheum* **52(12)**:3685–92.

5 American College of Rheumatology Ad Hoc Committee on Clinical Guidelines. (1996) Guidelines for the initial evaluation of the adult patient with acute musculoskeletal symptoms. *Arthritis Rheum* **39(1)**:1–8.

6 American College of Rheumatology Subcommittee on Osteoarthritis Guidelines. (2000) Recommendations for the medical management of osteoarthritis of the hip and knee: 2000 update. *Arthritis Rheum* **43(9)**:1905–15.

7 McAlindon T, Formica M, Schmid CH *et al.* (2007) Changes in barometric pressure and ambient temperature influence osteoarthritis pain. *Am J Med* **120(5)**:429–34.

8 Roddy E, Zhang W, Doherty M *et al.* (2005) Evidence-based recommendations for the role of exercise in the management of osteoarthritis of the hip or knee: the MOVE consensus. *Rheumatology (Oxford)* **44(1)**:67–73.

9 Yocum DE, Castro WL, Cornett M. (2000) Exercise, education, and behavioral modification as alternative therapy for pain and stress in rheumatic disease. *Rheum Dis Clin North Am* **26(1)**:145–59, x–xi.

10 Fiechtner JJ, Brodeur RR. (2002) Manual and manipulation techniques for rheumatic disease. *Med Clin North Am* **86(1)**:91–103.

11 Ernst E. (2004) Musculoskeletal conditions and complementary/alternative medicine. *Best Pract Res Clin Rheumatol* **18(4)**:539–56.

12 Mason L, Moore RA, Edwards JE *et al.* (2004) Topical NSAIDs for acute pain: a meta-analysis. *BMC Fam Pract* **5**:10.

13 Bellamy N, Campbell J, Robinson V *et al.* (2005) Viscosupplementation for the treatment of osteoarthritis of the knee. *Cochrane Database Syst Rev* **2**:CD005321.

14 Tannenbaum H, Bombardier C, Davis P *et al.* (2006) An evidence-based approach to prescribing nonsteroidal antiinflammatory drugs. Third Canadian Consensus Conference. *J Rheumatol* **33(1)**:140–57.

15 Furlan AD, Sandoval JA, Mailis-Gagnon A *et al.* (2006) Opioids for chronic noncancer pain: meta-analysis of effectiveness and side effects. *CMAJ* **174**:1589–94.

16 Noble M, Treadwell JR, Tregear SJ *et al.* (2010) Long-term opioid management of chronic noncancer pain. *Cochrane Database Syst Rev* **20(1)**:1–70.

17 Lynch ME. (2008) The pharmacotherapy of chronic pain. *Rheum Dis Clin North Am* **34**:369–85.

Further reading

Chou R, Fanciullo GJ, Fine PG *et al.* (2009) Clinical guidelines for the use of chronic opioid therapy in chronic noncancer pain. *J Pain* **10(2)**:113–30.

Chapter 30

Headache

Stephen D. Silberstein

Jefferson Medical College, Thomas Jefferson University, Philadelphia, USA

Introduction

Headache is one of the most common medical complaints of humankind, accounting for more than 18 million outpatient visits per year in the United States. The International Headache Society (IHS) classification system (ICHD-2) [1] divides headache into primary and secondary disorders. In a primary headache disorder, headache is the disorder. In a secondary headache disorder, headache is attributable to another disorder.

Evaluation and diagnostic testing

Headache diagnosis is based on a history, physical and neurologic examination. Characteristics helpful in diagnosis include age at onset; headache frequency, duration, location and severity; factors associated with initiation, exacerbation or remission; accompanying symptoms; and preceding conditions.

Recurrent episodic severe headaches with onset in adolescence or early adulthood suggests a primary headache disorder. A sudden-onset severe (thunderclap) headache suggests a subarachnoid hemorrhage (SAH). In patients over 50 years of age,

Clinical Pain Management: A Practical Guide, 1st edition.
Edited by Mary E. Lynch, Kenneth D. Craig and
Philip W.H. Peng.
© 2011 Blackwell Publishing Ltd.

tenderness on palpation of the temporal arteries accompanied by scalp tenderness, jaw claudication or visual changes suggests giant cell arteritis (GCA). Neck stiffness may indicate meningeal irritation due to infection or SAH hemorrhage. Papilledema indicates increased intracranial pressure. Focal neurologic symptoms or mental status changes typically accompany structural lesions. History may suggest the cause of headache: for example, recent head trauma, hemophilia, alcoholism or anticoagulant therapy may suggest a subdural hematoma.

Testing serves to exclude organic causes of headache, rule out coexistent diseases that could complicate treatment, and establish a baseline for and exclude contraindications to drug treatment.

Patients require urgent computed tomography (CT) or magnetic resonance imaging (MRI) when any of the following is present:
- Sudden-onset thunderclap headache;
- Altered mental status, including seizure;
- Focal neurologic deficits;
- Papilledema; or
- Severe hypertension.

A normal CT scan does not rule out SAH, meningitis or encephalitis; lumbar puncture is indicated when they are suspected. Patients with unusual persistent headaches may also require lumbar puncture.

Symptoms requiring prompt imaging include a change in prior headache pattern, new-onset headache after age 55, systemic symptoms (e.g. weight loss), secondary risk factors (e.g. cancer, HIV, head trauma) or chronic unexplained headache. MRI, magnetic resonance angiography (MRA) and/or magnetic resonance venography (MRV) are preferred; these tests can show many causes of headache (e.g. carotid dissection, cerebral vein thrombosis, pituitary apoplexy, vascular malformations, cerebral vasculitis, Chiari type I malformation) that can be missed on CT.

Other tests are used if specific disorders are suspected (e.g. erythrocyte sedimentation rate for GCA).

Migraine

Migraine is a chronic neurologic disease characterized by episodic attacks of headache and associated symptoms [2]. In the United States about 17.6% of women and 6% of men had one migraine attack in the previous year [3].

Description of the migraine attack

The migraine attack can consist of premonitory, aura, headache and resolution phases. Premonitory symptoms may include psychological, neurologic, constitutional or autonomic features (depression, cognitive dysfunction and food cravings) and can occur hours to days before headache onset.

The migraine aura consists of focal neurologic symptoms that precede, accompany or (rarely) follow an attack. Aura usually develops over 5–20 minutes, lasts less than 60 minutes, can be visual, sensory or motor, and may involve language or brainstem disturbances [1]. Headache usually follows within 60 minutes of the end of the aura.

The typical headache is unilateral, of gradual onset, throbbing, moderate to marked in severity and aggravated by movement [1]. It lasts 4–72 hours in adults and 2–48 hours in children [1].

Anorexia is common. Nausea occurs in almost 90% of patients, while vomiting occurs in about one-third. Sensory hypersensitivity results in patients seeking a dark quiet room [2,4]. Patients may experience blurry vision, nasal stuffiness, anorexia, hunger, tenesmus, diarrhea, abdominal

Table 30.1 Migraine without aura.

A At least five attacks
B Headache attacks last 4–72 hours and occur <15 days/month or unsuccessfully treated
C Headache has at least two of the following characteristics:
1 Unilateral location
2 Pulsating quality
3 Moderate or severe intensity
4 Aggravation by or causing avoidance from routine physical activity
D During headache at least one of the following:
1 Nausea and/or vomiting
2 Photophobia and phonophobia
E Not attributed to another disorder

Table 30.2 Migraine with typical aura.

A At least two attacks
B Fully reversible visual and/or sensory and/or speech symptoms but no motor weakness
C Homonymous or bilateral visual symptoms including positive features (i.e. flickering lights, spots, lines) or negative features (i.e. loss of vision) and/or unilateral sensory symptoms including positive features (i.e. visual loss, pins and needles) and/or negative features (i.e. numbness)
D At least one of two:
1 At least one symptom develops gradually over ≥5 minutes and/or different symptoms occur in succession
2 Each symptom lasts ≥5 minutes and ≤60 minutes
E Headache that meets criteria B–D for migraine without aura (Table 30.1), begins during the aura or follows aura within 60 minutes
F Not attributed to another disorder

cramps, polyuria, facial pallor, sensations of heat or cold, and sweating. Depression, fatigue, anxiety, nervousness, irritability and impairment of concentration are common.

The ICHD-2 divides migraine into migraine without aura (Table 30.1) and migraine with aura (Table 30.2) [1]. Migraine persisting for more than 3 days defines "status migrainosus." Migraine occurring 15 or more days per month is called chronic migraine (CM) (Table 30.2).

Basilar-type migraine aura features brainstem symptoms: ataxia, vertigo, tinnitus, diplopia, nausea and vomiting, nystagmus, dysarthria, bilateral paresthesia, or a change in level of consciousness and cognition [1]. Hemiplegic migraine can be sporadic or familial [2,4]. Familial hemiplegic migraine (FHM) is an autosomal dominant disorder associated with attacks of migraine, with and without aura, and hemiparesis.

Pathophysiology

The migraine aura is probably caused by cortical spreading depression (CSD). Headache probably results from activation of meningeal and blood vessel nociceptors combined with a change in central pain modulation. Headache and its associated neurovascular changes are subserved by the trigeminal system. Stimulation results in the release of substance P and calcitonin gene-related peptide (CGRP) from sensory C-fiber terminals and neurogenic inflammation. Neurogenic inflammation sensitizes nerve fibers (peripheral sensitization), which now respond to previously innocuous stimuli, such as blood vessel pulsations, causing, in part, the pain of migraine. Brainstem activation also occurs in migraine without aura, in part bcause of increased activity of the endogenous antinociceptive system. The migraine aura can trigger headache: CSD activates trigeminovascular afferents. In the absence of aura, CSD may occur in silent areas of the cortex or the cerebellum.

Treatment

Migraine treatment begins with making a diagnosis, explaining it to the patient and developing a treatment plan that considers comorbid conditions [2,4]. Treatment may be acute or preventive, and patients may require both approaches. Acute treatment attempts to relieve the pain and impairment once an attack has begun. Preventive therapy is given to reduce the frequency, duration or severity of attacks. Additional benefits include improved responsiveness to acute attack treatment, improved function and reduced disability.

Acute treatment can be specific (dihydroergotamine [DHE] and triptans) or non-specific (analgesics and opioids). Non-specific medications control the pain of migraine or other pain disorders, while specific medications are effective in migraine (and certain other) headache attacks but are not useful for non-headache pain disorders. Analgesics are used for mild to moderate headaches. Triptans or DHE are first line drugs for severe attacks and for less severe attacks that do not adequately respond to analgesics. Early intervention prevents escalation and may increase efficacy. Limiting acute treatment to 2–3 days a week can prevent medication overuse headache. When headaches are very frequent, early intervention may not be appropriate.

Treatment occasionally fails and patients need to have rescue medications (opioids, neuroleptics and corticosteroids) available. These provide relief, but often limit function because of sedation or other adverse events.

Preventive treatment

Preventive treatment may prevent the progression of episodic to chronic migraine. However, prevention is not being utilized to nearly the extent it should be; only 5% of all migraineurs currently use preventive therapy to control their attacks [5].

Indications for preventive treatment include the following:
• Migraine that significantly interferes with the patient's daily routine despite acute treatment;
• Failure of, contraindication to, or troublesome adverse events from acute medications;
• Acute medication overuse;
• Very frequent headaches (>1 per week);
• Patient preference;
• Special circumstances, such as hemiplegic.

Preventive medication groups include beta-adrenergic blockers, antidepressants, calcium channel antagonists, anticonvulsants and non-steroidal anti-inflammatory drugs (NSAIDs). Choice is based on efficacy, adverse events and coexistent conditions. The drug is started at a low dose and increased slowly until therapeutic effects develop or the ceiling dose is reached. A full

Table 30.3 Chronic migraine.

A Headache on 15 or more days per month for at least 3 months
B Patient has had at least five attacks fulfilling criteria B–D for migraine without aura (Table 30.1)
C On 8 or more days per month for at least 3 months headache has fulfilled criteria for migraine without aura (Table 30.1) except for duration or treated and relieved by triptan(s) or ergot
D No medication overuse and not attributed to another disorder

Table 30.4 Tension-type headache.

Frequent episodic tension-type headache
A At least 10 episodes fulfilling criteria B–E. Number of days with such headache = 1 day per month and < 15 days per month for at least 3 months
B Headache lasting from 30 minutes to 7 days
C At least two of the following pain characteristics:
  1 Pressing/tightening (non-pulsating) quality
  2 Mild or moderate intensity (may inhibit but does not prohibit activities)
  3 Bilateral location
  4 No aggravation by walking stairs or similar routine physical activity
D Both of the following:
  1 No nausea or vomiting (anorexia may occur)
  2 Photophobia and phonophobia are absent, or one but not the other may be present
E Not attributed to another disorder

Chronic tension-type headache
A At least 10 episodes fulfilling criteria B–F. Number of days with such headache ≥15 days per month for at least a 3-month period (≥180 days per year)
B Headache lasts hours or may be continuous
C At least two of the following pain characteristics:
  1 Pressing or tightening quality
  2 Mild or moderate severity (may inhibit but does not prohibit activities)
  3 Bilateral location
  4 No aggravation by walking stairs or similar routine physical activity
D Both of the following:
  1 No more than one of the following: photophobia, phonophobia or mild nausea
  2 No moderate or severe nausea and no vomiting
E No medication overuse
F Not attributed to another disorder

therapeutic trial may take 2–6 months. If headaches are well controlled, medication can be tapered and discontinued. The preventive medications with the best documented efficacy are beta-blockers, valproic acid and topiramate.

Although monotherapy is preferred, it is sometimes necessary to combine preventive medications. Antidepressants are often used with beta-blockers or calcium channel blockers, and topiramate or valproic acid may be used in combination with any of these medications. Coexistent diseases have important implications for treatment. In some instances, two or more conditions may be treated with a single drug.

Behavioral and psychological interventions used for prevention include relaxation training, thermal biofeedback combined with relaxation training, electromyography biofeedback and cognitive behavioral therapy.

Chronic daily headache

Chronic daily headache (CDH) refers to headache disorders experienced 15 or more days a month [1]. The major primary disorders are chronic migraine (CM) (Table 30.3), hemicrania continua (HC), chronic tension-type headache (CTTH) (Table 30.4) and new daily persistent headache (NDPH).

Most patients with CM are women. Patients often report a process of transformation characterized by headaches that become more frequent over months to years, with the associated symptoms of photophobia, phonophobia and nausea becoming less severe and less frequent. The head-

aches resemble a mixture of tension-type headache and migraine.

Medication overuse headache

Patients with frequent headaches often overuse analgesics, opioids, ergotamine and triptans (Table 30.5). Although stopping the acute medication may result in withdrawal symptoms and increased headache, subsequent headache improvement usually occurs. Acute drug overuse may interfere

Table 30.5 Headache attributed to medication overuse.

A Headache present on >15 days/month
B Regular overuse for >3 months of one or more acute and/or symptomatic treatment drugs
1 Ergotamine, triptans, opioids or combination analgesic medications on ≥10 days/month on a regular basis for >3 months
2 Simple analgesics or any combination of ergotamine, triptans, analgesics opioids on ≥15 days/month on a regular basis for >3 months without overuse of any single class alone
C Headache has developed or markedly worsened during medication overuse

Table 30.6 Cluster headache.

A At least five attacks fulfilling
B Severe or very severe unilateral orbital, supraorbital and/or temporal pain lasting 15–180 minutes if untreated
C Headache is accompanied by at least one of the following:
1 Ipsilateral conjunctival injection and/or lacrimation
2 Ipsilateral nasal congestion and/or rhinorrhea
3 Ipsilateral eyelid edema
4 Ipsilateral forehead and facial sweating
5 Ipsilateral miosis and/or ptosis
6 A sense of restlessness or agitation
D Attacks have a frequency from one every other day to eight per day
E Not attributed to another disorder

with the effectiveness of preventive headache medications. Prolonged use of large amounts of medication may cause renal or hepatic toxicity in addition to tolerance, habituation or dependence.

Treatment

Patients with CDH can be difficult to treat, especially when complicated by medication overuse. First, exclude secondary headache disorders; second, diagnose the specific primary headache disorder; and third, identify comorbid conditions and exacerbating factors. Limit acute medications and start preventive medication, with the understanding that the drugs may not become fully effective until medication overuse has been eliminated. Detoxification options include outpatient infusion in an ambulatory infusion unit. If outpatient treatment proves difficult or is dangerous, hospitalization may be required.

Tension-type headache

Tension-type headache (TTH) (Table 30.6) is very common, with a lifetime prevalence of 69% in men and 88% in women. Episodic TTHs (ETTH) are now classified as either infrequent (<1 day/month or 12 days/year) or frequent (>1 but <15 days/month or >12 but <180 days/year) [6]. The pain is a dull achy non-pulsatile feeling of tightness, pressure or constriction, and it is usually mild to moderate in intensity. Most patients have bilateral pain; some have neck or jaw discomfort. There is no prodrome and, with the exception of occasional anorexia, there are no associated autonomic or gastrointestinal symptoms. Many TTH patients also have migraine [1].

Management

Patients with TTH usually self-medicate with over-the-counter analgesics, with or without caffeine. If they are not effective, prescription NSAIDs or combination analgesic preparations can be used. Patients with both migraine and TTHs benefit from specific migraine medication, such as triptans or DHE [6].

Medications used for TTH prevention include antidepressants, beta-blockers and anticonvulsants. Antidepressants, the medication of first choice, should be started at a low dose and increased slowly every 3–7 days. The addition of biofeedback therapy or beta-blocking agents may improve its therapeutic benefit [6].

Cluster headache and other trigeminal autonomic cephalgias

The short-lasting primary headache syndromes with autonomic activation include cluster headache (Table 30.6), paroxysmal hemicrania (episodic or chronic) and short-lasting unilateral neuralgiform headache with conjunctival injection and tearing (SUNCT syndrome).

With an incidence of 0.01–1.5% in various populations, cluster headache prevalence is lower than that of migraine or TTH. Men have a higher prevalence than women. The most common form of cluster headache is episodic cluster. Cluster headache generally begins in the late twenties.

Patients with cluster headache have multiple episodes of short-lived but severe, unilateral, orbital, supraorbital or temporal pain. At least one associated symptom must occur: conjunctival injection, lacrimation, nasal congestion, rhinorrhea, facial sweating, miosis, ptosis or eyelid edema. Episodic cluster consists of headache periods of 1 week to 1 year, with remission periods lasting at least 14 days, whereas chronic cluster headache has either no remission periods or remissions that last less than 14 days.

The pain of a cluster attack rapidly increases to excruciating levels within 15 minutes. The attacks often occur at the same time each day and frequently awaken patients from sleep. The attacks usually last from 30–90 minutes. During an attack, patients often feel agitated or restless. The attack frequency varies from one every other day to eight a day, occurring in periods that last a week to a year. Remissions between cluster periods generally last 6 months to 2 years.

Management

Effective acute treatments include oxygen, sumatriptan and DHE. Inhaled oxygen, 7–10 L/min for 10 minutes following headache onset, is 70% effective and is often the first choice treatment. Parenteral injections of sumatriptan or DHE provide significant relief for about 80% of patients [7,8].

Cluster headaches require preventive treatment; drugs include calcium channel blockers, lithium, corticosteroids, valproic acid, topiramate, melatonin and capsaicin. If medical therapy fails completely, surgical intervention may be beneficial. The surgery consists of neuronal ablation procedures directed toward the sensory input of

the trigeminal nerve and autonomic pathways, and is effective in 75% of patients [9].

Trigeminal neuralgia

Trigeminal neuralgia is a painful disorder occurring in the maxillary and mandibular divisions of the trigeminal nerve. It is typically evoked by trivial stimuli. It is a disorder of the elderly, often causes severe disability, and has a relapsing remitting course. It is characterized by brief severe electric shock-like pain and is limited to one or more divisions of the trigeminal nerve. The pain generally lasts seconds, although it can last up to 2 minutes. Multiple attacks may occur daily. Most individuals have short periods of pain-free time between spikes of pain. Symptomatic trigeminal neuralgia is caused by a structural lesion, such as an acoustic neuroma, or multiple sclerosis. Patients are usually started with a drug regimen that includes phenytoin, carbamazepine, oxcarbazepine and baclofen. Candidates for surgical therapy are patients who have failed medical therapy (which occurs approximately 30% of the time) or who became intolerant to medical therapy. Approximately 50% of those with trigeminal neuralgia will require surgery.

Conclusions

Headache is one of the most common medical complaints of humankind. Headache diagnosis is based on a history, physical and neurologic examination. Testing serves to exclude organic causes of headache. Migraine is a chronic neurologic disease characterized by episodic attacks of headache and associated symptoms. Migraine treatment begins with making a diagnosis, explaining it to the patient and developing a treatment plan. Acute treatment attempts to relieve or stop the progression of an attack or the pain and impairment once an attack has begun. Preventive therapy is given in an attempt to reduce the frequency, duration or severity of attacks. Preventive treatment may prevent episodic migraine's progression to chronic migraine. CDH refers to headache disorders experienced 15 or more days a month.

Patients with frequent headaches often overuse analgesics, opioids, ergotamine and triptans. TTH is the most common type of headache disorder. Patients with TTH usually self-medicate with over-the-counter analgesics. Patients with cluster headache have multiple episodes of short-lived but severe, unilateral, orbital, supraorbital or temporal pain. The pain of a cluster attack rapidly increases to excruciating levels within 15 minutes. Effective acute treatments include oxygen, sumatriptan and DHE. Most patients with cluster headache require preventive treatment. Trigeminal neuralgia is a painful disorder in the distribution of the trigeminal nerve that is typically evoked by trivial stimuli. Both medical and surgical modalities may be used as treatment. Approximately 50% of patients with trigeminal neuralgia will require surgery.

References

1 Headache Classification Committee. (2004) International Classification of Headache Disorders, 2nd edition. *Cephalalgia* **24(Suppl 1)**:1–160.

2 Lipton RB, Scher AI, Silberstein SD *et al.* (2008) Migraine diagnosis and comorbidity. In: Silberstein SD, Lipton RB, Dodick DW, eds. *Wolff's Headache and Other Head Pain*, 8th edn. Oxford University Press, New York. pp. 153–76.

3 Lipton RB, Diamond S, Reed M *et al.* (2001) Migraine diagnosis and treatment: results from the American Migraine Study II. *Headache* **41**:638–45.

4 Silberstein SD, Freitag FG, Bigal ME. (2008) Migraine treatment. In: Silberstein SD, Lipton RB, Dodick DW, eds. *Wolff's Headache and Other Head Pain*, 8th edn. Oxford University Press, New York. pp. 177–292.

5 Lipton RB, Scher AI, Kolodner K *et al.* (2002) Migraine in the United States: epidemiology and patterns of health care use. *Neurology* **58**:885–94.

6 Silberstein SD. (2005) Transformed and chronic migraine. In: Goadsby PJ, Silberstein SD, Dodick DW, eds. *Chronic Daily Headache for Clinicians.* BC Decker, Hamilton. pp. 21–56.

7 Silberstein SD. (1994) Pharmacological management of cluster headache. *CNS Drugs* **2(3)**:199–207.

8 Goadsby PJ, Tfelt-Hansen P. (2009) Cluster headaches: introduction and epidemiology. In: Olesen J, Goadsby PJ, Ramadan N *et al.*, eds. *The Headaches*, 3rd edn. Lippincott, Williams & Wilkins, Philadelphia. pp. 743–5.

9 Jarrar RG, Black DF, Dodick DW *et al.* (2003) Outcome of trigeminal nerve section in the treatment of chronic cluster headache. *Neurology* **60(8)**:1360–2.

Chapter 31

Orofacial pain

Barry J. Sessle[1], Lene Baad-Hansen[2] & Peter Svensson[2,3]

[1] Faculties of Dentistry and Medicine, University of Toronto, Toronto, Canada
[2] Department of Clinical Oral Physiology, Aarhus University, Aarhus, Denmark
[3] Department of Maxillofacial Surgery, Aarhus University Hospital, Aarhus, Denmark

Introduction

The orofacial region is the site of some of the most common acute and chronic pain conditions. This region also has special psychological, social and emotional meaning and importance in eating, drinking, sexual behaviour, speech and expression of emotions. The orofacial tissues are densely innervated by nociceptive afferents and have an extensive somatosensory representation in the central nervous system (CNS). These features also account for why many people find it unpleasant and painful to go for a routine dental examination.

This chapter first highlights the peripheral and central neurobiological mechanisms underlying orofacial pain, and then outlines the clinical features of some of the most common or perplexing orofacial pain conditions.

Orofacial nociceptive processes

Primary afferent mechanisms

The rich innervation of the orofacial region is almost exclusively by branches of the trigeminal nerve. Many trigeminal primary afferent fibers terminate in these tissues as free nerve endings and function as nociceptors. The nociceptive afferents are either small-diameter, myelinated (A-delta) afferents or even smaller (and slower conducting) unmyelinated (C) afferents. Their primary afferent cell bodies occur in the trigeminal ganglion.

Like analogous afferent endings and ganglion cell bodies of spinal nerves (Chapter 3), trigeminal nociceptive afferents are subject to considerable modulation because a peripheral substrate exists for complex interactions between the neural, immune, cardiovascular and endocrine systems [1–3]. Tissue damage, and inflammation if present, cause the release of chemical mediators, some of which can activate the nociceptive endings whereas others produce so-called nociceptor or peripheral sensitization. This sensitization can be reflected in a lowered activation threshold, increased responsiveness to subsequent noxious stimuli and spontaneous activity of the nociceptive endings that contribute, respectively, to the allodynia, hyperalgesia and spontaneous pain that are features of acute and many persistent orofacial pain conditions [1–3]. The chemical mediators may also spread through the tissues and act on the endings of adjacent nociceptive afferents, and thus contribute to the spread of orofacial pain. Injury or inflammation of peripheral tissues, including nerves, may also lead to phenotypic changes, sprouting or abnormal discharges of the

Clinical Pain Management: A Practical Guide, 1st edition.
Edited by Mary E. Lynch, Kenneth D. Craig and
Philip W.H. Peng.
© 2011 Blackwell Publishing Ltd.

nociceptive afferents and be of pathophysiological significance in certain pain conditions.

Facial skin, oral mucosa, temporomandibular joint (TMJ), craniofacial muscle and periodontal tissues are supplied by nociceptive afferents with properties generally analogous to those of spinal nociceptive afferents although corneal and cerbrovascular nociceptive afferents do have some special properties as do those supplying the tooth pulp [2,3]. The tooth pulp is a highly vascular and richly innervated tissue which is exceptionally sensitive to stimulation and a frequent source of dental pain. The dentine encasing the pulp is also very sensitive despite its sparse innervation, and it appears that activation of intradentinal afferents is brought about by a hydrodynamic mechanism. Injury to the tooth and pulpal inflammation (e.g. as a result of dental caries) can induce peripheral sensitization of intradental afferents, which may result in extremely intense toothache, because inflammation of the pulp occurs in a non-compliant environment (it is encased by dentine) with a high extracellular tissue pressure. This is thought to be an important factor accounting for the great sensitivity of pulp afferents when the pulp is inflamed [2,3].

Brainstem mechanisms

From the trigeminal ganglion, trigeminal afferents project into the brainstem and terminate on neurons especially in the trigeminal brainstem sensory nuclear complex which consists of the trigeminal main sensory and the trigeminal spinal tract nucleus. The latter is subdivided into three subnuclei: oralis, interpolaris and caudalis (Figure 31.1). The subnucleus caudalis is a laminated structure with many morphological and functional similarities to the dorsal horn of the spinal cord; indeed, it is often termed the medullary dorsal horn. Based on its anatomic, neurochemical and physiological features and the effects of brainstem lesions, caudalis is now considered the principal brainstem relay site of trigeminal nociceptive information, although the other subnuclei (interpolaris, oralis) may contribute to the brainstem mechanisms of orofacial pain [4–6].

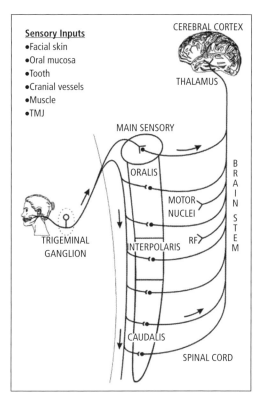

Figure 31.1 Major somatosensory pathway from the orofacial region. Trigeminal primary afferents project via the trigeminal ganglion to second-order neurons in the trigeminal brainstem sensory nuclear complex comprising the main sensory nucleus and the subnuclei oralis, interpolaris and caudalis of the spinal tract nucleus. These neurons may project to neurons in higher levels of the brain (e.g. thalamus) or in brainstem regions such as cranial nerve motor pools or the reticular formation (RF). Not shown are the projections of some cervical nerve and cranial nerve VII, X and XII afferents to the trigeminal complex and the projection of many VII, IX and X afferents to the solitary tract nucleus. TMJ, temporomandibular joint. *Source*: Reproduced with permission from Sessle [4].

Some caudalis nociceptive neurons respond only to stimulation of a cutaneous or mucosal mechanoreceptive field and, as a consequence, they are thought to have an important role in our ability to localize, detect and discriminate superficial noxious stimuli. However, most can also be activated by peripheral afferent input from other tissues (e.g. tooth pulp, TMJ, jaw muscle or cerebrovasculature). Such features are thought to contribute to the very common clinical findings of poor localization and referral of pain from deep tissues or from one tooth to another.

Neurons in caudalis and other components of the trigeminal brainstem complex project to the thalamus either directly or indirectly by polysynaptic pathways (e.g. via the reticular formation) (Figure 31.1). Some of the latter projections, as well as those to the cranial nerve motor nuclei, provide part of the central substrate underlying autonomic, endocrine and muscle reflex responses to orofacial stimuli. Some neurons have only intrinsic projections such that their axons do not leave the trigeminal brainstem complex but instead terminate within it (e.g. interneurons in lamina II of caudalis, the so-called substantia gelatinosa).

Thalamocortical mechanisms

Orofacial somatosensory information is relayed from the brainstem to the lateral thalamus (e.g. ventrobasal complex; the ventroposterior nucleus in humans) and medial thalamus (e.g. medial nuclei) which contain nociceptive neurons with properties generally similar to those described for nociceptive neurons in the subthalamic relays such as subnucleus caudalis [6]. Those in ventrobasal thalamus have properties and connections with the overlying somatosensory cerebral cortex which point to a role in localization and discrimination of orofacial noxious stimuli, whereas those in the more medial thalamic nuclei project to other higher brain areas (e.g. hypothalamus, anterior cingulate cortex) which are involved more in affective or motivational dimensions of pain.

Modulatory influences

Pain is modulated by a variety of influences that regulate perceptual, emotional, autonomic and neuroendocrine responses to noxious stimuli by utilizing several excitatory and inhibitory neurochemicals. Some of these modulatory influences may be expressed at thalamic and cortical levels, but the intricate organization of each subdivision of the trigeminal brainstem complex, coupled with the variety of inputs to each of them from peripheral tissues or descending from some parts of the brain (e.g. in the thalamus, reticular formation, limbic system and cerebral cortex), provides a rich substrate for numerous interactions between the various inputs that can result in the modulation of orofacial nociceptive transmission [4,6]. This means that the neural circuitry underlying nociceptive transmission, including that in the trigeminal system is "plastic" and not "hard-wired."

The descending influences are activated by a variety of behavioral and environmental events and can modify pain. Orofacial nociceptive transmission is also subject to modulation by so-called segmental or afferent influences, which can be evoked by peripheral stimulation and involve the interneuronal circuitry existing with subnucleus caudalis. Segmental or descending inhibitory substrates are thought to contribute to the efficacy of several analgesic approaches (e.g. drugs such as morphine, carbamazepine, tricyclic antidepressants [TCAs]).

Trigeminal nociceptive transmission can, as in the spinal system, also be enhanced by alterations to the peripheral afferent inputs to the CNS as a result of trauma or inflammation to peripheral tissues or nerves. Trauma or inflammation produces a barrage of nociceptive primary afferent inputs into the CNS that may lead to prolonged neuroplastic alterations in subnucleus caudalis (and spinal dorsal horn) which collectively have been termed central sensitization. Trigeminal central sensitization is reflected in an increased excitability of caudalis nociceptive neurons, manifested as an increase in spontaneous activity, mechanoreceptive field expansion, lowering of activation threshold, and enhancement of peripherally evoked nociceptive responses of the neurons [4,6]. These neuroplastic changes are thought to contribute to persistent orofacial pain and its common characteristics of spontaneous pain, pain spread and referral, allodynia and hyperalgesia. Several membrane receptor mechanisms, ion channels and intracellular signaling processes are involved in trigeminal central sensitization, and include purinergic and neurokinin as well as N-methyl-D-aspartate (NMDA) and non-NMDA glutamatergic receptor mechanisms. Trigeminal central sensitization occurs not only in subnucleus caudalis but also in subnucleus oralis and higher brain regions such as ventrobasal thalamus; nonetheless, caudalis has been shown to be responsible for the expression of central sensitization in these structures by way of its projections to both.

Clinical aspects

Orofacial pain covers a wide range of conditions with different clinical manifestations. There have been several attempts to provide comprehensive classifications [7–10]; however, the following focuses on some of the most common and most perplexing of these conditions. Because of their complexity, plus the special emotional and psychosocial meaning of the orofacial region, the diagnostic work-up and management strategy will often require a substantial interdisciplinary approach between the medical profession, dentists, psychologists and specialists in orofacial pain.

Temporomandibular disorders

Temporomandibular disorders (TMD) are a family of related pain conditions in the jaw muscles, TMJ and associated structures. They can be divided into three main categories:
1 Myofascial pain;
2 Disc displacements; and
3 TMJ arthralgia, osteoarthrosis and osteoarthritis.
TMD is very common in the population (3–15%) and is 1.5–2 times more prevalent in women than in men, with a peak around 20–45 years. Osteoarthrosis increases over the lifespan. The incidence of TMD pain is 2–4%, with the persistent types being 0.1%. Generalized pain conditions such as fibromyalgia, whiplash-associated disorders, tension-type headache, low-back pain and general joint laxity have been found to be comorbid with TMD pain conditions.

There are three cardinal symptoms of TMD:
1 Pain in the jaw muscles and/or TMJ;
2 Sounds from the TMJ (clicks, crepitation); and
3 Limitation in range of jaw motion [9].
Pain is moderate to intense, fluctuating during the day with exacerbations during jaw movements.

Myofascial TMD pain is described as a deep ache, tender and diffuse, often with referral to the TMJ, ear, temple and teeth. TMJ arthralgia is more localized around the TMJ, with a sharp component and pain referrals to the ear region. Typically, the jaw muscles and the TMJ will be painful on palpation. Clicking in the TMJ is rarely a problem but may be unpleasant for the patient. The TMJ disc position may cause limitation in the range of motion (TMJ locking). TMD diagnosis is based on a systematic history and clinical examination, and in some cases imaging of the TMJ (e.g. magnetic resonance imaging [MRI] or computed tomography [CT]) [11].

The pathophysiology of TMD pain is unclear but both peripheral and central sensitization is believed to be involved, with contributions from anatomic, psychological–psychosocial and neurobiological factors (see above). There is also evidence of a less effective activation of endogenous pain-inhibitory systems in TMD patients, and recent studies suggest that there may be genetic risk factors involved in complex TMD pain conditions.

TMD cannot be causally treated but only managed with the primary goal of pain alleviation and restoring of function [12]. Various physical strategies (e.g. stretching, relaxation, oral splints) can be used but there is a limited evidence basis for these. The number-needed-to-treat (NNT) values for oral splints range 3–4 for management of myofascial TMD and around 5–6 for TMJ arthralgia, and there is good evidence that self-care instructions and monitoring can provide at least as good pain relief as usual dental approaches. Evidence-driven recommendations for pharmacological procedures are also needed. Non-steroidal anti-inflammatory drugs (NSAIDs) such as ibuprofen in combination with diazepam can be used for short-term management of TMD pain. Gabapentin appears to have some effect on myofascial TMD pain and tenderness, as does cyclobenzaprine or flupirtine. Low doses of TCAs may be an option for persistent TMD pain. Naproxen is effective in management of TMJ arthralgia. Intra-articular morphine increases the pressure pain thresholds and jaw-opening capacity and reduces TMJ pain but probably has limited clinical application.

Botulinum toxin cannot at present be recommended because of inconclusive evidence.

Tooth pain

Tooth pain is a very common, usually acute condition. Prevalence estimates range 7–66%, depending on criteria and the population studied [11]. The most frequent local causes are presented in Table 31.1. Acute tooth pain is very intense, disturbs sleep and may be confused with trigeminal neuralgia and various headache conditions such as migraine (Chapter 29).

Tooth pain is also present after dental procedures or oral surgery and as with all postoperative pain must be managed using appropriate analgesia to maximize pain control which will facilitate comfort and healing. As with other postoperative pain it is also possible that better pain control at the time of the procedure will diminish the chances of persistent postoperative pain.

Neuropathic orofacial pain

Traumatic injury to trigeminal nerve branches may occasionally result in neuropathic orofacial pain (NOP). The trigeminal system is often stated to have unique features compared to the spinal system with respect to its lower propensity to develop neuropathic pain following a nerve injury [11]; however, direct comparative studies are lacking. Tooth extraction or root canal treatment entails deafferentation of the nerve supply to the tooth pulp [13] and may lead to development of NOP. The presence of chronic infections and inflammatory reactions in the tooth pulp or periapical region may in some cases increase the risk. Third molar surgery causes 4–6% of patients to have somatosensory disturbances in the inferior alveolar or lingual nerves after 1 week but persists only in 0.7–1% after 2 years (for review see Svensson & Baad-Hansen [11]). Orthognathic surgery is used for correction of craniofacial abnormalities and many patients develop injuries to the maxillary or mandibular divisions of the trigeminal nerve. Depending on specific type of osteotomy, patient age, intraoperative variables

and somatosensory assessment techniques, nerve injury prevalence data vary 10–85%, but < 5% of such cases eventually develops NOP [11]. Dental implant insertion and other surgical procedures may also contribute to risk for trigeminal nerve injuries. Zygomatico-orbital fractures are common facial injuries and occur in about 1 of every 10,000 people, with frequent (~ 50%) acute involvement of the somatosensory function of the infraorbital nerve but only 3–4% with chronic NOP [11]. Dental injections carry a very small risk (e.g. 1 out of 26,762 mandibular blocks) for the development of NOP; the proposed mechanisms are direct needle trauma, formation of hematoma or neurotoxicity of the local anesthetic [11].

Patients with NOP report a constant burning, dull aching or sharp and/or shooting pain with a traumatic onset. Pain can be triggered by mechanical stimuli applied to the skin or oral mucosa or by normal oral functions. Clinical inspection reveals no signs of inflammation but there may be somatosensory dysfunction. Quantitative sensory testing (QST) reveals both hypoesthesia and hyperesthesia. Advanced electrophysiological tests are also of potential value [13]. In the differential diagnosis, it is crucial to rule out odontogenic pains, sinusitis, sialoadenitis, atypical facial pain and atypical odontalgia. It has been suggested that QST could be important to differentiate between some of these conditions. Trigeminal neuralgia must also be considered but the clinical presentation is usually very different (Chapter 29).

The pathophysiology of NOP is likely to involve basic mechanisms similar to those linked with spinal nerve lesions. However, recovery appears to be faster in the trigeminal system, autonomic responses differ (e.g. no sprouting of sympathetic terminals on trigeminal ganglion cells), and the neuropeptide content and the specific patterns of upregulation and downregulation of sodium channels are different between the two systems, and these differences have potential implications for clinical characteristics [3]. In the absence of specific guidelines for management of NOP, the same principles as for other neuropathic pain conditions should be followed (Chapter 33). However, an important point is to avoid further trauma to the

Table 31.1 Causes of acute tooth pain.

Condition	Features	Cause/comments	Treatment
Caries	May cause both spontaneous and stimulus-evoked pain		Treat the carious lesion Treat pain with appropriate analgesics
Dentine hypersensitivity	Sharp or shooting pain with mechanical or thermal stimulation of dentinal surface	Caused by hydrodynamic activation of intradental afferents	Local application of fluoride gel or a desensitizing agent [24] Use of a soft toothbrush
Cracked tooth syndrome	Sharp, poorly localized pain evoked by mastication, simple test is to have patient bite on a cotton roll	Incomplete fracture of a vital tooth that may extend into the pulp Radiography does not reveal the pathology	Restorative dental procedure If severe: endodontic treatment or extraction
Reversible pulpitis	No spontaneous pain Evoked by hot or cold liquids or food items	Caused by pulpal inflammation which resolves with treatment or time	Treat the pain evoking stimulus (e.g. carious lesion) If NSAIDs are ineffective a stronger analgesic may be required
Irreversible pulpitis	Spontaneous pain and pain evoked by hot or cold liquids or food items	Caused by pulpal inflammation with changes in pulpal nociceptors and central connections resulting in sensitization	Endodontic treatment and appropriate analgesia*
Apical periodontitis	Often asymptomatic but when present, symptoms include pain, tooth elevation, sensitivity to percussion and swelling	An inflammatory condition of the apical periodontium caused by necrosis of the tooth pulp with accumulation of bacteria and inflammatory mediators in the root canal with spread into periapical tissues	Endodontic treatment If an abscess is present it must be drained and systemic antibiotics may be indicated
Referred pain	Experienced as pain involving the teeth and surrounding tissues	Pain can be referred to the teeth from structures outside of the mouth: • maxillary sinuses • jaw muscles • heart/angina	Rule out dental pathology and TMD, image sinuses, perform EKG, refer to specialist as appropriate

EKG, electrocardiogram; NSAID, non-steroidal anti-inflammatory drug; TMD, temporomandibular disorder.
* Appropriate analgesia refers to treatment required to assist the patient with adequate pain control and is reviewed in chapters on pharmacotherapy.

area (e.g. by avoiding further explorative oral surgery).

Persistent idiopathic facial pain

Persistent idiopathic facial pain (PIFP) includes atypical facial pain (AFP) and atypical odontalgia (AO). AFP is defined as a "persistent facial pain that does not have the characteristics of the cranial neuralgias … and is not attributed to another disorder." The term AO is used for a continuous pain that occurs in a tooth or a tooth socket after extraction and that has no clear identifiable cause. AO has also been called "phantom tooth pain" or idiopathic toothache. Controversy exists regarding these terms; for example, AFP is not included in the International Association for the Study of Pain (IASP) classification [7] but still is used in the International Headache Society (IHS) classification [8]. In this chapter, the terms AO and AFP are used, not because the authors endorse them, but because of the lack of internationally accepted alternatives.

AFP and AO are estimated to be more frequent than trigeminal neuralgia (TN: 0.7/100,000) and less common than TMD. AO may occur in 3–12% of patients having undergone endodontic treatment [14–16]. In this sense the term "idiopathic" may be inappropriate, although the exact mechanisms underlying AO are still unclear. AFP particularly affects middle-aged or older women whereas AO affects both sexes and all adult ages with a predominance of women in their mid-forties. The symptoms can be deep, poorly localized, mostly unilateral (in two-thirds of patients) pain in the mid-face but the pain can also be superficial [17–20]. The pain often starts soon after dental surgery or a trauma, is confined to a defined zone of the face (e.g. the nasolabial groove) but may spread in a fashion that does not follow the distribution of the trigeminal nerve [7]. The pain is present every day, most of the day and is not associated with somatosensory loss or visible signs of pathology. Words like diffuse, drawing, burning, stabbing or throbbing are used to characterize AFP and AO. There is a marked comorbidity especially with psychiatric disorders and other pain conditions (e.g. headache and back pain [20]).

AFP and AO are conditions with suggested risk factors that include psychological factors, hormonal factors, minor nerve trauma and infection of the sinuses or teeth. Tooth pain is excluded by oral and dental examinations with relevant radiography. Diagnostic local anesthetic blocks can be useful when dental pathology is suspected. Pain originating from the maxillary sinuses can be ruled out by nasal endoscopy, radiography or CT of the sinuses. TMD pain also needs to be considered. Trigeminal neuralgia can usually be distinguished from AFP and AO by the symptomatology: patients with trigeminal neuralgia are pain-free most of the

time and have attacks with short-lasting shock-like pain, whereas AFP and AO pain is constant and non-paroxysmal. Patients with some forms of primary headaches may also present with symptoms like AFP and AO.

The management of AFP and AO is challenging. The first step is to educate the patient to accept the fact that there is no infection or "bad tooth" causing the pain. The next step is pharmacological treatment where the first choice is TCAs such as amitriptyline. Anticonvulsants such as gabapentin may also be useful. Other types of treatments (e.g. acupuncture, transcutaneous electrical nerve stimulation [TENS], biofeedback) lack sufficient evidence, whereas hypnosis appears effective [21]. Opioids and NMDA receptor antagonists are not promising agents in AO treatment [22].

Burning mouth syndrome

Burning mouth syndrome (BMS) is an intraoral burning sensation for which no dental or medical cause is evident. Other terms such as glossodynia and stomatodynia have been used [23]. Its prevalence is 0.7–15% but may be confounded by inclusion of burning mouth as a *symptom* rather than a *syndrome*. BMS increases with age and women aged 60–69 have the highest prevalence. BMS is characterized by daily moderate to severe burning pain, sometimes with dysesthetic qualities, in the mouth (tongue, palate, lips, gingiva) persisting for most of the day. The oral mucosa looks normal and no pathology can be detected. Symptoms are usually bilateral and may be associated with taste changes and dry mouth. There is significant comorbidity with depression and anxiety but for most patients these are likely the result of having a constant pain condition of unknown cause.

The etiology and pathophysiology of BMS are unknown; however, recent studies have demonstrated intraoral small-fiber changes, (subclinical) somatosensory changes, and abnormal brainstem reflex responses, which suggest dysfunction in the periphery or CNS.

In the differential diagnosis, it is important to appreciate that burning mouth symptoms could be caused by systemic or local conditions, including anemia, vitamin B, folic acid or iron deficiency, untreated diabetes, hormonal disturbances, oral candidiasis, hyposalivation, Sjögren's syndrome, oral lichen planus, systemic lupus erythematosus, medication side effects and certain allergies.

Management consists of patient education, avoidance of spicy foods and some patients experience pain relief while sucking (sugar-free) pastilles. Pharmacological treatment of BMS is generally disappointing. Antidepressants are not more effective than placebo. Topical clonazepam may have some clinical use.

References

1 Meyer RA, Ringkamp M, Campbell JN *et al.* (2006) Peripheral mechanisms of cutaneous nociception. In: McMahon SB, Koltzenburg M, eds. *Wall and Melzack's Textbook of Pain*, 5th edn. Elsevier, Amsterdam. pp. 3–34.

2 Matthews B, Sessle BJ. (2008) Peripheral mechanisms of orofacial pain. In: Sessle BJ, Lavigne GL, Lund JP *et al.*, eds. *Orofacial Pain*, 2nd edn. Quintessence, Chicago. pp. 27–43.

3 Sessle BJ. (2009) Role of peripheral mechanisms in craniofacial pain conditions. In: Cairns BE, ed. *Peripheral Receptor Targets for Analgesia: Novel Approaches to Pain Management*. Wiley, New York. pp. 3–20.

4 Sessle BJ. (2000) Acute and chronic craniofacial pain: brainstem mechanisms of nociceptive transmission and neuroplasticity, and their clinical correlates. *Crit Rev Oral Biol Med* **11**:57–91.

5 Woda A. (2003) Pain in the trigeminal system: from orofacial nociception to neural network modeling. *J Dent Res* **82**:764–8.

6 Sessle BJ, Iwata K, Dubner R. (2008) Central nociceptive pathways. In: Sessle BJ, Lavigne GL, Lund JP *et al.*, eds. *Orofacial Pain*, 2nd edn. Quintessence, Chicago. pp. 35–43.

7 Merskey H, Bogduk N. (1994) *Classification of Chronic Pain*, 2nd edn. IASP Press, Seattle.

8 Headache Classification Committee. (2004) International Classification of Headache Disorders, 2nd edn. *Cephalalgia* **24(Suppl 1)**: 1–160.

9 Okeson JP. (2005) *Bell's Orofacial Pains*, 6th edn. Quintessence, Chicago.

10 McNeil C, Dubner R, Woda A. (2008) What is pain and how do we classify orofacial pain? In: Sessle BJ, Lavigne GL, Lund JP *et al.*, eds. *Orofacial Pain*, 2nd edn. Quintessence, Chicago. pp. 3–11.

11 Svensson P, Baad-Hansen L. (2008) Facial pain. In: Wilson P, Watson PJ, Haythornthwaite JA *et al.*, eds. *Clinical Pain Management: Chronic Pain*, 2nd edn. Hodder Arnold, Cornwall. pp. 467–83.

12 Schindler H, Svensson P. (2007) Myofascial temporomandibular disorder pain. In: Turp JC, Sommer C, Hugger A, eds. *The Puzzle of Orofacial Pain: Pain and Headache*. Karger, Basel. pp. 91–123.

13 Svensson P, Sessle BJ. (2004) Orofacial pain. In: Miles TS, Nauntofte B, Svensson P, eds. *Clinical Oral Physiology*. Quintessence, Chicago. pp. 93–139.

14 Woda A, Pionchon P. (1999) A unified concept of idiopathic orofacial pain: clinical features. *J Orofac Pain* **13**:172–84.

15 Clark GT. (2006) Persistent orodental pain, atypical odontalgia and phantom tooth pain: when are they neuropathic disorders? *J Calif Dent Assoc* **34**:599–609.

16 Lynch ME. (1996) The role of sympathetic activity in orofacial pain. *J Orofac Pain* **10**:297–305.

17 Campbell RL, Parks KW, Dodds RN. (1990) Chronic facial pain associated with endodontic therapy. *Oral Surg Oral Med Oral Pathol* **69**:287–90.

18 Marbach JJ, Raphael KG. (2000) Phantom tooth pain: a new look at an old dilemma. *Pain Med* **1**:68–77.

19 Polycarpou N, Ng YL, Canavan D *et al.* (2005) Prevalence of persistent pain after endodontic treatment and factors affecting its occurrence in cases with complete radiographic healing. *Int Endod J* **38**:169–78.

20 Baad-Hansen L. (2008) Atypical odontalgia: pathophysiology and clinical management. *J Oral Rehabil* **35**:1–11.

21 Abrahamsen R, Baad-Hansen L, Svensson P. (2008) Hypnosis in the management of persist-

ent idiopathic orofacial pain: clinical and psychosocial findings. *Pain* **136**:44–52.

22 Baad-Hansen L, Juhl GI, Brandsborg B *et al.* (2007) Differential effect of intravenous S-ketamine and fentanyl on atypical odontalgia and capsaicin-evoked pain. *Pain* **129**:46–54.

23 Forssell H, Svensson P. (2006) Facial pain: atypical facial pain and burning mouth syndrome. In: Cervero F, Jensen TS, eds. *Handbook of Clinical Neurology*, 3rd series. Elsevier, Amsterdam. pp. 573–96.

24 Orchardson R, Gillam DG. (2006) Managing dentin hypersensitivity. *J Am Dent Assoc* **137**:990–8.

Chapter 32

Visceral pain

Klaus Bielefeldt[1,2] & Gerald F. Gebhart[1,3]

[1] Center for Pain Research, University of Pittsburgh Medical Center, Pittsburgh, USA
[2] Department of Medicine, University of Pittsburgh Medical Center, Pittsburgh, USA
[3] Department of Anesthesiology, University of Pittsburgh Medical Center, Pittsburgh, USA

Introduction

Visceral pain is a common clinical problem and manifests in a wide spectrum of illnesses from acute myocardial infarction to dysmenorrhea or irritable bowel syndrome. Not surprisingly, severity, duration, location and character of pain as well as associated symptoms vary tremendously. Despite these obvious differences, visceral pain syndromes share some characteristics. Sherrington defined visceral sensations as introceptive. Such introceptive signals provide important homeostatic information and are closely linked to autonomic function. Introception is also associated with a strong motivational dimension. For example, hunger triggers complex behavioral responses that ultimately result in food intake. The level of complexity increases even further as motivation and emotion are closely related, which may explain why humans rate the unpleasantness of visceral events (e.g. rectal distension) higher than that of similarly intense somatic stimuli (e.g. local pressure) [1].

Visceral pain is associated with changes in autonomic function that may be cause and/or consequence of the underlying painful disorder

and often complicate treatment. This interrelationship affects pain management, as medications may also influence organ function (e.g. constipation with opioids). The affective dimensions of pain are quite prominent, especially if essential and typically pleasant activities of daily life such as eating become triggers of pain or other unpleasant sensations.

Basic mechanisms of visceral pain

Investigating pain mechanisms largely focuses on nociception, which links a noxious stimulus to perception and behavioral responses. While this concept is not entirely correct, it enables us to investigate and treat components that contribute to pain.

Molecular mechanisms of visceral sensation

Based on the link between activation of peripheral afferents and perception, we should be able to blunt or even block pain by interfering with the molecules that translate a noxious stimulus into action potentials discharged by nociceptive neurons. Several candidate molecules have emerged. Using pharmacologic tools or experiments with knockout animals, three members of the transient receptor potential family of ion channels (TRPV1, TRPV4, TRPA1) appear to have

Clinical Pain Management: A Practical Guide, 1st edition.
Edited by Mary E. Lynch, Kenneth D. Craig and
Philip W.H. Peng.
© 2011 Blackwell Publishing Ltd.

an important role in responses to high intensity mechanical stimulation during visceral distension [2]. Purinergic receptors, which are activated by ATP, may also contribute to visceral sensation and pain. These receptors require ATP release from neighboring cells, thus functionally linking the nervous system to other structures, such as the epithelium. The importance of epithelial signals has long been recognized in gastrointestinal physiology, with specialized enteroendocrine cells releasing mediators, which in turn activate primary afferent neurons. The best-characterized signaling cascade involves the release of serotonin, which initiates local reflexes and activates extrinsic afferents that may lead to conscious perception of visceral stimuli [3]. Recent evidence points to endocannabinoids as another signaling system that modulates visceral sensation and function. Animal experiments and human data have clearly established a role for cannabinoid receptors in regulation of gastrointestinal motility and transit, which may have therapeutic potential but also contribute to adverse effects. While effective as antiemetics, cannabinoid agonists have not yet demonstrated analgesic properties in visceral pain in humans [4].

Structural elements of visceral sensation

The density of visceral afferent innervation is relatively low. Many sensory neurons have multiple receptive fields within one organ. Most visceral afferents are polymodal, meaning they respond to more than one stimulus modality. These anatomic and physiologic findings correlate with the clinical observation that visceral sensations are poorly localized and do not reliably reflect the underlying stimulus modality.

Except for pelvic structures, all viscera receive a dual sensory innervation with spinal and vagal afferents. Pelvic organs are also innervated by two distinct sensory pathways, which both project to the spinal cord via the lower splanchnic and pelvic nerve, respectively. The cell bodies of vagal sensory fibers are located in the nodose and the slightly more rostral jugular ganglion, with central termination projecting directly to brainstem nuclei.

Vagal afferent input has a role in the regulation of autonomic and homeostatic functions and is important in nausea, cough and dyspnea, or complex sensations, such as hunger or satiety, but likely contributes little to acute pain. Spinal afferents have their cell bodies in dorsal root ganglia and project to second order neurons within the spinal cord, which will send information rostrally through the spinothalamic tract and dorsal column. Second order neurons in the spinal cord typically receive convergent input from cutaneous sites, which provides the structural basis for pain referral.

Central processing of visceral sensation

Perception requires the activation of higher cortical structures. Detailed psychophysical experiments coupled with functional brain imaging revealed a matrix of structures activated by painful stimuli, discussed in more detail in Chapter 3. Despite similarities, some differences are emerging between visceral and somatic sensation. Visceral sensations typically activate the anterior portion of the insular cortex with relatively limited activity in the somatosensory cortex. Consistent with the more significant emotional impact, visceral pain is associated with more activity in the rostral cingulate cortex and amygdyla [5].

Sensitization and visceral pain

We can typically describe the relationship between a stimulus and the related sensory response as a stimulus response function. More than 30 years ago, clinical studies in patients with irritable bowel syndrome (IBS) first demonstrated a shift of this stimulus–response function to greater sensitivity. Many subsequent studies suggest that sensitization of sensory pathways and processing contributes to the pathogenesis of chronic visceral pain syndromes. Sensitization can be caused by peripheral and/or central mechanisms. Experimentally induced gastrointestinal inflammation increases the excitability of primary afferent neurons. A variety of mediators have been identified as likely contributors, including prostaglandins, bradykinin, interleukins, cytokines and also several neurotrophic factors. Considering the importance of neurotrophic factors in maintaining or modulating the function of nerve cells, these signaling pathways may have a special role in chronic pain syndromes. Extensive experimental data show changes in the properties of second order spinal neurons and more rostrally located areas of the central nervous system, which are at least in part mediated through glutamate acting on N-methyl -D-aspartate (NMDA) receptors.

More than 10 years ago, researchers suggested that two distinct mechanisms contribute to the development of visceral hyperalgesia: hypersensitivity, as described above, and hypervigilance [6]. Hypervigilance is defined by a focus on visceral symptoms, typically driven by anxiety and cognitive appraisal of symptoms (e.g. catastrophizing), which results in enhanced perception of visceral input (see also Chapter 4).

Pain without peripheral input

The mechanisms of hypersensitivity described above are all based on shifts in the causal relationship between a noxious stimulus, its perception and the reaction of the organism. However, the model fails to explain chronic pain that is present without any peripheral input. While such a scenario runs counter to our training and practice, it is clinically quite relevant. For example, patients with IBS reported visceral pain in response to a visual stimulus that had previously been linked to painful colorectal distension. Functional brain imaging performed during such "conditioned" pain showed activation patterns that were quite similar to those seen during actual painful visceral stimulation [7]. Neuroaxial blocks to the point of complete surgical anesthesia eliminated pain in less than 50% of patients with chronic pancreatitis.

Evidence-based treatment strategies

The multiple organ systems that may be directly or indirectly involved in visceral pain syndromes often lead to very different symptoms, from palpitation or shortness of breath to nausea or constipa-tion. Despite the resulting complexity, several strategies have been tested across different patient groups.

Interventions targeting peripheral pathways

A variety of strategies have been developed to block the signal transduction and transfer of nociceptive neurons, with mixed and inconclusive results. Considering the preferential distribution of the vanilloid receptor TRPV1 on likely nociceptive neurons, antagonists and receptor desensitization through agonist application have been used in preclinical studies and/or small clinical studies. While promising, the approach is not ready for routine use. Rather than targeting a specific ion channel or a subgroup of nerve endings, one could less selectively suppress afferent input, for example by using local anesthetics. Topical administration of lidocaine has demonstrated some benefit in small studies. However, the need for repeated administration (e.g. lidocaine enemas) limits its utility in the management of chronic visceral pain syndromes [8]. Peripherally acting k-opioid receptor agonists of the arylamide family have been shown to block sodium channels and have decreased visceral hypersensitivity in animal studies. However, clinical studies do not show a convincing analgesic effect in patients with visceral pain. Pregabalin and gabapentin interact with the $\alpha_2\delta$ subunit of voltage-sensitive calcium channels and thus target peripheral and central nociception. Available evidence suggests improved responses to acute experimental visceral pain, but no significant change in disease-related chronic pain ratings [9].

The complexity of visceral innervation with bilateral afferent input and spinal as well as vagal sensory pathways complicates the practical use of regional blocks. Depending on the primary location and presumed etiology of the pain syndrome, three anatomically distinct areas are currently treated through such blocks, even though evidence supporting their efficacy is still limited. Small case series suggest a potential benefit of stellate ganglion block in select patients with refractory angina symptoms [10]. Splanchnic or celiac blocks have been examined more extensively, mostly in patients with advanced pancreatic adenocarcinoma. Current evidence supports a significant, albeit transient, improvement in pain control with decreased opioid use (Chapter 19). Uterine nerve ablation and/or presacral neurectomy are used in women with chronic pelvic pain associated with dysmenorrhea [11]. A single small randomized controlled trial suggests a small increase in efficacy of this approach compared with medical management, but will require confirmation through a larger study with longer follow-up.

Interventions targeting visceral contractions

Intermittent visceral pain is often associated with changes in smooth muscle activity, which may secondarily increase afferent input. Reducing contractility, for example with anticholinergics, has demonstrated some benefit in patients with IBS [5]. Considering the importance of prostaglandins in uterine contractions, non-steroidal anti-inflammatory drugs (NSAIDs) are helpful in alleviating uterine cramps. One trial showed benefit of inhaled beta-adrenergic agonists in proctalgia fugax, a disorder characterized by intense anal pain, mediated by internal anal sphincter contractions. Considering the importance of serotonin in gastrointestinal physiology, several drugs interfering with serotonin receptor signaling have been examined, but none showed convincing effects on visceral pain.

Interventions targeting central processing

Centrally acting analgesics

Opioids certainly blunt visceral pain. Yet, concerns about dependence, abuse and long-term effects certainly argue against their widespread use in common benign disorders. In addition, opioid side effects from nausea to constipation target visceral function. Nevertheless, opioids remain the mainstay of medical therapy for acute visceral pain and chronic pain associated with pancreatitis or pancreatic cancer.

Antidepressants

Based on studies showing a potential benefit in neuropathic pain, tricyclic antidepressants (TCAs) were employed in patients with visceral pain syndromes. While several studies reported changes in sensory thresholds or global improvement, results varied [12]. Consistent with meta-analyses, the largest trial did not show a significant benefit of desimipramine for patients with IBS when examined based on an intention-to-treat analysis, which may in part be because of the high incidence of adverse effects and patient withdrawals. In a "per-protocol analysis" antidepressants were superior to placebo, providing some, albeit less than convincing rationale for their use in clinical practice [13]. With the advent of newer agents, selective serotonin reuptake inhibitors (SSRIs) have also been tested in the management of patients with chronic visceral pain. Results were mixed but do not support significant benefit of SSRIs in visceral pain. To date, only one serotonin/norepinephrine reuptake inhibitor (venlafaxine) has been systematically examined in patients with chronic visceral pain and was not found to be superior to placebo [14].

Psychologically based interventions

Based on the importance of anxiety and depression in chronic visceral pain syndromes, psychological interventions may have an important role in their management. Several studies have examined the effects of cognitive behavioral therapy and hypnotherapy in different patient groups. While the effects on pain rating vary, most investigations demonstrate an improvement in global well-being scores that may be maintained for years after completion of treatment [15].

Alternative and complementary therapies

With the limited treatment options and often persistent symptoms, the use of alternative medical approaches from dietary changes to therapeutic writing is widespread [16]. Very few studies have systematically evaluated the effectiveness of these

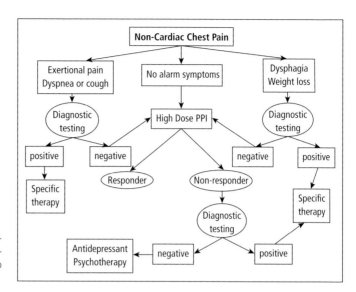

Figure 32.1 Diagnostic and therapeutic approach in patients with non-cardiac chest pain. PPI, proton pump inhibitor.

interventions in visceral pain. Of the different herbal remedies, only peppermint oil and capsaicin have some empiric support, suggesting utility in IBS or functional dyspepsia, respectively. While many case series indicate a potential benefit of acupuncture, a large and well-designed trial did not demonstrate any benefit compared to sham treatment [17]. Considering the likely interaction between luminal contents and visceral function and sensation, dietary intervention or alterations of the microbial flora within the gastrointestinal tract are intuitively attractive for patients with IBS or functional dyspepsia. Initial evidence supports a potential benefit of probiotics or restrictive diets in some patient subgroups [18]. However, results are inconclusive and such strategies should not yet be included in the routine treatment of visceral pain syndromes.

Management of common visceral pain syndromes

By the time patients seek specialized help to manage pain or discomfort most of the affected individuals have already been evaluated extensively and tried a variety of different treatment approaches. Consensus or evidence-based treatments have typically been exhausted. Nevertheless, we outline algorithms for the more common visceral pain syndromes to provide some guidance for a rational approach in these patients.

Non-cardiac chest pain

Non-cardiac chest pain (NCCP) is typically an intermittent non-exertional pain that is not associated with dyspnea or other symptoms suggesting a cardiac etiology. The most common cause of NCCP is gastroesophageal acid reflux. Thus, the most cost-effective approach is an empiric trial of high dose acid suppression, which may even function as a diagnostic tool. If this step fails, compliance, appropriate dosing and timing of medication use should be checked before contemplating further steps, which will depend on the presence of associated symptoms (Figure 32.1) [19].

Functional dyspepsia

Dyspeptic symptoms are quite common with an estimated prevalence of up to 15% in the general population. Pain or discomfort are primarily localized in the epigastric area and typically show an association with food intake. Considering the

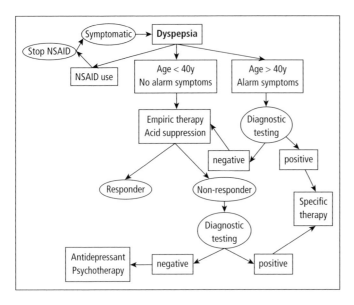

Figure 32.2 Diagnostic and therapeutic approach in patients with dyspeptic symptoms in countries with low prevalence of *Helicobacter pylori* infection. NSAID, non-steroidal anti-inflammatory drug.

importance of gastric acidity in foregut disorders, therapies primarily rely on empiric acid suppression, unless alarm symptoms, such as weight loss or bleeding, are present. While infections with *Helicobacter pylori* may contribute to chronic dyspeptic symptoms, the low prevalence in Western countries argues against a practice that routinely looks for infectious gastritis as the initial step (Figure 32.2) [20].

Chronic pancreatitis

Chronic pancreatitis typically causes significant pain, which may decrease with the development of atrophy during disease progression. Most patients will receive opioids, which is problematic considering the importance of substance abuse (i.e. alcoholism) as the most common cause for chronic pancreatitis in Western countries. While localized nerve blocks can be performed relatively easily, they only provide transient if any benefit. Strategies to improve pain by inhibiting pancreatic stimulation through oral administration of pancreatic enzymes are often used but have not consistently shown benefit [21]. A recent well-designed study suggests a significant benefit of antioxidants [22]. While promising, the results cannot be generalized

as most patients had an idiopathic form of pancreatitis, which is relatively rare in most developed countries.

Irritable bowel syndrome

IBS is the most common gastrointestinal disease associated with discomfort and pain. The clinical manifestations vary substantially, including patients with severe diarrhea as well as individuals with significant constipation. Independent of the clinical scenario, dietary adjustments and lifestyle modification may benefit patients with IBS. While this consensus is largely based on expert opinion, costs and risks of thorough dietary assessment and counseling are minimal. Beyond such general advice, most specific treatment strategies should be based on the dominant complaint. Diarrhea-predominant IBS may benefit from antidiarrheals or cholestyramine. In refractory patients, other options exist, but generally require close monitoring or more extensive testing, and should thus be guided by gastroenterologists. If the patient primarily complains about constipation, laxatives generally improve bowel patterns. If pain persists or is the dominant symptom, current evidence provides some, although not very convincing, support

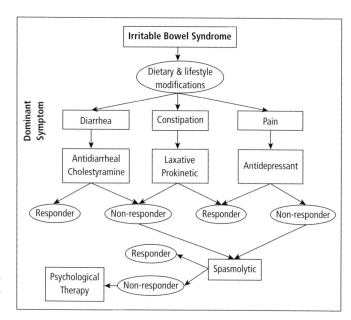

Figure 32.3 Diagnostic and therapeutic approach in patients with irritable bowel syndrome (IBS).

for the use of antidepressant medication. The choice should depend on patient symptoms and comorbid conditions. For example, the constipating effects of TCAs may be desirable in patients with diarrhea, but detrimental if constipation is present. Discomfort may also respond to spasmolytics, such as antimuscarinic agents or peppermint oil. While good evidence supports the use of psychological therapies, well-designed programs are difficult to find, limiting the ability to use them more frequently (Figure 32.3) [23].

Chronic pelvic pain

Chronic pelvic pain encompasses multiple different disorders from myofascial pain to dysmenorrhea or interstitial cystitis. Overall, relatively few well-designed trials have been conducted to examine the efficacy of different diagnostic or therapeutic strategies in patients with chronic pelvic pain and the best approach is to follow the general principles of chronic pain management found in other chapters in this book utilizing a multidisciplinary biopsychosocial approach. If diagnostic evaluations suggest an inflammatory component (e.g. chronic prostatitis), NSAIDs may

be beneficial. Although operative interventions are often used, the true efficacy of surgical approaches has not been systematically examined with adequate follow-up [11].

Conclusions

Chronic visceral pain, from non-cardiac chest pain to IBS, is common. The underlying cause and/or associated changes in visceral function vary tremendously. Compared with somatic pain syndromes, visceral pain carries a more significant emotional burden. Treatment is complicated by the fact that many of the medications used for management of chronic pain exhibit a high incidence of adverse effects on autonomic function. As with all chronic pain conditions, a multidisciplinary approach is required treating pain, clinical manifestation of organ or organ system dysfunction as well as psychosocial factors.

References

1 Strigo IA, Bushnell MC, Boivin M *et al.* (2002) Psychophysical analysis of visceral and cutaneous pain in human subjects. *Pain* **97(3)**:235–46.

2 Robinson DR, Gebhart GF. (2008) Inside information: the unique features of visceral sensation. *Mol Interv* **8(5)**:242–53.

3 Gershon MD, Tack J. (2007) The serotonin signaling system: from basic understanding to drug development for functional GI disorders. *Gastroenterology* **132(1)**:397–414.

4 Fioramonti J, Bueno L. (2008) Role of cannabinoid receptors in the control of gastrointestinal motility and perception. *Exp Rev Gastroenterol Hepatol* **2(3)**:385–97.

5 Knowles CH, Aziz Q. (2009) Basic and clinical aspects of gastrointestinal pain. *Pain* **141(3)**:191–209.

6 Naliboff BD, Munakata J, Fullerton S *et al.* (1997) Evidence for two distinct perceptual alterations in irritable bowel syndrome. *Gut* **41(4)**:505–12.

7 Yáguez L, Coen S, Gregory LJ *et al.* (2005) Brain response to visceral aversive conditioning: a functional magnetic resonance imaging study. *Gastroenterology* **128(7)**:1819–29.

8 Verne GN, Robinson ME, Vase L *et al.* (2003) Reversal of visceral and cutaneous hyperalgesia by local rectal anesthesia in irritable bowel syndrome (IBS) patients. *Pain* **105(1-2)**:223–30.

9 Houghton LA, Fell C, Whorwell PJ *et al.* (2007) Effect of a second-generation $\alpha_2\delta$ ligand (pregabalin) on visceral sensation in hypersensitive patients with irritable bowel syndrome. *Gut* **56(9)**:1218–25.

10 Moore R, Groves D, Hammond C *et al.* (2005) Temporary sympathectomy in the treatment of chronic refractory angina. *J Pain Symptom Manage* **30(2)**:183–91.

11 Cheong Y, William Stones R. (2006) Chronic pelvic pain: aetiology and therapy. *Best Pract Res Clin Obstetr Gynaecol* **20(5)**:695–711.

12 Quartero AO, Meineche-Schmidt V, Muris J *et al.* (2005) Bulking agents, antispasmodic and antidepressant medication for the treatment of irritable bowel syndrome. *Cochrane Database Syst Rev* **2**:CD003460.

13 Drossman DA, Toner BB, Whitehead WE *et al.* (2003) Cognitive-behavioral therapy versus education and desipramine versus placebo for moderate to severe functional bowel disorders. *Gastroenterology* **125**:19–31.

14 van Kerkhoven LAS, Laheij RJF, Aparicio N *et al.* (2008) Effect of the antidepressant venlafaxine in functional dyspepsia: a randomized, double-blind, placebo-controlled trial. *Clin Gastroenterol Hepatol* **6(7)**:746–52.

15 Lackner JM, Mesmer C, Morley S *et al.* (2004) Psychological treatments for irritable bowel syndrome: a systematic review and meta-analysis. *J Consult Clin Psychol* **72**:1100–13.

16 Tillisch K. (2006) Complementary and alternative medicine for functional gastrointestinal disorders. *Gut* **55(5)**:593–6.

17 Lembo AJ, Conboy L, Kelley JM *et al.* (2009) A treatment trial of acupuncture in IBS patients. *Am J Gastroenterol* **104**:1489–97.

18 Camilleri M, Chang L. (2008) Challenges to the therapeutic pipeline for irritable bowel syndrome: end points and regulatory hurdles. *Gastroenterology* **135(6)**:1877–91.

19 Fass R, Sifrim D. (2009) Management of heartburn not responding to proton pump inhibitors. *Gut* **58**:295–309.

20 Tack J, Bisschops R, Sarnelli G. (2004) Pathophysiology and treatment of functional dyspepsia. *Gastroenterology* **127(4)**:1239–55.

21 Winstead NS, Wilcox CM. (2009) Clinical trials of pancreatic enzyme replacement for painful chronic pancreatitis: a review. *Pancreatology* **9**:344–50.

22 Bhardwaj P, Garg PK, Maulik SK *et al.* (2009) A randomized controlled trial of antioxidant supplementation for pain relief in patients with chronic pancreatitis. *Gastroenterology* **136(1)**: 149–59.

23 Mayer EA. (2008) Irritable bowel syndrome. *N Engl J Med* **358(16)**:1692–9.

Chapter 33

Pelvic and urogenital pain

Anjali Martinez[1] & Fred M. Howard[2]

[1] Obstetrics and Gynecology, George Washington University, Washington DC, USA
[2] Obstetrics and Gynecology, University of Rochester School of Medicine, Rochester, USA

Introduction

Chronic pelvic pain is a common disorder in women, with a prevalence of about 4% [1]; similar to the prevalence of migraine headaches and asthma. It is a frequent reason for outpatient visits to doctors. Women with chronic pelvic pain not infrequently also have limited function or disability, marital problems or divorce, and often have been subjected to multiple surgical treatments without much benefit.

Chronic pelvic pain is defined as non-cyclic pelvic or lower abdominal pain of greater than 3–6 months' duration. Traditionally, chronic vulvar pain is not included based on its anatomic location, but it is discussed in this chapter as part of genital pain. Note that a specific diagnosis is not necessary for the diagnosis of chronic pelvic pain, and indeed sometimes chronic pain itself is the only or best diagnosis. Chronic pelvic or urogenital pain may have multiple etiologies, and often multiple etiologies exist at once. Some of these disorders have no cure so naturally lead to the chronic nature of chronic pelvic pain, but why other etiologies lead to chronic pain are less understood.

Clinical Pain Management: A Practical Guide, 1st edition.
Edited by Mary E. Lynch, Kenneth D. Craig and Philip W.H. Peng.
© 2011 Blackwell Publishing Ltd.

Although most etiologies of pelvic pain may start as visceral or somatic nociceptive pain, neuropathic pain or centralization of pain may occur, so that the pain is maintained regardless of the status of the original source of pain.

The differential diagnoses of the disorders associated with chronic pelvic pain are very broad. Visceral sources of pain include the gastrointestinal tract, the urologic system and the reproductive system. Somatic sources of chronic pain in this area include the musculoskeletal system and the neurologic system. In a large British primary care study, chronic pelvic pain was more often related to the gastrointestinal tract and urinary system than to the reproductive system [1]. Although many etiologies of chronic pelvic pain are not gender-specific, this discussion focuses on chronic pelvic pain in women. Disorders that have strong evidence of a causal relationship with chronic pelvic pain include interstitial cystitis, irritable bowel syndrome (IBS), constipation, endometriosis and abdominal wall myofascial pain. For many disorders, there is only limited evidence that the disease leads to chronic pain. For a list of diagnoses commonly associated with chronic pelvic pain see Table 33.1.

Diagnosis is mostly based on a thorough history and physical examination. Because the etiologies of pain are diverse, both the history and examination must cover multiple organ systems. A good

Table 33.1 Conditions that may cause or exacerbate pelvic and urogenital pain, by level of evidence.

Level of evidence	Gastrointestinal	Gynecologic	Urologic	Musculoskeletal
Level A	Irritable bowel syndrome	Endometriosis	Interstitial cystitis	Abdominal wall Myofascial pain (trigger points)
	Constipation	Gynecologic malignancies	Bladder malignancy	Pelvic floor tension myalgia
	Inflammatory bowel disease	Ovarian retention syndrome (residual ovary syndrome)	Radiation Cystitis	Neuralgia of iliohypogstric, ilioinguinal, and/or genitofemoral nerve
	Carcinoma of the colon	Ovarian remnant syndrome		Peripartum pelvic pain syndrome
		Pelvic congestion syndrome		
		Pelvic inflammatory disease		
		Vestibulodynia		
		Vulvodynia		
Level B		Adhesions	Urethral diverticulum	Neoplasia of spinal cord or sacral nerve
		Benign cystic mesothelioma		Coccygodynia
		Leiomyomata		Lumbar disk herniation
		Postoperative peritoneal cysts		
Level C	Colitis	Adenomyosis	Chronic urinary tract infection	Compression of lumbar vertebrae
	Chronic intermittent bowel obstruction	Atypical dysmenorrhea	Recurrent acute cystitis	Degenerative joint disease
	Diverticulosis	Adnexal cysts	Recurrent acute urethritis	Hernias (ventral, inguinal, femoral, spigelian)
		Cervical stenosis	Urolithiasis	Thoracolumbar facet syndrome
		Chronic endometritis		
		Residual accessory ovary		
		Genital prolapse		
		Endosalpingiosis		

Level A: good and consistent scientific evidence of causal relationship to chronic pelvic pain.
Level B: limited or inconsistent scientific evidence of causal relationship to chronic pelvic pain.
Level C: causal relationship to chronic pelvic pain based on expert opinions.

history will include details of the pain itself including quality, severity, timing and location, preferably mapped by the patient on a diagram of the body; a psychosocial history; questions regarding bowel and bladder symptoms and a depression screen.

The physical examination is performed to identify any anatomic sources of the patient's pain. It is important to isolate and examine the musculoskeletal, gastrointestinal, urinary, reproductive and neurological systems during the evaluation to pinpoint specific diagnoses if present. In particular, the pelvic examination for chronic pelvic pain is different from the traditional bimanual pelvic examination in that it is performed with one finger of one hand so that focal areas of tenderness that reproduce the patient's baseline pain can be sought in bony, nervous, muscular and visceral structures (referred to as a "pain-mapping exam"). For details on conducting the physical examination, see Clinical Gynecologic Series: an Expert's View on Chronic Pelvic Pain [2].

Presentations of some of the most common disorders associated with chronic pelvic pain are outlined here. IBS is the most common diagnosis in women with chronic pelvic pain. Diagnosis is based on history but laboratory data may help differentiate it from an infectious or inflammatory process. Symptoms must include chronic abdominal pain and abnormal bowel habits. Because these symptoms are often subjective and vary greatly among individuals, it may be useful to use standardized criteria for the diagnosis of IBS such as the Rome criteria. The most recent criteria (Rome III) are recurrent abdominal pain or discomfort for at least 3 days per month in the last 3 months associated with two or more of the following: pain improves with defecation, onset of pain is associated with a change in frequency of stool or onset of pain is associated with a change in form or appearance of stool [3].

The diagnostic criteria for interstitial cystitis, now often referred to as painful bladder syndrome or bladder pain syndrome, are somewhat controversial. Most often it is a clinical diagnosis characterized as pelvic pain, pressure or discomfort related to the bladder, associated with a persistent urge to void or urinary frequency in the absence of infection or other urinary tract pathology. Patients with interstitial cystitis usually have nocturia as well as daytime frequency. The finding of bladder mucosal hemorrhages or glomerulations at the time of cystoscopy with hydrodistention has traditionally been considered the gold standard for diagnosis, but there is clear evidence that both false negative and false positive findings are relatively common with cystoscopic hydrodistention. An office screening test for interstitial cystitis is the potassium sensitivity test; a patient's symptoms

are evaluated after intravesical instillation of water and then with 40 mL potassium chloride. Most people with interstitial cystitis will have pain and urgency with the potassium instillation. Many clinicians currently make the diagnosis based on clinical criteria only, without performing either cystoscopy or potassium sensitivity testing.

Endometriosis is the presence of histologically confirmed endometrial glands and/or stroma outside of the endometrium and myometrium. Endometriosis-associated pelvic pain usually begins as cyclic menstrual pain or dysmenorrhea but can progress to constant pain with premenstrual and menstrual exacerbations. Patients may also present with an adnexal mass (endometrioma) or infertility. Physical examination is often normal, but sometimes shows evidence of scarring with malposition of the uterus or cervix, palpable tender endometriotic nodules or an adnexal mass.

Vestibulodynia (also called provoked localized vulvodynia or vulvar vestibulitis) is a chronic recurrent vulvar pain with abnormal vestibular tenderness to cotton-tip applicator palpation (positive "Q-tip test") at the minor vestibule, external to the hymeneal ring. Frequently, the woman is unable to use tampons and unable to have coitus because of pain. Pain with speculum insertion is almost always present. The "Q-tip test" consists of gentle palpation of the external genitalia and vagina with a cotton swab; tenderness is limited to the vestibule in patients with vestibulodynia. It is important that candidiasis or dermatoses are excluded during the evaluation.

Many of the diagnoses associated with chronic pelvic pain need no diagnostic laboratory or imaging studies, so routine testing, such as barium enemas, colonoscopy, laparoscopy or intravenous pyelography, is not always necessary. Diagnostic testing should be based on the history and physical examination evaluations. For example, diagnostic laparoscopy is valuable if chronic pain is thought to be caused by endometriosis or pelvic adhesive disease, but not if interstitial cystitis or IBS seem to be the most likely associated disorders. A negative laparoscopy should never be used to tell a patient that she has no diagnosis or that her pain is not real.

Like many sources of chronic pain, treatment options for chronic pelvic or urogenital pain are usually not curative. Instead, the goal of treatment is control of symptoms and for improved function and activity. Treatment can be pain-specific for chronic pain itself or disease-specific, meaning it targets the diagnoses that are contributing to the patient's pain. A patient's treatment regimen may often include both of these treatment options.

Pain-specific treatment

Education, reassurance and a good patient–physician relationship go a long way in treating chronic pain conditions. Often, a patient with chronic pelvic pain has been to many doctors and simply listening to their story and believing their symptoms benefits them. Medical treatment for chronic pain includes analgesics such as aspirin, acetaminophen, non-steroidal anti-inflammatory medications and opiates. Opiates for chronic pain should be used after other analgesics have failed and when there is a need to improve the patient's level of functioning or activity. Opiates used for chronic pain should be taken on a regular schedule instead of as needed. Medical management may also include antidepressants, especially tricyclic antidepressants because they can help improve pain tolerance and sleep habits separately from their antidepressive qualities. Anticonvulsants such as gabapentin or pregabalin are often used in medical treatment, especially if neuropathic pain is a possible component of the patient's pain. Further detail is summarized in a recent review on the management of chronic pelvic pain [4].

Disease-specific treatment

For brevity, specific treatment options for only the most common disorders causing chronic pelvic or urogenital pain are discussed here.

Endometriosis

Endometriosis can be treated medically and surgically. Medical treatment usually involves hormonal suppression of ovarian cycling, with the goal of suppressing growth and activity of endometriosis lesions. The most extensively studied medical treatment for endometriosis is of gonadotropin-releasing hormone agonists (GnRH-a). In a randomized controlled trial of empiric treatment with the GnRH-a depot leuprolide, patients with suspected endometriosis based on extensive clinical evaluation (without laparoscopies) were treated with leuprolide or placebo for 3 months [5]. Some 81% of patients on leuprolide had pain relief, compared with 39% of patients who received placebo. Most of the patients in this study had confirmation of the diagnosis of endometriosis when laparoscopies were carried out after the 3 month trial. Duration of treatment with GnRH agonists is associated with loss in bone mineral density over time. Treatment should be limited to 6 months at a time to limit adverse affects or add-back therapy of estrogens and/or progesterone can be used concurrently to minimize loss of bone density. Add-back therapy limits bone density loss but may lead to side effects such as breakthrough bleeding and pain symptoms. Combination oral contraceptives are often used to treat endometriosis in either cycling or continuous form, but are not as well studied in clinical trials for this purpose. Progestin only treatment is another option and its efficacy has been confirmed in clinical trials. Norethindrone acetate and medroxyprogesterone acetate are the progestins that have been shown to be effective in clinical trials of treatment of endometriosis-associated pelvic pain. Medical treatments are only effective while the woman is actively taking the medicine; effects wear off soon after discontinuing treatment. In summary, medical treatment options include daily oral progestins, cyclic or continuous oral contraceptives, or GnRH agonists alone for up to 6 months or longer with add-back therapy.

Surgical treatment options include laparoscopic treatment of endometriosis. Laparoscopy may also be diagnostic, as biopsies taken during laparoscopy may confirm the diagnosis. Two blinded randomized controlled trials have been carried out confirming the efficacy of conservative surgical treatment of endometriosis for alleviating pelvic pain [6,7]. Performing presacral neurectomy at the time of endometriosis surgery has been shown to slightly improve pain relief with conservative surgery [8]. Uterosacral nerve ablation has not been shown to improve pain symptoms compared to traditional surgical treatment [9,10].

There is no study directly comparing medical and surgical treatments for endometriosis, but comparing Ling's [5] outcomes in the leuprolide study and Sutton *et al.*'s [6] findings in the surgery study suggest that efficacy may be similar.

Irritable bowel syndrome

Dietary modification is usually recommended as first line therapy for IBS but has not been well studied [3]. A trial of eliminating lactose should be attempted because of the similar symptoms of lactose intolerance and IBS and their frequent overlap. Artificial sweeteners and fructose may also contribute to symptoms and should be avoided. Patients with gas and bloating symptoms should try to eliminate drinking carbonated beverages, chewing gum and smoking to decrease the amount of swallowed air and to decrease the intake of gas-producing foods. In patients with predominantly gas and bloating symptoms fiber may exacerbate symptoms, but in patients with constipation increased fiber may help. Medical management targets the patient's most bothersome symptoms. Antispasmodics such as peppermint oil or dicyclomine can help with gas and bloating and antidiarrheals such as loperamide are helpful in patients with predominantly symptoms of diarrhea.

Interstitial cystitis

Behavioral and diet modifications are often the first recommended treatments for painful bladder syndrome, but have not been well studied. Foods or beverages such as alcohol, caffeine and acidic foods that exacerbate symptoms should be avoided. Sodium pentosan polysulfate is the only Food and Drug Administration approved oral medication for interstitial cystitis. Based on a systematic review, it was shown to be more effective than placebo at relieving pain and other symptoms with a relative risk of 1.78 [11] and a number-needed-to-treat of about 3.8. A randomized controlled study showed that 4-month treatment with amitriptyline helped with pain and urgency symptoms in interstitial cystitis or painful bladder syndrome but was not statistically significant in improving urinary frequency when compared with placebo [12].

Vestibulodynia/provoked localized vestibular pain

Medical treatment of localized provoked vestibulodynia include topical treatments such as 5% lidocaine and systemic medications such as tricyclic antidepressants. About half the women who self-treated with topical lidocaine reported a 50% improvement in symptoms [13]. The most effective treatment for localized provoked vestibulodynia is surgery in the form of a vulvar vestibulectomy; success rates are between about 60% and 90%. The efficacy of surgical treatment has been confirmed by a randomized clinical trial [14]. However, because surgical therapy is more invasive, it is often offered only if medical management is ineffective.

Conclusions

Because chronic pelvic pain is relatively common among women and the differential diagnoses are so broad, it is important for healthcare providers across many specialties to be familiar with the commonly associated disorders and the idea that chronic pain itself may be the most important or possibly the only diagnosis. Having a physician listen and then validate the patient's chronic pelvic pain is an important component of treatment. Finally, first line treatment may often be offered regardless of the provider's specialty, decreasing the time the woman searches for care before she starts getting help for her chronic pain.

References

1 Zondervan KT, Yudkin PL, Vessey MP *et al.* (1999) Patterns of diagnosis and referral in women consulting for chronic pelvic pain in UK primary care. *Br J Obstet Gynaecol* **106**:1156–61.

2 Howard, F. (2003) Chronic pelvic pain. *Obstet Gynecol* **101(3)**:594–611. Clinical Gynecologic Series: An Expert's View.

3 Longstreth GF, Thompson WG, Chey W *et al.* (2006) Functional bowel disorders. *Gastroenterology* **130(5)**:1480–91.

4 Fall M, Baranowski AP, Elniel S *et al.* (2010) EAU guidelines on chronic pelvic pain. *Eur Urol* **57**:35–48.

5 Ling FW. (1999) Randomized controlled trial of depot leuprolide in patients with chronic pelvic pain and clinically suspected endometriosis. Pelvic Pain Study Group. *Obstet Gynecol* **93**: 51–8.

6 Sutton CJG, Ewen SP, Whitelaw N *et al.* (1994) Prospective, randomized, double-blind trial of laser laparoscopy in the treatment of pelvic pain asociated with minimal, mild and moderate endometriosis. *Fertil Steril* **62**:696–700.

7 Abbott JA, Hawe J, Clayton RD *et al.* (2003) The effects and effectiveness of laparoscopic excision of endometriosis: a prospective study with 2–5 year follow-up. *Hum Reprod* **18(9)**:1922–7.

8 Zullo F, Palomba S, Zupi E *et al.* (2003) Effectiveness of presacral neurectomy in women with severe dysmenorrhea caused by endometriosis who were treated with laparoscopic conservative surgery: a 1-year prospective randomized double-blind controlled trial. *Am J Obstet Gynecol* **189(1)**:5–10.

9 Sutton C, Pooley A, Jones K *et al.* (2001) A prospective, randomized, double-blind contolled trial of laparoscopic uterine nerve ablation in the treatment of pelvic pain associated with endometriosis. *Gynaecol Endosc* **10(4)**:217–22.

10 Vercellini P, Aimi G, Busacca M *et al.* (2003) Laparoscopic uterosacral ligament resection for dysmenorrhea associated with endometriosis: results of a randomized, controlled trial. *Fertil Steril* **80(2)**:310–9.

11 Dimitrakov J, Kroenke K , Steers WD *et al.* (2007) Pharmacologic managment of painful bladder syndrome/interstitial cystitis: a systematic review. *Arch Intern Med* **167(18)**:1922–9.

12 van Ophoven A, Pokupic S, Heinecke A *et al.* (2004) A prospective, randomized, placebo controlled, double-blind study of amitriptyline for the treatment of interstitial cystitis. *J Urol* **172(2)**:533–6.

13 Landry T, Bergeron S, Dupuis MJ *et al.* (2008) The treatment of provoked vestibulodynia: a critical review. *Clin J Pain* **24(2)**:155–71.

14 Bergeron S, Binik Y, Khalife S *et al.* (2001) A randomized comparison of group cognitive-behavioral therapy, surface electromyographic biofeedback and vestibulectomy in the treatment of dyspareunia resulting from vulvar vestibulitis. *Pain* **91**:297–306.

Chapter 34

Neuropathic pain

Maija Haanpää[1] & Rolf-Detlef Treede[2]

[1] Rehabilitation Orton, Helsinki, Finland; Department of Neurosurgery, Helsinki University Hospital, Helsinki, Finland
[2] Medical Faculty Mannheim, University of Heidelberg, Mannheim, Germany

Introduction

Neuropathic pain (NP), defined as "pain arising as a direct consequence of a lesion or disease affecting the somatosensory system" [1] is a challenge to healthcare providers as it is common, often under-diagnosed, under-treated and, when severe, associated with suffering, disability and impaired quality of life. Standard treatment with conventional analgesics does not typically provide effective relief of pain.

In population-based studies the prevalence of pain with neuropathic characteristics is 7–8%, including mild cases with no need for symptomatic treatment. The most common reasons for NP are radiculopathy, diabetic polyneuropathy and nerve trauma including postoperative neuralgia. As the prevalence of diabetes is expected to double over the next two decades, the prevalence of painful diabetic neuropathy is presumably increasing. Herpes zoster, degeneration of the spine and stroke are common in the elderly and cause chronic NP in a substantial number of people. As the proportion and number of elderly is

increasing worldwide, the prevalence of these NP conditions is rising.

Unlike nociceptive pain, which is caused by physiological activation of peripheral nociceptive nerve terminals to threat of tissue damage, chronic NP has no beneficial effect. It can arise from damage to the nerve pathways at any point from the terminals of the peripheral nociceptors to the cortical neurons in the brain. NP is classified as central (originating from damage of brain or spinal cord) or peripheral (originating from damage in peripheral nerves, plexus or roots). NP is also classified on the basis of the character of the insult to the nervous system (e.g. inflammatory, metabolic, vascular or mechanical). Only a small minority (5%) of patients with peripheral nerve injury develop NP, whereas in spinal cord injury the percentage is at least 50%. It is not known why the same condition is painful in some patients and painless in others.

Currently, a mechanism-based classification of NP is not possible, as the detailed pain mechanisms in an individual case cannot be identified. Furthermore, one mechanism can be responsible for many different symptoms, and the same symptom in two patients can be caused by different mechanisms [2]. As NP can coexist with nociceptive pain, clinicians should try to identify different pain components and treat each of them according to the best available evidence.

Clinical Pain Management: A Practical Guide, 1st edition.
Edited by Mary E. Lynch, Kenneth D. Craig and
Philip W.H. Peng.
© 2011 Blackwell Publishing Ltd.

Basic mechanisms

Damage to the somatosensory system leads to negative sensory symptoms (feeling of numbness) and signs (sensory loss to the somatosensory submodalities touch, proprioception, thermoreception, nociception or visceroreception). Damaged neurons, however, can also develop spontaneous activity (e.g. by altered expression of ion channels at a neuroma or in the dorsal root ganglion). When ectopically generated action potentials are transmitted to the nociceptive network in the brain, this results in a pain sensation that is projected to the receptive field of the damaged neural structure (Figure 34.1). Peripheral nerve damage can also lead to secondary changes within the central nervous system, including altered synaptic connectivity and receptive field reorganization. These secondary changes involve local excitatory and inhibitory neurons, ascending and descending

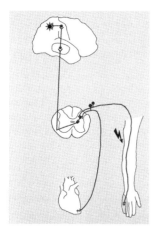

Nerve damage

Impulse conduction

Brain activation

Pain projection

Figure 34.1 Projected pain. Damage to a peripheral nerve may lead to action potential generation at the site of damage. When these action potentials reach the nociceptive network in the brain, the resulting pain sensation is projected into the peripheral receptive field of the damaged nerve, where this activity would normally originate. Thus, pain in a body part may result from damage to that body part itself, or to any site along the neural pathways connecting that body part with the brain. Based on Treede (2001) Kapitel A3, In: Zenz, Jurna (Hrsg.) Lehrbuch der Schemerztherapie, Fig. 11.

pathways, as well as microglia and astrocytes [3]. When the neural damage is partial, the remaining neural connections may be facilitated as a result of these secondary changes, leading to positive sensory symptoms (paraesthesia and spontaneous pain) and signs (hyperalgesia and allodynia, mostly to mechanical or cold stimuli). (For further discussion of mechanisms see Chapter 3.)

The coexistence of negative and positive sensory phenomena within the same region is prototypical for patients with NP. The spatial distribution of these symptoms and signs and the distribution of the projected pain sensation provide information on the neuroanatomic site of neural damage. Current and future therapies for NP are directed at central and peripheral nociceptive signal processing (centrally and peripherally acting analgesics, modulators of endogenous pain control systems), ectopic impulse generation (local anesthetics) and at the pathophysiological processes of degeneration, regeneration and reorganization [4]. In general, systemic NP medication has to pass the blood–brain barrier in order to reach its target. Such a barrier is also present in the peripheral nervous system, but the blood–nerve barrier is leaky in the dorsal root ganglion and in peripheral nerve inflammation.

Clinical picture

NP can be spontaneous (stimulus-independent) or elicited by a stimulus (stimulus-evoked pain). Spontaneous pain is often described as a constant burning sensation [5], but it may also include intermittent shooting lancinating sensations, electric shock-like pain and dysesthesia (i.e. an unpleasant abnormal sensation). The pain may also be accompanied by paresthesia, an abnormal sensation that is not unpleasant. Stimulus-evoked pains are elicited by mechanical, thermal or chemical stimuli. Hyperalgesia consists of an increased pain response to a stimulus that is normally painful and activates peripheral nociceptive terminals, whereas allodynia has been introduced as a term to describe pain sensation from a stimulus that does not normally provoke pain and that does not activate nociceptors (such as gentle stroking by a brush), and thus implies a change in central neural process-ing [6]. Additionally, there may be other symp-toms and clinical findings (e.g. motor paresis, muscle cramps, autonomic nervous system signs) depending on the site of the lesion. It is not possi-ble to conclude the etiology of NP from the clinical characteristics of pain.

Once present, NP pain tends to be long-lasting. However, some patients may recover from their pain completely, and others may obtain relief by pharmacotherapy or learn to cope with their symp-toms by attending interdisciplinary treatment or self-management programs.

Clinical examination

Assessment of a patient with suspected NP aims at: (i) recognition of NP; (ii) localizing of the lesion as far as possible (peripheral or central and further whether the lesion is in the brain hemisphere, brainstem, spinal cord, nerve root, plexus, periph-eral nerve or its branches); and (iii) diagnosing the causative disease or event. In addition, assessment of psychosocial aspects is necessary for an individ-ually tailored management strategy. Possible comorbidities such as impaired sleep, anxiety, depression, disability and secondary impairment in work, family and social life should also be taken into account [7].

The clinical examination of the patient present-ing with NP is the same as that described for any patient presenting with chronic pain (Chapters 7 and 9). The neurosensory examination is particu-larly important. Sensory testing at the bedside can be accomplished with simple tools [8]. Touch is tested with a finger or cotton wool, pinprick with a wooden cocktail stick, warm and cold with a cold and a warm object, and vibration with a tuning fork. The response to each stimulus can be graded as normal, decreased or increased. The findings in the painful area are compared with the findings in the contralateral area in unilateral pain, and in other sites on the proximal–distal axis in bilat-eral pain.

Identifying a neurological disease or a nervous system lesion is based on a systematic search of neurological abnormalities in the clinical examina-tion. In the neurological examination the signs are repeatable, and the location of lesion is concluded on the basis of the neurological signs. In addition to the sensory examination, the motor assessment (muscle strength, tonus, coordination and fluency of movements), examination of tendon reflexes and examination of cranial nerves are performed. Assessment of the peripheral autonomic nervous function (warmth and color of skin, sudomotor function) is important especially when a complex regional pain syndrome is suspected.

Other diagnostic procedures

Sometimes the diagnosis is straightforward (e.g. NP after an obvious nerve lesion during surgery or post-herpetic neuralgia after shingles). In these cases no additional tests are needed. If a patient has stocking and glove-type pain location (Figure 34.2), then one might consider nerve conduction studies (NCS) and electromyography (EMG). As presented in more detail in Chapter 9, EMG and NCS evaluate large myelinated axons and because neuropathic pain is often caused by disease of small myelinated Aδ and C fibers these tests may be normal in patients whose condition principally affects the small fibers. The cause of polyneuropa-thy may be identified further using laboratory tests (e.g. full blood count, sedimentation rate, glucose, creatinine, alanine transaminase [ALT], glucose tolerance test, vitamin B_{12}, serum protein immu-noelectrophoresis and thyroid function). If the NCS and EMG are normal it is possible that the patient may have pure thin fiber polyneuropathy. In this case additional investigations include quan-titative sensory testing (QST) (Chapter 9), laser evoked potential (LEP) and skin biopsy to assess small-caliber (C, Aδ) sensory fibers. These tests are not yet available in many centers and one must often rely on bedside testing and very good clinical examination in order to substantiate the diagnosis. The most common cause for thin-fiber painful polyneuropathy is impaired glucose tolerance.

In general, the decision about a consultation with a specialist should be individualized and depends on the clinical picture, the experience and training of the clinician, and the availability of

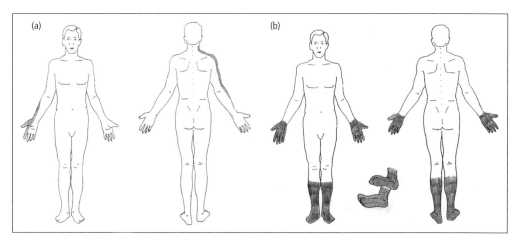

Figure 34.2 Examples of pain drawings of neuropathic pain patients. (a) Radicular pain of the right C6 dermatome. (b) Painful polyneuropathy.

specialists with relevant expertise. Patients suspected to have NP should be seen by a physician who is experienced in assessing somatosensory system function. When referring to the neurological clinic for further assessment, care should be taken to ask for tests of small peripheral fiber and spinothalamic tract system functions, because these tests are not yet part of their standard repertoire. Tests in a specialized center may include conventional electrophysiological procedures, quantitative somatosensory testing, neuroimaging, blood and cerebrospinal fluid samples and less conventional laboratory tools to assess the nociceptive pathways in the peripheral and central nervous systems. For more detailed information, neurological handbooks are recommended.

Management of neuropathic pain

As reviewed in previous chapters, the first step is to educate the patient about the cause of their pain and approaches to management, which include correction of the pathology where possible, self-management strategies, interdisciplinary approaches including therapeutic exercise, addressing of psychosocial issues and pharmacotherapy. As pain is usually regarded as a threat, explaining the character of NP (unnecessary nuisance instead of a warning sign) helps the patient to cope with the situation. The causative disease may warrant specific treatment (e.g. decompression of a peripheral nerve entrapment or a nerve root compression, medication to reach normoglycemia for diabetics to prevent progression of neuropathy and other complications, or immunomodulatory treatment of multiple sclerosis) or secondary prevention (e.g. commencement of antithrombotic medication and control of risk factors of atherosclerosis after a stroke).

Pharmacotherapy of neuropathic pain

Pharmacotherapy of NP must be individualized. NP is treated mainly with antidepressants and antiepileptics, whereas simple analgesics have not shown efficacy on NP. Complete pain relief is usually not achieved. In meta-analyses, patients with at least 50% pain relief are classified as responders. Reduction of pain with at least 30% is considered clinically relevant. The etiology of NP, concomitant chronic medical conditions and their medications, individual risks (e.g. previous abuse or suicidal history) and costs of treatment need to be considered. In addition to pain relief, medication may provide better sleep, improved mood or relief of anxiety. In many cases the side effect profile guides drug selection.

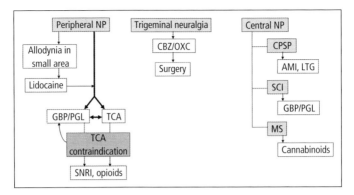

Figure 34.3 Evidence-based treatment algorithm for neuropathic pain (NP). For peripheral NP, tricyclic antidepressants (TCAs) and gabapentinoids (e.g. gabapentin [GBP] or pregabalin [PGL]) are first line, unless TCAs are contraindicated. Topical lidocaine (with local effect) is recommended for patients with dynamic mechanical allodynia in a small area. Serotonin-noradrenalin reuptake inhibitor (SNRI) drugs (duloxetine and venlafaxine) and opioids are second choice. For trigeminal neuralgia the sodium channel blockers carbamazepine (CBZ) and oxcarbazepine (OXC) are first line. If they fail, surgery is recommended. For central post stroke pain (CPSP), amitriptyline (AMI) is first line, but if it fails lamotrigine (LTG) can be tried. Gabapentinoids have shown efficacy for spinal cord injury (SCI) pain, and cannabinoids for multiple sclerosis (MS).

Recent evidence-based guidelines, based on randomized controlled trials, recommend topical lidocaine, tricyclic antidepressants (TCAs), gabapentinoids (gabapentin and pregabalin) and serotonin-noradrenalin reuptake inhibitors (SNRIs; duloxetine and venlafaxine) as the first line choices for NP (Figure 34.3) [9,10]. Carbamazepine and oxcarbazepine are drugs of choice for trigeminal neuralgia. When the first line drugs fail to provide acceptable pain relief for NP other than trigeminal neuralgia, tramadol and strong opioids are recommended, providing the patient has no contraindications for opioid use. Recent observations of opioid-induced endocrine changes and the increase in opioid abuse and diversion have reduced the eagerness to prescribe them. Cannabinoids have demonstrated efficacy in randomized controlled trials of NP in multiple sclerosis, HIV and in NP associated with allodynia [11] but are generally reserved as third line agents or second line when there are additional symptoms such as spasticity or nausea associated with the pain (Chapter 18). In refractory patients, combination therapy using two agents with synergistic mechanisms of action may offer greater pain relief. However, while there is compelling animal evidence for combination therapy, few human studies evaluating the efficacy of various drug combinations have been published. In addition, the risk of side effects may increase with combination therapies. A combination of gabapentin and an opioid (oxycodone or morphine) achieved better analgesia for neuropathic pain than either drug alone [12], as did a combination of nortriptyline with gabapentin [13] but the dosage may need to be adjusted to improve tolerability.

Mechanisms of action and dosing of the first line NP drugs and opioids are presented in Table 34.1. Adverse drug reactions, precautions and contraindications of drugs recommended for NP are summarized in Table 34.2 [14].

For patients with NP refractory to pharmacological therapy [15] neuromodulation may be considered (Chapter 20). Spinal cord stimulation (SCS) is recommended as a possible treatment for adults with chronic pain of neuropathic origin if they continue to experience chronic pain (measuring at least 50 mm on a 0–100 mm visual analog scale) for at least 6 months despite standard treatments, and have had a successful trial of SCS as part of an

Table 34.1 Mechanisms of action and dosing of the first line drugs and opioids for neuropathic pain.

Medication	Mechanism of action	Starting dose	Titration	Maximum recommended dose
TCAs				
Nortriptyline, desipramine, (amitriptyline, imipramine)*	Serotonin and noradrenalin reuptake inhibition, sodium channel block, NMDA-receptor antagonist	10–25 mg at bedtime	Increase by 10–25 mg every 3–7 days as tolerated	150 mg daily; further titration guided by blood concentration of the drug and its active metabolite
SNRIs				
Duloxetine	Serotonin and noradrenalin reuptake inhibition	30 mg once daily	Increase to 60 mg once daily after 1 week	120 mg daily
Venlafaxine	Serotonin and noradrenalin reuptake inhibition	37.5 mg once or twice daily	Increase by 75 mg each week	225 mg daily
Gabapentinoids				
Gabapentin	A calcium channel $\alpha_2\delta$ ligand, which reduces release of presynaptic transmitters	100–300 mg at bedtime	Increase by 100–300 mg three times daily every 1–7 days as tolerated	3600 mg daily (divided into 3 doses)
Pregabalin	A calcium channel $\alpha_2\delta$ ligand, which reduces release of presynaptic transmitters	75 mg twice daily	Increase to 300 mg daily after 3–7 days, then by 150 mg/day every 3–7 days as tolerated	600 mg daily (divided into 2–3 doses)
Topical lidocaine				
5% lidocaine patch	Block of peripheral sodium channels and thus of ectopic discharges	Maximum 3 patches daily for a maximum of 12 h	None needed	Maximum 3 patches daily for a maximum of 12 h
Sodium channel blockers[†]				
Carbamazepine	Sodium channel block	100 mg twice daily	Increase by 100 mg twice daily every 3–7 days as tolerated	1200 mg daily; further titration guided by blood concentration of the drug
Oxcarbazepine	Sodium channel block	150 mg twice daily	Increase by 150 mg twice daily every 3–7 days as tolerated	1800 mg daily; further titration guided by blood concentration of the drug
Opioid agonists				
Tramadol	μ-opioid receptor agonist and serotonin and noradrenalin reuptake inhibition	50 mg once or twice daily	Increase by 50–100 mg daily in divided doses every 3–7 days as tolerated	400 mg daily; in patients older than 75, 300 mg daily
Morphine, oxycodone, methadone, lenorphanol Fentanyl		10–15 mg morphine every 4 h or as needed (equianalgesic dosage should be used for other opioid analgesics)	Increase by 50–100 mg daily in divided doses every 3–7 days as tolerated	Evaluation by pain specialist is highly recommended at relatively high dosage (e.g. 120–180 mg morphine daily; equianalgesic dosage should be used for other opioid analgesics)

NMDA, N-methyl-D-aspartate; SNRIs, serotonin-noradrenalin reuptake inhibitors; TCA, tricyclic antidepressant.

* Secondary amine TCAs (notriptyline, desipramine) are preferred because of better tolerability. Use of a tertiary amine TCA (amitriptyline, imipramine) is recommended only if a secondary amine TCA is not available.

[†] Recommended for trigeminal neuralgia.

Source: After Haanpää *et al*. [14].

Table 34.2 Adverse drug reactions, precautions and contraindications of drugs recommended for neuropathic pain.

Medication	Major side effects	Precautions	Contraindications	Comments, recommendations
TCAs				
Nortriptyline, desipramine, (amitriptyline, imipramine)	Cardiac conduction block, sedation, confusion, anticholinergic effects (dry mouth, constipation, urinary retention, blurred vision), orthostatic hypotension, weight gain	Use with caution in patients with history of seizures, prostatic hypertrophy, urinary retention, chronic constipation, narrow-angle glaucoma, increased intraocular pressure or suicidal ideation. Use with caution in patients with concomitant SSRI, SNRI or tramadol treatment	Recovery phase after myocardial infarction. Arrhytmias, particularly heartblock of any degree. Concomitant use of MAO inhibitors. Porphyria	ECG screening recommended in persons over 40 years of age. Heart rate and blood pressure follow-up (both supine and standing measurements) recommended with dose escalation. ECG and blood concentration follow-up recommended at doses > 150 mg daily. Follow-up of weight recommended especially in diabetics
SNRIs				
Duloxetine	Nausea, loss of appetite, constipation, sedation, dry mouth, hyperhidrosis, anxiety	Use with caution in patients with history of mania, seizures, bleeding tendency or those on anticoagulants. Use with caution in patients with concomitant SSRI or tramadol treatment	Concomitant use of MAO inhibitors Uncontrolled hypertension	Blood pressure follow-up recommended in patients with known hypertension and/or other cardiac disease, especially during the first month of treatment. Smokers have almost 50% lower plasma concentrations of duloxetine compared to non-smokers
Venlafaxine	Nausea, loss of appetite, hypertension, sedation, insomnia, anxiety, dry mouth, hyperhidrosis, constipation	Use with caution in patients with hypertension. Use with caution in patients with concomitant SSRI or tramadol treatment	Concomitant use of MAO inhibitors	Blood-pressure follow-up recommended
Gabapentinoids				
Gabapentin	Sedation, dizziness, weight gain, edema, blurred vision	Simple antacids reduce bioavailability		Follow-up of weight recommended especially in diabetics
Pregabalin	Sedation, dizziness, weight gain, edema, blurred vision			Follow-up of weight recommended especially in diabetics

Continued

Table 34.2 *(continued)*

Medication	Major side effects	Precautions	Contraindications	Comments, recommendations
Sodium channel blockers				
Carbamazepine	Somnolence, dizziness, headache, ataxia, nystagmus, diplopia, blurred vision, nausea, rash, hyponatremia, leucopenia, thrombocytopenia, hepatotoxicity	Consider risk of pharmacokinetic interactions with concomitant medications	Atrioventricular block Concomitant use of MAO inhibitors Porphyria	Liver enzymes, blood cells, platelets and sodium levels should be monitored for at least 1 year. Induction of microsomal enzymes may influence of metabolism of several drugs
Oxcarbazepine	Somnolence, dizziness, headache, diplopia, nausea, fatigue, hyponatremia, ataxia	25–30% risk of cross-allergy with carbamazepine		Does not entail enzymatic induction. Sodium levels should be controlled during the first months of the treatment
Opioid agonists				
Tramadol	Nausea, dizziness, sedation, headache, constipation, dry mouth, hyperhidrosis, seizures, orthostatic hypotension	Risk of dependence and abuse. Potential to cause withdrawal with abrupt discontinuation. Use with caution in patients with history of seizures. Use with caution in patients with concomitant SSRI or SNRI treatment	Concomitant use of MAO inhibitors	Potential to cause withdrawal with abrupt discontinuation
Morphine, oxycodone, methadone, lenorphanol, pethidine	Somnolence, nausea, constipation, itch, hyperhidrosis, dry mouth, myoclonus, respiratory depression	Risk of dependence and abuse. Potential to cause withdrawal with abrupt discontinuation. Use with caution in patients with history of seizures or impaired respiratory function	Respiratory depression. Concomitant use of MAO inhibitors	"Opioid agreement" recommended Coadministration of pre-emptive stool softeners recommended. Pretreatment ECG screening and follow-up recommended for methadone. Pethidine is contraindicated because of the potential for pethidine toxicity with chronic dosing, nicularly in renal impairment

ECG, electrocardiogram; MAO, monamine oxidase; SNRI, serotonin-noradrenalin reuptake inhibitor; SSRI, selective serotonin reuptake inhibitor; TCA, tricyclic antidepressant.

Source: After Haanpää *et al.* [14].

assessment by a specialist team. Treatment with SCS should only be given after the person has been assessed by a specialist team experienced in assessing and managing people receiving treatment with SCS [16]. Motor cortex stimulation (MCS) may be considered for patients with refractory central post-stroke and well preserved motor cortex, and facial NP [17]. In NP the evidence for SCS is sound but for MCS limited. Neuroablative procedures are used only for patients with cancer pain and limited survival expectancy.

Conclusions

In conclusion, neuropathic pain is caused by a lesion or disease affecting the somatosensory system. It is often under-diagnosed and under-treated and when severe is associated with significant suffering and disability. An approach to the diagnosis and management of NP has been reviewed. The first step is to educate the patient about the cause of their pain as well as possible and review approaches to management which include correction of the pathology where possible, self-management strategies, interdisciplinary approaches including addressing of psychosocial issues, pharmacotherapy and, where appropriate, consideration of neuromodulatory approaches.

References

1 Treede R, Jensen T, Campbell J et al. (2008) Redefinition of neuropathic pain and a grading system for clinical use: consensus statement on clinical and research diagnostic criteria. *Neurology* **70**:1630–5.

2 Woolf CJ, Mannion RJ. (1999) Neuropathic pain: aetiology, symptoms, mechanisms and management. *Lancet* **353**:1959–64.

3 Scadding JW, Koltzenburg M. (2005) Neuropathic pain. In: McMahon SB, Koltzenburg M, eds. *Wall and Melzack's Textbook of Pain*. Churchill Livingstone, Edinburgh. pp. 973–99.

4 Campbell JN, Basbaum AI, Dray A et al., eds. (2006) *Emerging Strategies for the Treatment of Neuropathic Pain*. IASP Press, Seattle.

5 Bennett MI, Attal N, Backonja MM et al. (2007) Using screening tools to identify neuropathic pain. *Pain* **127**:199–203.

6 Loeser JD, Treede RD. (2008) The Kyoto Protocol of IASP basic pain terminology. *Pain* **137**:473–7.

7 Haanpää M, Backonja M, Bennett M et al. (2009) Assessment of neuropathic pain in primary care. *Am J Med* **122**:S13–21.

8 Cruccu G, Anand P, Attal N et al. (2004) EFNS guidelines on neuropathic pain assessment. *Eur J Neurol* **11**:153–62.

9 Attal N, Cruccu G, Haanpää M et al. (2006) EFNS guidelines on pharmacological treatment of neuropathic pain. *Eur J Neurol* **13**:1153–69.

10 Dworkin RH, O'Connor A, Backonja M et al. (2007) Pharmacologic management of neuropathic pain: evidence-based recommendations. *Pain* **132**:237–51.

11 Lynch M. (2008) Drug treatment for chronic pain. In: Rashiq S, Schopflocher D, Taenzer P, eds. *Chronic Pain: A Health Policy Perspective*. Wiley-Blackwell, Edmonton, Alberta. pp. 101–20.

12 Gilron I, Bailey JM, Tu D et al. (2005) Morphine, gabapentin, or their combination for neuropathic pain. *N Engl J Med* **352**:1324–34.

13 Gilron I, Bailey M, Dongsheng Tu et al. (2009) Nortriptyline and gabapentin, alone and in combination for neuropathic pain: a double-blind, randomised controlled crossover trial. *Lancet* **374**:1252–61.

14 Haanpää M, Gourlay GK, Kent JL et al. (2010). Treatment considerations for patients with neuropathic pain with medical comorbidities and other medical conditions. *Mayo Clin Proc* **85**(3 Suppl):S15–25.

15 Hansson P, Attal N, Baron R et al. (2009) Toward a definition of pharmacoresistant neuropathic pain. *Eur J Pain* **13**:439–40.

16 National Institute for Health and Clinical Excellence (NICE). (2008) Pain (chronic neuropathic or ischaemic): spinal cord stimulation. NICE Technology Appraisal No 159. www.nice.org.uk/Guidance/TA159. Accessed September 25, 2009.

17 Cruccu G, Aziz L, Garcia-Larrea L et al. (2007) EFNS guidelines on neurostimulation therapy for neuropathic pain. *Eur J Neurol* **14**:952–70.

Chapter 35

Complex regional pain syndrome

Michael Stanton-Hicks

Pain Management Department, Center for Neurological Restoration; Children's Hospital CCF Shaker Campus, Pediatric Pain Rehabilitation Program, Cleveland Clinic, Cleveland, USA

Introduction

Complex regional pain syndrome (CRPS) embodies a number of painful disorders where the symptoms both exceed the magnitude and duration of the clinical course that would normally be expected from such an inciting event. The presentation, in most instances, occurs distally in one or more extremities but may also occur at another site in the body [1,2]. Invariably, motor dysfunction, sensory dysfunction and an inflammatory process develop with progression of the syndrome. Other clinical features include spontaneous pain, allodynia/hyperalgesia, edema and autonomic abnormalities. These signs and symptoms precede secondary changes in superficial and deep tissues.

CRPS I (formerly reflex sympathetic dystrophy) is typically triggered by a minor injury such as a sprain or insect bite, but may also occur after fractures. CRPS II (formerly causalgia) occurs in association with injury to a peripheral nerve.

The epidemiology reported in two recent studies, one from the USA and the other from the Netherlands, suggests an incidence in the American study of 5.5 per 100,000 persons and a prevalence

of 21 per 100,000 (IASP criteria) [3]. The European study determined there to be an incidence of 26.2 per 100,000 but used slightly different diagnostic criteria [4]. Female adults are more often affected than males in a ratio of 2:1. In adolescents and children this increases to 4:1 [3–5].

This chapter describes the diagnostic assessment and subsequent management of CRPS based on a best evidence approach. A number of mechanisms underlying sensory, motor, inflammatory and autonomic disturbances are addressed in the context of treatment and management strategies. While the International Association for the Study of Pain (IASP) diagnostic criteria lacked clinical validity, their introduction was meant to provide a clearly descriptive set of observations that could be applied to the diagnosis of CRPS. It was also anticipated that criteria would be subjected to internal and external validation to improve specificity while maintaining sensitivity [6]. Table 35.1 shows the IASP criteria for CRPS.

Development of the validation process

For the symptoms and signs that constitute each group in the IASP criteria to be internally valid, they must be statistically derived. In the light of these studies, it became obvious that the IASP criteria could be improved if a fourth group of signs and

Clinical Pain Management: A Practical Guide, 1st edition. Edited by Mary E. Lynch, Kenneth D. Craig and Philip W.H. Peng.
© 2011 Blackwell Publishing Ltd.

Table 35.1 International Association for the Study of Pain (IASP) diagnostic criteria for complex regional pain syndrome.

> **1** The presence of an initiating noxious event, or a cause of immobilization
> **2** Continuing pain, allodynia or hyperalgesia with which the pain is disproportionate to any inciting event
> **3** Evidence at some time of edema, changes in skin blood flow or abnormal sudomotor activity in the region of pain
> **4** This diagnosis is excluded by the existence of conditions that would otherwise account for the degree of pain and dysfunction
> Type I: without evidence of major nerve damage
> Type II: with evidence of major nerve damage

Source: Modified from Merskey & Bogduk (1994) *Classification of Chronic Pain*, 2nd edn. IASP Task Force on Taxonomy, IASP Press, Seattle.

symptoms were added. These include decreased range of motion, motor dysfunction and trophic changes (Table 35.2). Internal validation with factor analysis of 123 patients showed that the patients indeed clustered into four statistically distinct subgroups [7].

CRPS and genetics

Many diseases with an inflammatory component, such as multiple sclerosis and celiac disease, have a genetic association with the human leucocyte antigen (HLA) system. CRPS patients may have a similar inflammatory genetic profile. Human studies have suggested a link to the HLA system [8]. Genetic analysis of fluid from artificial blisters in CRPS patients has determined polymorphisms for potential mediators of inflammation such as tumor necrosis factor α (TNFα) [9]. The demography of CRPS following Colles fracture or sprain in children is similar to the development of neuropathic pain following injury of the nervous system. These findings, and those from animal studies in knockout mice, have demonstrated a high probability that there is a genetic predisposition in individuals who develop CRPS either spontaneously or as a result of injury. There are now many studies describing the compromised immune response or

Table 35.2 Proposed diagnostic criteria for complex regional pain syndrome (CRPS).

> Must display continuing pain disproportionate to any inciting event
> Must report one symptom in three of the four following categories
> Must display one sign in two or more of the following categories at the time of evaluation
> There must be no other diagnosis that better explains the signs and symptoms

Categories	Signs and symptoms
1 Sensory	Allodynia (to light touch, deep pressure or joint movement)
	Hyperalgesia (to pinprick)
2 Vasomotor	Temperature asymmetry
	Skin color change
	Skin color asymmetry
3 Sudomotor	Edema
	Sweating change
	Sweating asymmetry
4 Motor/trophic	Decreased range of motion
	Motor dysfunction (weakness, tremor, dystonia)
	Trophic changes (hair, nails, skin)

Source: Adapted from Harden *et al*. [53], p. 330.

autoimmune pathology in CRPS [10]. Antibodies and autoantibodies have been found in 40% of CRPS patients in comparison to only 5% in other neuropathies.

Sensory characteristics and pathophysiology of CRPS

It is the peripheral manifestation of sensory abnormalities that declare the syndrome of CRPS [3,11,12]. Although intense pain is a characteristic, pain may increase and decrease throughout the clinical course of the syndrome. Research shows that there is a considerable loss of Aδ and C fibers, many with abnormal branches, in CRPS patients. Axonal density is reduced by 29% in affected skin [11,12], resembling that seen in other neuropathic pain conditions. These findings underscore a poorly studied potential mechanism of neuroplasticity with associated sensitization. As a result, a normally non-painful stimulus becomes painful (allodynia). Animal studies suggest that the N-methyl-D-aspartate (NMDA), the neurokinin-1 (NK-1) and α-amino-3-hydroxy-5-methyl-4-isoxazole propionic acid (AMPA) receptors are involved [13]. The proportion with which each of these mechanisms may contribute to CRPS in humans is speculative.

There is evidence that both pyramidal and extrapyramidal disturbances occur in CRPS. These involve range of motion, involuntary movements, tremor and dystonia. Also, cortical reorganization of motor units correlates with the extent of motor dysfunction with increased activation of primary motor and supplementary motor cortices [14]. Transcranial stimulation has revealed hyperexcitability of the sensory and motor cortex. As a result of these findings, mirror therapy with graded motor imagery has been found helpful as a treatment modality. It teaches patients to reconcile their motor output and sensory feedback [15].

Autonomic nervous system

A disturbance of the sympathetic component of the autonomic nervous system has always been associated with CRPS. The alteration in sweating, vasoconstriction-related fluctuations in temperature and the phenomenon of sympathetically maintained pain (SMP) has been considered synonymous with CRPS [13]. Pain sensation is exaggerated by sympathetic afferent coupling in the periphery, where α_1-adrenoceptors are expressed on primary afferent nerve endings [16]. Vasoconstriction can be a result of sympathetic hyperactivity, abnormal sensitivity or upregulation of adrenergic receptors [16]. SMP is a symptom that may be demonstrated by sympatholysis in patients who have neuropathic disorders. It is not a prerequisite for a diagnosis of CRPS. Patients can be separated into those having SMP and those with sympathetically independent pain (SIP) [17].

Inflammatory characteristics

Inflammation is characterized by the "inflammatory soup" of mediators. In the case of CRPS, the levels of the inflammatory markers, such as interleukin-6 (IL-6), TNFα, bradykinin, messenger RNA (mRNA), IL-2 levels and tryptase are increased in comparison with the contralateral side [18]. Neurogenic inflammatory mediators including substance P and calcitonin gene-related protein (CGRP) are also elevated in CRPS [19].

Behavioral–premorbid psychological aspects

While pre-existing psychological factors were considered highly possible in the etiology of CRPS, a number of studies have since dispelled this notion [20,21]. There is evidence to show that the behavior of patients with CRPS reflects an accompanying reaction to the stress and anxiety [22]. There is no such thing as a CRPS personality as once described [23]. A recent study undertook a prospective analysis of psychological patterns in patients with upper extremity radius fracture. Patients who had an uncomplicated course after their fracture were compared with a similar group of patients who developed CRPS. The overall medical and psychological picture in both groups was identical [24].

Functional restoration

Because CRPS involves the entire nervous system it is associated with measurable central and peripheral pathophysiology. The impact of dysfunctional changes in an effected extremity requires the immediate implementation of physiotherapeutic maneuvers. This is to apprehend further loss of function, set the stage for general rehabilitation and achieve the remission of clinical signs and symptoms [25,26]. Because pain is central to the diagnosis of CRPS, its response varies within individuals, particularly in terms of comorbidity and other variables [27,28]. Its expression, depending on its origin from deep tissues or superficial tissues and allodynia, must be addressed if one is to achieve functional improvement.

For the best possible outcome, a comprehensive interdisciplinary approach that rapidly capitalizes on restoration of function, managing pain and addressing all of the physical and psychological impediments engendered by the syndrome must be incorporated.

Many of the central nervous system changes, sometimes described as altered central processing or neglect, must be allayed if functional restoration is to be achieved [29]. Mirror therapy, as an adjunct to treatment, has been used to address the sensory missmatch between sensory input and motor output in the treatment of CRPS. Such provocative studies may re-establish function while decreasing or eliminating pain [30].

Operant-based movement phobia (kinesophobia) or fear of movement must be overcome to achieve an improvement in function [31]. Figure 35.1 illustrates a physiotherapeutic algorithm to facilitate progress along the longitudinal course of functional restoration.

Pharmacologic and interventional therapies

Management of CRPS in adults

When CRPS is recognized within a few weeks of its onset, treatment can be directed at relieving pain, addressing the inflammatory component and determining whether there is autonomic dysfunction. The administration of prednisone, 30 mg/day over a period of 7 days, has a well-demonstrated efficacy in almost 75% of patients [32]. While tricyclic antidepressants have been studied extensively for the treatment of neuropathic pain, there are no studies undertaken for CRPS patients [33]. While their efficacy is not yet established, anecdotal evidence would suggest that their use is at least associated with a reduction in symptoms and improvement in sleep. A small study of the serotonin norepinephrine reuptake inhibitor venlafaxine demonstrated efficacy for neuropathic pain [34]. Anticonvulsants, particularly gabapentin, have been used for the treatment of neuropathic pain [35]. One controlled study supports its use in CRPS [36].

A number of drugs that regulate calcium metabolism such as bisphosphonates have been shown to reduce pain, edema and improve the range of movement in acute CRPS [37]. NMDA receptor blocking agents including ketamine, dextromethorphan and memantine have been used in the treatment of painful diabetic neuropathy but controlled trials have not confirmed these drugs to be as effective in the management of CRPS. Subanesthetic and anesthetic intravenous ketamine infusion is concurrently under study in anesthetic (coma) and subanesthetic doses. Several case series have been reported for patients with refractory CRPS with good success. Recent randomized controlled trials also suggested similar findings, although the duration of effect was limited to 12 weeks [38].

The gamma-aminobutyric acid (GABA) agonist baclofen, administered intrathecally, is effective in the treatment of dystonia found in CRPS [39]. While oral baclofen may be used to address the myofascial syndrome and tremor in CRPS, it is doubtful whether this route of administration can achieve sufficient cerebrospinal fluid levels to be therapeutically effective.

Opioids are used to assist the management of pain in CRPS. The use of opioids should be considered in the context of the physiotherapeutic algorithm and primarily as an adjunct to facilitate restoration of function.

Free radicle scavengers have been used in the management of CRPS I. A small randomized controlled trial showed some benefit with topically applied dimethyl sulfoxide. These agents are more effective in "warm" CRPS [40].

Blocks of the sympathetic nervous system have been an integral component of therapy for CPRS for decades. A positive response, with reduction or elimination of pain after a sympathetic block, implies the presence of SMP, a term introduced by Roberts suggesting sensitization of wide dynamic range neurons in the dorsal horn [41]. A negative response is termed SIP. This is neither a requirement for the diagnosis of CRPS, nor is it a standard of treatment [42]. The use of intravenous regional anesthesia has undergone a number of studies. All except one did not support any benefit of this procedure [43,44].

Surgical sympathectomy has been undertaken in patients with CRPS [45]. There is little to commend its continued use.

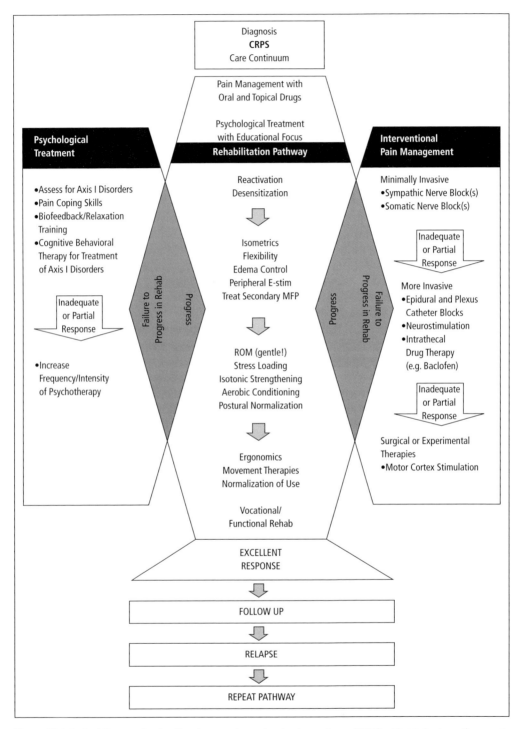

Figure 35.1 Revised therapeutic algorithm for complex regional pain syndrome (CRPS) with emphasis on therapeutic options in response to patient's clinical progress in the rehabilitation pathway. Adapted from Stanton-Hicks *et al.* (1998) Complex Regional Pain Syndrome: Guidelines for Therapy. *Clin J Pain* **14(2)**: 155–66.

Long-acting local anesthetics may be delivered to the epidural space or certain regional sites such as the axillary, brachial plexus or popiteal nerves, to provide analgesia for exercise therapy. These techniques can be used for days or weeks when employed under controlled circumstances and are associated with a very low incidence of infection. A chart review of 19 patients was published in 2002 by Moufawad *et al.* [46]. The authors commented that because this series was retrospective in nature, a Type 1 error should be entertained.

The use of spinal cord stimulation (SCS) to manage symptoms of CRPS is supported by a randomized controlled long-term follow-up study [47]. The study by Health Technology Assessment Programme (NIHR) by Simpson *et al.* [48] demonstrated the effectiveness of SCS for CRPS in reducing neuropathic pain and reducing the cost of conventional medical management over a projected 4-year period. The Neuromodulation Therapy Access Coalition reported supportive evidence for the use of SCS in the treatment of CRPS. Prager & Chang [49] reported the early use of SCS to support an interdisciplinary rehabilitation program.

A recent review identified 41 randomized controlled trials regarding the treatment of CRPS. It concluded that only biphosphonates appear to offer clear benefits for patients with CRPS [37]. However, even this agent is now in question! [50].

CRPS in children

There is still a delay in recognizing CRPS in children. At the present time, a diagnosis is not reached before a mean of 4 months. However, this represents a significant improvement from 10 years ago when the mean delay in recognizing the syndrome was 1 year [51]. CRPS I is most prevalent in children and only rarely is a case of CRPS II seen.

It is the response to treatment that immediately distinguishes children from their adult counterparts. In general, in our experience at the Cleveland Clinic, exercise therapy with behavioral management will achieve almost 97% remission. While acknowledging that its pathophysiology remains poorly understood, there are features that strongly support a neurologic basis for the disease. The main features distinguishing children from adults are lower prevalence of edema, hyperpathia, hypesthesia, paresis and tremor. Only rarely are trophic changes seen and the affected extremity is usually vasodilatated and warm. Pseudoparalysis and myoclonus is more common than in the adult [52]. The factors that distinguish children from adults are most likely due to a coalition of endocrine, behavioral, developmental and environmental factors. The rapid remission of CRPS in children is most likely a consequence of all these factors. Most children respond to coordinated exercise and behavioral therapy. In a few cases, it may be necessary to use some form of intervention such as a sympathetic block, a continuous regional anesthesia technique or an externalized SCS trial to facilitate participation in an exercise program.

Conclusions

Tremendous strides have been made in understanding the pathophysiology underlying CRPS. These insights have helped to sharpen the diagnosis and improve criteria that describe the essential signs and symptoms that make up the diagnosis.

Genetic factors, particularly as they influence the inflammatory process both neurogenic and regional, reveal many features of this syndrome that have parallels with other well-described autoimmune conditions.

The sensory characteristics have their foundation in dysfunction of both the peripheral and central nervous systems. The peripheral manifestations of sensory disturbance are both cause and effect of spinal and supratentorial changes in patients with CRPS. Autonomic dysfunction is integral with these central and peripheral nervous system neuropathologies and helps to explain the clinical picture.

Behavioral aspects of CRPS would appear to be reactive and intimately involved with the clinical expression of the syndrome, particularly the severe pain, dysfunction and attendant disability. The syndrome in children is similar but has characteristics peculiar to the age group which depend on endocrine, environmental and other growth factors that distinguish their presentation from that in the adult.

Treatment is directed towards what pathophysiology is known and in particular to providing the relief of pain, managing psychological fallout while concentrating on the restoration of function.

References

1 Janig W, Baron R. (2003) Complex regional pain syndrome: mystery explained? *Lancet Neurol* **2(11)**:687–97.

2 Baron R, Fields HL, Janig W *et al.* (2002) National Institutes of Health Workshop. Reflex sympathetic dystrophy/complex regional pain syndromes: state-of-the-science. *Anesth Analg* **95(6)**:1812–6.

3 Sandroni P, Benrud-Larson LM, McClelland RL *et al.* (2003) Complex regional pain syndrome type I: incidence and prevalence in Olmsted County, a population-based study. *Pain* **106(1–2)**:209–10.

4 deMos M, de Bruijn AG, Huygen FJ *et al.* (2007) The incidence of complex regional pain syndrome: a population based study. *Pain* **129(1–2)**:2–20.

5 Sherry DD, Wallace CA, Kelley C *et al.* (1999) Short and long term outcomes of children with complex regional pain syndrome type I treated with exercise therapy. *Clin J Pain* **15(3)**:218–23.

6 Harden RN, Bruehl S, Galer BS *et al.* (1999) Complex regional pain syndrome: are the IASP diagnostic criteria valid and sufficiently comprehensive? *Pain* **83(2)**:211–19.

7 Bruehl S, Harden RN, Galer BS *et al.* (2002) Complex regional pain syndrome: are there distinct subtypes and sequential stages of the syndrome? *Pain* **95**:119–24.

8 Mailis A, Wade J. (1994) Profile of Caucasian women with the possible genetic predisposition to reflex sympathetic dystrophy: a pilot study. *Clin J Pain* **10**:210–17.

9 Huygen FJ, DeBruijn AG, DeBruijn MJ *et al.* (2002) Evidence for local inflammation in complex regional pain syndrome type I. *Mediators Inflamm* **11**:47–51.

10 Blaes F, Schmitz K, Tschernatsch M *et al.* (2004) Autoimmune etiology of complex regional pain syndrome (M. Sudek). *Neurology* **65**:1734–6.

11 Albrecht PJ, Hines S, Eisenberg E *et al.* (2006) Pathologic alterations of cutaneous innervation and vasculature in affected limbs from patients with complex regional pain syndrome. *Pain* **120**:244–66.

12 Oaklander AL, Rissmiller JG, Gelman LB *et al.* (2006) Evidence of focal small-fiber axonal degeneration in complex regional pain syndrome-I (reflex sympathetic dystrophy). *Pain* **120**:235–43.

13 Ji RR, Kohno T, Moore KA *et al.* (2003) Central sensitization and LTP: do pain and memory share similar mechanisms? *Trends Neurosci* **26**:696–705.

14 van Rijn MA, Marinus J, Putter H *et al.* (2007) Onset and progression of dystonia in complex regional pain syndrome. *Pain* **130**:287–93.

15 Vladimir Tichelaar YIG, Geertzen JH *et al.* (2007) Mirror box therapy added to cognitive behavioral therapy in three chronic complex regional pain syndrome type I patient: a pilot study. *Int J Rehabil Res* **30**:181–8.

16 Drummond PD, Finch PM, Skipworth S *et al.* (2001) Pain increases during sympathetic arousal in patients with complex regional pain syndrome. *Neurology* **57**:1296–303.

17 Raja SN, Treede RD, Davis KD *et al.* (1991) Systemic alpha-adrenergic blockade with phentolamine: a diagnostic test for sympathetically maintained pain. *Anesthesiology* **74(4)**:691–8.

18 Heijmans-Antonissen C, Wesseldijk F, Munnikes RJ *et al.* (2006) Multiplex bead array assay for detection of 25 soluble cytokines in blister fluid of patients with complex regional pain syndrome type 1. *Mediators Inflamm* **1:28398**:1–8.

19 Gradl G, Finke B, Schattner S *et al.* (2007) Continuous intra-arterial application of substance P induces signs and symptoms of experimental complex regional pain syndrome (CRPS) such as edema, inflammation and mechanical pain but no thermal pain. *Neuroscience* **148**:757–65.

20 Rauis AL. (1999) Psychological aspects: a series of 104 posttraumatic cases of reflex sympathetic dystrophy. *Acta Orthop Belg* **65**:86–90.

21 Janig W, Baron R. (2006) Is CRPS I a neuropathic pain syndrome? *Pain* **120**:227–9.

22 Harden RN, Rudin NJ, Bruehl S *et al.* (2004) Increased systemic catecholamines in complex regional pain syndrome and relationship to psychological factors: a pilot study. *Anesth Analg* **99**:1478–85.

23 Covington EC. (1996) Psychological issues in reflex sympathetic dystrophy. In: Janig W, Stanton-Hicks M, eds. *Reflex Sympathetic Dystrophy: A Reappraisal. Progress in Pain Research and Management.* IASP Press, Seattle. pp. 192–216.

24 Puchalski P, Zyluk A. (2005) Complex regional pain syndrome type 1 after fractures of the distal radius: a prospective study of the role of psychological factors. *J Hand Surg (Br)* **30(6)**:574–80.

25 Oerlemans HM, Oostendorp RA, de Boo T *et al.* (2000) Adjuvant physical therapy versus occupational therapy in patients with reflex sympathetic dystrophy type I. *Arch Phys Med Rehabil* **81(1)**:49–56.

26 Uher EM, Vacariu G, Schneider B *et al.* (2000) Comparison of manual lymph drainage with physical therapy in complex regional pain syndrome, type I: a comparative randomized controlled therapy study. *Wien Klin Wochenschr* **112(3)**:133–7.

27 Fordyce WE, Fowler RS, Lehmann JF. (1973) Operant conditioning in the treatment of chronic pain. *Arch Phys Med Rehabil* **54**: 399–408.

28 Bruehl S, Chung OY. (2006) Psychological and behavioral aspects of complex regional pain syndrome management. *Clin J Pain* **22(5)**: 430–7.

29 Mosely GL. (2006) Guided motor imagery for pathologic pain: a randomized controlled trial. *Neurology* **67(12)**:2129–34.

30 McCabe CS, Haigh RC, Blake DR. (2008) Mirror visual feedback for the treatment of complex regional pain syndrome (Type-I) *Curr Pain Headache Rep* **12**:103–7.

31 Lee BH, Scharff L, Sethna NF *et al.* (2002) Physical therapy and cognitive behavioral treatment for complex regional pain syndromes. *J Pediatr* **141(1)**:135–40.

32 Braus DF, Krauss JK, Strobel J. (1994) The shoulder-hand syndrome after stroke: a prospective clinical trial. *Ann Neurol* **36**,728–33.

33 Bowsher D. (1997) The effects of pre-emptive treatment of postherpetic neuralgia with amitriptyline: a randomized, double-blind, placebo-controlled trial. *J Pain Symptom Manage* **13(6)**:327–31.

34 Sindrup CD, Jensen TS. (1999) Efficacy of pharmacological treatments of neuropathic pain: an update and effect related to mechanism of drug action *Pain* **83**:389–400.

35 Mellick GA, Mellick LB. (1997) Reflex sympathetic dystrophy treated with gabapentin *Arch Phys Med Rehabil* **78**:98–105.

36 van de Vusse AC, Stomp-van den Berg SG, Kessels AH *et al.* (2004) Randomized control trial of gabapentin in complex regional pain syndrome type 1 [ISRCTN84121379]. *BMC Neurol* **4**:13.

37 Adami S, Fossaluzza V, Gatti D *et al.* (1997) Bisphosphonate therapy of reflex sympathetic dystrophy syndrome. *Ann Rheum Dis* **56(3)**:201–4.

38 Sigtermans MJ, van Hilten JJ, Bauer MCR *et al.* (2009) Ketamine produces effective and long-term pain relief in patients with complex regional pain syndrome type 1. *Pain* **145**:304–11.

39 van Rijn MA, Munts AG, Marinus T *et al.* (2009) Intrathecal baclofen for dystonia of complex regional pain syndrome. *Pain* **143**: 41–7.

40 Perez RS, Zuurmond WW, Bezemer PD *et al.* (2003) The treatment of complex regional pain syndrome type I with free radical scavengers: a randomized controlled study. *Pain* **102(3)**: 297–307.

41 Roberts W. (1986) A hypothesis on the physiological basis for causalgia and related pains. *Pain* **24**:297–311.

42 Davis KD, Treede RD, Raja SN *et al.* (1991) Topical application of clonidine relieves

hyperalgesia in patients with sympathetically maintained pain. *Pain* **47(3)**:309–17. [see comments]

43 Jadad AR, Carroll D, Glynn CJ *et al.* (1995) Intravenous regional sympathetic blockade for pain relief in reflex sympathetic dystrophy: a systematic review and a randomized, double-blind crossover study. *J Pain Symptom Manage* **10(1)**:13–20.

44 Hord AH, Rooks MD, Stephens BO *et al.* (1992) Intravenous regional bretylium and lidocaine for treatment of reflex sympathetic dystrophy: a randomized, double-blind study. *Anesth Analg* **74(6)**:818–21.

45 Singh B, Moodley J, Shaik AS *et al.* (2003) Sympathectomy for complex regional pain syndrome. *J Vasc Surg* **37(3)**:508–11.

46 Moufawad S, Malak O, Mekhail NA. (2002) Epidural infusion of opiates and local anesthetics for complex regional pain syndrome. *Pain Pract* **2**:81–6.

47 Kemler MA, Barendse GA, van Kleef M *et al.* (2000) Spinal cord stimulation in patients with chronic reflex sympathetic dystrophy. *N Engl J Med* **343**:618–24.

48 Simpson EL, Duenas A, Holmes MW *et al.* (2009) Spinal cord stimulation for chronic pain of neuropathic and ischemic origin: systematic review and economic evaluation. *Health Technol Assess* **13**:1–179.

49 Prager JP, Chang JH (2000) Transverse tripolar spinal cord stimulation produced by a percutaneously placed triple lead system. Paper presented at: Worldwide Pain Conference, Meeting of International Neuromodulation, North American Neuromodulation Society, and World Institute of Pain, July 15–21, 2000.

50 Brunner F, Schmid A, Kissling R, Held U, Bachmann LM (2009) Biophosphonates for the therapy of complex regional pain syndrome I – systematic review. *Eur J Pain* **13(1)**:17–21.

51 Tran DQ, Duong S, Bertini P *et al.* (2010) Treatment of complex regional pain syndrome: a review of the evidence. *Can J Anesth* **57(2)**: 149–66.

52 Tan EC, Zijlstra B, Essink M *et al.* (2008) Complex regional pain syndrome Type I in children. *Acta Paediatr* **97**:875–9.

53 Harden RN, Bruehl S, Stanton-Hicks M *et al.* (2007) Proposed new diagnostic criteria for complex regional pain syndrome. *Pain Med* **8(4)**:326–31.

Chapter 36

Cancer pain management

David Hui & Eduardo Bruera

Department of Palliative Care & Rehabilitation Medicine Unit 1414, University of Texas M.D. Anderson Cancer Center, Houston, USA

Introduction

Pain is one of the most common and distressing symptoms among cancer patients, with increasing frequency and severity as disease progresses. Approximately 30–50% of newly diagnosed cancer patients report having pain. This proportion increases to 35–96% in terminally ill cancer patients [1]. Despite significant progress in research and education on pain management, there remain multiple barriers to effective pain control. These include inconsistent pain assessment, insufficient training and knowledge, misconceptions about opioids and financial challenges [2]. In addition to overcoming these obstacles, it is important to recognize that the diagnosis of cancer is associated with significant physical, psychological and spiritual distress, all of which can contribute to worsening pain. Thus, effective management of cancer pain necessitates an interprofessional approach customized to the individual's needs.

Basic mechanisms

Patients with cancer may experience pain from progressive disease, diagnostic procedures, cancer

Clinical Pain Management: A Practical Guide, 1st edition.
Edited by Mary E. Lynch, Kenneth D. Craig and Philip W.H. Peng.
© 2011 Blackwell Publishing Ltd.

treatments and/or other comorbidities. Table 36.1 provides an overview of cancer pain mechanisms. The basic mechanism of nociception is reviewed in Chapter 3 and is not discussed in this chapter. Cancer is a life-threatening disease, and is frequently associated with psychosocial distress. Although the pathway of neurotransmission from noxious stimuli to somatosensory cortex is similar between cancer pain and non-cancer pain, how cancer patients perceive, and ultimately express, their pain may be quite different from patients with non-cancer diagnoses (Figure 36.1).

An understanding of the unique circumstances associated with the diagnosis of cancer has important implications for both assessment and treatment of cancer pain. First, cancer patients typically have a heavy symptom burden, as a result of progressive cancer, cancer treatments and/or comorbidities. Using the Memorial Symptom Assessment Scale, one study demonstrated that advanced cancer patients have an average of 11 ± 6 symptoms [3]. Because many of these symptoms are closely related, effective management of pain in the context of malignancy requires concurrent management of other complaints (e.g. coughing and chest pain, vomiting and abdominal pain). Second, polypharmacy is a common issue among cancer patients, with a high potential for drug interactions. For instance, the level of methadone may be affected by concurrent use of various CYP3A4 inducers and/or inhibitors. Third, the diagnosis of

Table 36.1 Cancer pain mechanisms.

Type	Clinical features	Examples
Nociceptive-somatic	Well localized	Bone metastasis Pathologic fracture Surgical incision pain
Nociceptive-visceral	Poorly localized Deep, squeezing, pressure, referred pain	Liver metastasis Pancreatitis Bowel obstruction
Neuropathic	Poorly localized Dysesthetic, constant burning, radiating pain Neuralgic/lancinating	Compression of nerve roots by tumor Spinal cord compression Chemotherapy-induced peripheral neuropathy Radiation-induced brachial plexopathy

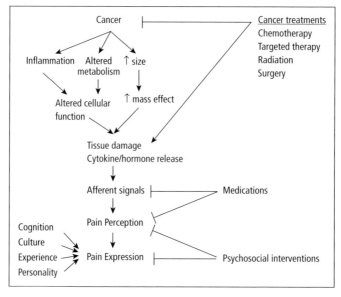

Figure 36.1 Pathophysiology of cancer pain. Cancer progression can result in increasing mass effect and altered cellular function, leading to tissue damage and cytokine/hormone release. Afferent signals are transmitted to the central nervous system, and eventually the somatosensory cortex where the pain is perceived. In addition to nociceptive input, how the patient expresses his/her symptom(s) is affected by other factors, such as culture, personal experience, personality and cognition. Cancer therapies, various supportive care medications and psychosocial interventions all have a role in alleviation of pain.

cancer is associated with various psychological, social and financial stresses, which could lead to significant depression and anxiety, contributing to an altered expression of pain (Figure 36.1). Finally, end-of-life is associated with unique issues such as delirium, dehydration, decreased oral intake and existential distress, which could have an impact of pain control practices.

Clinicians caring for cancer patients should be cognizant of the concept of "total pain," defined as the sum of four components: physical, psychological, social and spiritual. This framework highlights the complex interconnectedness between the body, mind and spirit. For instance, a patient may experience 4 out of 10 shoulder pain caused by the nociceptive input from bone metastasis, while another patient with similar level of noxious physical stimuli may rate his/her pain as 10 out of 10 because of significant psychosocial (e.g. recent bad news) or spiritual (e.g. punishment from God) distress. Pain for the first patient can easily be managed with analgesics, while pain for the second patient warrants comprehensive assessment with multidisciplinary input.

Poorly controlled pain can result in reduced sleep, decreased function, altered mood and significantly compromise patients' quality of life. When a patient requires ever-increasing doses of analgesics without adequate pain control, it is important to step back and look for specific risk factors (Table 36.2) before prescribing more medications. This not only helps to minimize the amount of analgesics and thus the associated side effects, but also provides a more effective pain control strategy.

Assessment

Effective management of cancer pain begins with regular and frequent screening, which would allow clinicians to diagnose pain early, to initiate treatment in a timely fashion and to monitor the effectiveness of therapy.

In addition to a focused pain history and physical examination, it is critical to assess common factors that may affect pain management. At our center, we routinely screen patients for various physical and psychological symptoms, delirium and history of alcoholism, using validated instruments such as the Edmonton Symptom Assessment Scale (ESAS; Figure 36.2) [4], the Memorial Delirium Assessment Scale (MDAS) [5] and the CAGE questionnaire [6], respectively. This information can help clinicians to formulate the pain diagnosis, and assess the need to utilize specific pain manage-

Table 36.2 Risk factors for refractory cancer pain.

Risk factors	Specific solutions
Disease-related factors	
Progressive cancer (compression, obstruction, infiltration)	Cancer treatments (radiation, chemotherapy)
Cancer related complications	Supportive measures
Ischemia	Antibiotics
Infections	Surgery
Fractures	
Treatment related complications	Opioid rotation, dose reduction, adjuvants for opioid-sparing effect
Opioid-induced neurotoxicity (e.g. hyperalgesia)	
Patient-related factors	
Delirium	Neuroleptics, non-pharmacologic treatments
Personality	Counseling
Psychosocial stressors	Counseling
Chemical coping	Limit opioids, emphasis on function, counseling
Secondary gain	Counseling

ment strategies. For instance, a delirious patient who keeps complaining of pain should be treated with neuroleptics rather than simply escalating the opioid dose. In another example, a patient with 10 out of 10 pain and severe symptoms in multiple other ESAS domains is likely to have a psychosocial component contributing to the overall experience of pain, and would benefit from further psychological assessments.

Recognizing the importance of these factors, the Edmonton Classification System for Cancer Pain (ECS-CP) is a pain assessment tool that has been validated in predicting pain management complexity. It consists of five clinical factors: pain mechanisms, incident pain, psychological distress, addictive behavior and cognitive impairment [7]. Regular assessment and documentation using ECS-CP will facilitate communication between members of the interprofessional team and help optimize pain control.

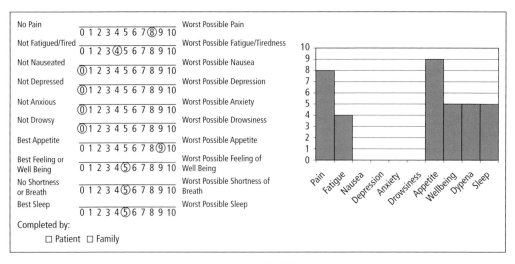

No Pain	0 1 2 3 4 5 6 7⑧9 10	Worst Possible Pain
Not Fatigued/Tired	0 1 2 3④5 6 7 8 9 10	Worst Possible Fatigue/Tiredness
Not Nauseated	⓪1 2 3 4 5 6 7 8 9 10	Worst Possible Nausea
Not Depressed	⓪1 2 3 4 5 6 7 8 9 10	Worst Possible Depression
Not Anxious	⓪1 2 3 4 5 6 7 8 9 10	Worst Possible Anxiety
Not Drowsy	⓪1 2 3 4 5 6 7 8 9 10	Worst Possible Drowsiness
Best Appetite	0 1 2 3 4 5 6 7 8⑨10	Worst Possible Appetite
Best Feeling or Well Being	0 1 2 3 4⑤6 7 8 9 10	Worst Possible Feeling of Well Being
No Shortness or Breath	0 1 2 3 4⑤6 7 8 9 10	Worst Possible Shortness of Breath
Best Sleep	0 1 2 3 4⑤6 7 8 9 10	Worst Possible Sleep

Completed by:
☐ Patient ☐ Family

Figure 36.2 The Edmonton Symptom Assessment Scale (ESAS). ESAS documents the average intensity of 10 symptoms over the past 24 hours. It has been validated in cancer populations, and is a useful for both screening purposes as well as longitudinal assessments. The left panel is a plot of a patient's ESAS score, which allows a quick visual examination of the patient's symptom profile, and facilitates comparison between assessments.

Management

In 1990, the World Health Organization proposed a three-step approach to management of cancer pain, which has notably increased the awareness and subsequent treatment of pain in cancer patients. Under this model, treatment of cancer pain begins with non-opioid analgesics, such as acetaminophen and non-steroidal anti-inflammatory drugs (NSAIDs). If pain persists, the second step consists of the addition of weak opioids such as codeine or hydrocodone. For patients who continue to experience significant pain, the use of strong opioids such as morphine, hydromorphone, oxycodone, oxymorphone, fentanyl and methadone is warranted. Adjuvant treatments such as antidepressants, anticonvulsants, bisphosphonates, radiation and chemotherapy may be added to the pain regimen at any time if indicated.

While some have questioned the need for starting weak opioids prior to initiation of strong opioids, the fact that weak opioids do not require a triplicate prescription in most countries means that they are generally more accessible, and thus represent a reasonable analgesic option for patients.

Opioid mechanism of action

Details of opioid action have been reviewed in Chapter 16. Opioids exert their analgesic effect through binding to various μ-, δ- and κ-receptors, both centrally and peripherally. Activation of μ1-receptors is responsible for the analgesic and euphoric effects of the opioid, while interaction with μ2-receptors is associated with various opioid-induced side effects such as respiratory depression, nausea and sedation. Methadone also has N-methyl-D-aspartate (NMDA) antagonist activity, which is associated with a theoretical benefit for neuropathic pain and opioid-resistance.

There is great interindividual variation in the degree of responsiveness to opioids, which is dependent on various pharmacodynamic and pharmacokinetic factors. These in turn are affected by the patient's age, sex, genetic makeup (i.e. opioid receptor expression and sensitivity, P450 enzymes), organ function, comorbidities, diet and concurrent medications. For instance, 8–10% of the Caucasian population have an inactive CYP2D6 variant and cannot convert codeine from its prodrug form to the active metabolite. The pharmacogenomics of opioid agents represents an area of active research.

Because pain expression is a subjective measure, psychosocial factors such as personality, past experience, culture and placebo effect may also affect the response.

Clinical use of opioids

Patients with moderate to severe cancer pain should be started on short-acting opioids around the clock, with as needed opioid (usually 10% of total daily dose) every 1–2 hours for breakthrough pain. While each opioid has a variable potency and activity spectrum, there is no evidence that any opioid is superior to another as first line therapy for cancer pain.

Because of the need to titrate the opioid dose initially, the use of long-acting formulations and transdermal fentanyl should be avoided until the pain is stabilized. In general, patients who require three or more breakthroughs per day should have their regular dosage increased, whereas patients who do not require any breakthrough medications may benefit from a dosage reduction. Once a stable dosage of pain medication has been achieved, patients may switch to long-acting formulations for convenience. Immediate release opioid every 4 hours, slow release formulations every 12 hours and transdermal fentanyl every 72 hours have similar efficacy. For patients who require parenteral opioids, continuous intravenous infusion, continuous subcutaneous infusion and intermittent subcutaneous injections all represent effective models of pain control [8,9].

Adverse effects of opioids

Common opioid-related adverse effects include sedation, nausea and vomiting, which tend to resolve within a few days as patients develop tolerance to opioids. However, constipation is likely to continue for the duration of treatment. Patients should be counseled regarding these common side effects, and prescribed antiemetics (e.g. metoclopramide 10 mg orally every 4 hours) and laxatives (e.g. 2 senna tablets orally at bed time) for prophy-

laxis. For patients with severe opioid-induced constipation, the use of μ-antagonists such as methylnaltrexone can be useful.

QTc prolongation may develop in patients on high doses of methadone (> 100 mg/day) or with pre-existing risk factors, such as structural cardiac diseases, electrolyte abnormalities or other medications associated with QTc prolongation. These individuals are at risk for development of torsade de pointes, ventricular arrhythmia and sudden cardiac death, and would benefit from regular electrocardiogram monitoring. Other adverse effects associated with long-term opioid use include hypogonadism, osteoporosis, sexual dysfunction, immunosuppression, altered renal function and peripheral edema [10].

Opioid-induced neurotoxicities (OIN) include delirium (agitation, tactile and visual hallucination), nightmares, myoclonus, hyperalgesia and seizures. Risk factors for OIN include high doses of opioids for prolonged periods of time, pre-existing cognitive impairment, renal failure and infections. Hyperalgesia should be suspected if patients have severe pain despite rapid escalation of opioid doses, and should be distinguished from inadequately controlled pain. The former is characterized by the presence of pain sensitivity, delirium and other OIN symptoms. Management of hyperalgesia includes opioid rotation, reduction of total opioid dose and use of other non-opioid analgesics such as acetaminophen, dexamethasone, lidocaine and ketamine [11].

Opioid rotation

Opioid rotation, the practice of switching from one opioid to another, is indicated for two reasons:
1 When pain persists despite escalating doses of an opioid; or
2 When opioid-induced neurotoxicity develops.
Because each opioid has a different spectrum of opioid receptor affinity and sensitivity, switching to a new opioid may allow for more effective pain control, taking advantage of incomplete cross-tolerance. By reducing the concentration of the previous opioid and its metabolites, opioid rotation can also help to mitigate neurotoxicity.

Table 36.3 Equianalgesic table.

Opioid	SC/IV opioid: SC/IV morphine	SC/IV opioid: oral opioid	Oral opioid: oral morphine	Oral morphine: oral opioid
Morphine	1	2–3	1	1
Hydromorphone	5	2–3	5	0.2
Oxycodone	1.5	2–3	1.5	0.7
Oxymorphone	0.10	10	3	0.3
Fentanyl*		See notes		
Methadone†	0.1	1–2	5–20	0.05–0.2

*For fentanyl, 25 µg/hour patch is equivalent to 90 mg of oral morphine per day; fentanyl 10 µg/hour IV infusion is equivalent 1 mg IV morphine.

† The potency of methadone increases with morphine equivalent daily dose (MEDD). The equianalgesic ratio for morphine to methadone conversion is 5 for MEDD < 99 mg, 8 for MEDD 100–299 mg, 12 for MEDD 300–499 mg, 15 for MEDD 500–999 mg and 20 or greater for MEDD > 1000 mg.

To calculate the equianalgesic dose

1. Take the total amount of opioid that effectively controls pain in the last 24 hours.
2. Multiply by conversion factor in table. Give 30% less of the new opioid to avoid partial cross-tolerance.
3. Divide by the number of doses/day.

Source: Modified from Reddy *et al.* [24].

A recent Cochrane review on opioid rotation included 14 prospective uncontrolled studies, 15 retrospective studies/audits and 23 case reports [12]. No randomized controlled trials were available. The majority of the studies used morphine as the first line opioid and methadone as the second line opioid. All reports except one concluded that opioid switching is a useful clinical maneuver for improving pain control and/or reducing opioid-related side-effects.

Opioid rotation is performed by determining the total morphine equivalent daily dose (MEDD), then calculating the dose of the new opioid using equianalgesic ratios (Table 36.3). A 30% dose reduction of the new opioid is generally applied, taking into account the incomplete cross-tolerance. However, for patients who require opioid rotation for improving pain control, no change in the total MEDD dose may be necessary. For patients who require opioid rotation for OIN, it is important to reduce the MEDD dose by 50%.

Chemical coping

Chemical coping is a common concern among patients and clinicians, and represents a key barrier to appropriate opioid use. While some believe that opioids are highly addictive and should be avoided at all cost, others think that opioids cannot be addictive as long as they are used for cancer pain.

Dependence is a normal pharmacophysiological effect with the development of withdrawal symptoms (e.g. agitation, pain, fever, sweats, tremor and tachycardia) if opioid is stopped abruptly after a prolonged period of use, while addiction is an abnormal psychopathological compulsion to use a substance affecting daily function. Opioid addiction causes considerable suffering for patients. It represents a source of distress for families and healthcare professionals, and results in disproportionate utilization of healthcare resources. For these reasons, identification of population at risk should be part of the daily practice of cancer pain management.

Predisposition to development of opioid addiction is likely through a combination of genetic and environmental factors. A positive history of substance abuse (i.e. alcohol and illicit drug use) indicates that the patient is at high risk of maladaptive chemical coping, including development of opioid addiction. The CAGE questionnaire is a validated tool for alcoholism, and consists of four questions:

Have you felt you needed to cut down on your drinking? Have you felt annoyed by criticism of your drinking? Have you felt guilty about drinking? Have you felt you needed a drink first thing in the morning (eye-opener)? An affirmative response to two or more questions indicates a high likelihood of alcoholism.

The Edmonton Staging System for Cancer Pain (ESS-CP) was developed in 1989 as a prognostic system for response to pain treatment, and included the mechanism of pain, characteristics of pain, previous narcotic exposure, cognitive function, psychological distress, tolerance and past history of drug addiction or alcoholism [13,14]. The ESC-CP represents the newest version of the ESS-CP. While addictive behaviour remains as one of the key factors in the ESC-CP, the predictability of this new classification system may have been reduced by the fact that it does not take into account addictive behavior if it occurred remotely [7]. Because people tend to employ the same coping mechanisms when dealing with stress, a history of alcoholism any time in the past should be relevant [15–17]. Patients with a history of substance abuse, even remotely, are more likely to develop opioid addiction. If unrecognized, these patients may be prescribed ever-escalating doses of opioid without adequate pain control, with increased risk of opioid-induced delirium, myoclonus, hyperalgesia and grand mal seizures. For such individuals, it is important to limit the use of opioids, to emphasize the use of opioids for improving function rather than pain control, and to provide interdisciplinary patient and family support.

Adjuvant therapies

While opioids are effective for management of cancer pain, adjuvant therapies or coanalgesics are indicated for specific pain syndromes for two reasons:
1 To enhance pain control through different mechanisms of action; and
2 To reduce the amount of opioid required (i.e. "opioid sparing").

Table 36.4 highlights a number of adjuvant therapies for common pain syndromes.

Table 36.4 Adjuvant treatments for specific cancer pain syndromes.

	Good evidence	Limited evidence
Bone pain	NSAIDs, COX-2 inhibitors	Steroids
	Bisphosphonates (Cochrane)	
	Palliative radiation (Cochrane)	
	Radionuclides (Cochrane)	
Neuropathic pain	Gabapentin	Steroids
	Tricyclic antidepressants	SSRI
	Carbamazepines	
	Serotonin-noradrenaline reuptake inhibitors (venlafaxine, duloxetin)	
	Lidocaine	
Pancreatic cancer pain	Celiac axis block	
Bowel obstruction	Anticholinergic agents	Steroids
	Octreotide	
Oral mucositis		Lidocaine viscous

COX, cyclo-oxygenase; NSAID, non-steriodal anti-inflammatory drug; SSRI, selective serotonin reuptake inhibitor.

For selected patients with good performance status and treatment sensitive disease, cancer therapies such as radiation, chemotherapy and targeted agents represent feasible options for effective pain control. However, tumor response is usually not observed until weeks later, and any clinical benefit tends to be for a short duration only. Furthermore, cancer therapies can be associated with significant morbidities. Thus, judicious use of antineoplastic therapies after careful consideration of the risks and benefits is warranted.

For neuropathic pain, tricyclic antidepressants [18], opioids [19], gabapentin/pregabalin [20], topical lidocaine and venlafaxine/duloxetine [18] have all been shown to be effective, with number-needed-to-treat (NNT) of 2.3, 2.7, 4.0, 4.4 and 5.1, respectively. Lidocaine is a sodium channel blocker with demonstrated efficacy for neuropathic pain [21]. It may be given as an infusion, with a loading dose of 1–3 mg/kg IV over 20 minutes, then continuous infusion at 0.5–2 mg/kg/hour. Lidocaine in a 5% patch may also be used. Intramuscular tetrodotoxin represents another novel therapeutic option, with its analgesic effect mediated through selective blockage of the sodium channel [22]. Given the wide selection of coanalgesics, the agent of choice depends on the patient's comorbidities and the agent's side effect profile.

Ketamine is an NMDA antagonist which represents an emerging option for cancer pain, although evidence supporting its efficacy is still limited [23]. Ketamine is typically given as a subcutaneous infusion at 0.1–0.2 mg/kg/hour, with a maximum dosage of 3.6 g/day. Alternatively, it may be administered orally at 10–25 mg every 8 hours, with a maximum dosage of 200 mg orally every 6 hours. Patients on ketamine should be monitored for excessive secretions and unpleasant hallucinations. Cannabinoids have also been used for selected patients with some effect (Chapter 18).

A number of complementary treatments such as music therapy and touch therapies also have an adjunctive role in cancer pain management. Involvement of other specialties such as intervention radiologists and anesthesiologists may also be indicated in specific circumstances, such as vertebroplasty/kyphoplasty for vertebral fractures, celiac plexus block for visceral abdominal pain and superior hypogastric plexus block for pelvic pain.

Continuity of care and multidisciplinary management

In addition to timely diagnosis and treatment of pain, it is important to provide continual education and counseling, to assess patients' adherence to the pain regimen, to follow-up on response to analgesics and to monitor side effects.

Throughout this chapter we emphasized that analgesics alone may not be adequate for pain management, particularly for patients who have complex psychosocial needs and existential suffering. A detail review of psychological assessment and counseling is beyond the scope of this chapter. However, consultation of palliative care specialists,

psychiatrists, clinical psychologists and other members of the interprofessional team in a timely fashion may help to minimize medication use and to optimize pain control.

References

1 Solano JP, Gomes B, Higginson IJ. (2006) A comparison of symptom prevalence in far advanced cancer, AIDS, heart disease, chronic obstructive pulmonary disease and renal disease. *J Pain Symptom Manage* **31**:58–69.

2 Oldenmenger WH, Sillevis Smitt PA, van Dooren S *et al.* (2009) A systematic review on barriers hindering adequate cancer pain management and interventions to reduce them: a critical appraisal. *Eur J Cancer* **45**:1370–80.

3 Portenoy RK, Thaler HT, Kornblith AB *et al.* (1994) Symptom prevalence, characteristics and distress in a cancer population. *Qual Life Res* **3**:183–9.

4 Bruera E, Kuehn N, Miller MJ *et al.* (1991) The Edmonton Symptom Assessment System (ESAS): a simple method for the assessment of palliative care patients. *J Palliat Care* **7**:6–9.

5 Breitbart W, Rosenfeld B, Roth A *et al.* (1997) The memorial delirium assessment scale. *J Pain Symptom Manage* **13**:128–37.

6 Ewing JA. (1984) Detecting alcoholism: the CAGE questionnaire. *JAMA* **252**:1905–7.

7 Fainsinger RL, Nekolaichuk CL. (2008) A "TNM" classification system for cancer pain: the Edmonton Classification System for Cancer Pain (ECS-CP). *Support Care Cancer* **16**:547–55.

8 Watanabe S, Pereira J, Tarumi Y *et al.* (2008) A randomized double-blind crossover comparison of continuous and intermittent subcutaneous administration of opioid for cancer pain. *J Palliat Med* **11**:570–4.

9 Parsons HA, Shukkoor A, Quan H *et al.* (2008) Intermittent subcutaneous opioids for the management of cancer pain. *J Palliat Med* **11**:1319–24.

10 Harris JD. (2008) Management of expected and unexpected opioid-related side effects. *Clin J Pain* **24(Suppl 10)**:S8–13.

11 de Leon-Casasola OA. (2008) Current developments in opioid therapy for management of cancer pain. *Clin J Pain* **24(Suppl 10)**:S3–7.

12 Quigle C. (2004) Opioid switching to improve pain relief and drug tolerability. *Cochrane Database Syst Rev* **3**:CD004847.

13 Bruera E, Schoeller T, Wenk R *et al.* (1995) A prospective multicenter assessment of the edmonton staging system for cancer pain. *J Pain Symptom Manage* **10**:348–55.

14 Bruera E, MacMillan K, Hanson J *et al.* (1989) The Edmonton Staging System for Cancer Pain: preliminary report. *Pain* **37**:203–9.

15 Bruera E, Moyano J, Seifert L *et al.* (1995) The frequency of alcoholism among patients with pain due to terminal cancer. *J Pain Symptom Manage* **10**:599–603.

16 Poulin C, Webster I, Single E. (1997) Alcohol disorders in canada as indicated by the CAGE questionnaire. *CMAJ* **157**:1529–35.

17 Moore RD, Bone LR, Geller G *et al.* (1989) Prevalence, detection, and treatment of alcoholism in hospitalized patients. *JAMA* **261**: 403–7.

18 Saarto T, Wiffen PJ. (2007) Antidepressants for neuropathic pain. *Cochrane Database Syst Rev* **4**:CD005454.

19 Eisenberg E, McNicol E, Carr DB. (2006) Opioids for neuropathic pain. *Cochrane Database Syst Rev* **3**:CD006146.

20 Wiffen PJ, McQuay HJ, Edwards JE *et al.* (2005) Gabapentin for acute and chronic pain. *Cochrane Database Syst Rev* **3**:CD005452.

21 Challapalli V, Tremont-Lukats IW, McNicol ED *et al.* (2005) Systemic administration of local anesthetic agents to relieve neuropathic pain. *Cochrane Database Syst Rev* **4**:CD003345.

22 Hagen NA, Fisher KM, Lapointe B *et al.* (2007) An open-label, multi-dose efficacy and safety study of intramuscular tetrodotoxin in patients with severe cancer-related pain. *J Pain Symptom Manage* **34**:171–82.

23 Bell R, Eccleston C, Kalso E. (2003) Ketamine as an adjuvant to opioids for cancer pain. *Cochrane Database Syst Rev* **1**:CD003351.

24 Reddy S. *et al.* (2008) Pain management. In: Elsayem A, Bruera E, eds. *The M.D. Anderson Supportive and Palliative Care Handbook*, 3rd edn. M.D. Anderson Cancer Center, Houston, TX, p. 35.

Further reading

Carr DB, Goudas LC, Balk EM *et al.* (2004) Evidence report on the treatment of pain in cancer patients. *J Natl Cancer Inst Monogr* **32**:23–31.

Dy SM, Asch SM, Naeim A *et al.* (2008) Evidence-based standards for cancer pain management. *J Clin Oncol* **26(23)**:3879–85.

Mantyh PW. (2006) Cancer pain and its impact on diagnosis, survival and quality of life. *Nat Rev Neurosci* **7(10)**:797–809.

McGeeney BE. (2008) Adjuvant agents in cancer pain. *Clin J Pain* **24(Suppl 10)**:S14–20.

Part 10

Special Populations

Chapter 37

Pain in older persons: a brief clinical guide

Thomas Hadjistavropoulos[1], Stephen Gibson[2] & Perry G. Fine[3]

[1] Department of Psychology and Center on Aging and Health, University of Regina, Regina, Canada
[2] National Aging Research Institute, Caulfield Pain Management Research Center, Royal Melbourne Hospital, Melbourne, Australia
[3] Pain Research Center, Department of Anesthesiology, School of Medicine, University of Utah, Salt Lake City, USA

Introduction

The point prevalence of acute pain is estimated at 5% of the adult community and does not appear to change as a function of age. The epidemiology of chronic pain is presented in Chapter 2, but here it is important to note that a consistent finding across all studies is a marked age-related increase in prevalence of chronic pain until 55–60 years old (reaching a peak at 30–65%) and then a slight decline into very advanced age [1]. Chronic pain is even more common in residential care settings, affecting as many as 80% of long-term care residents [2].

It has been demonstrated in several studies that patients with cognitive impairments tend to receive considerably less pain medication than their cognitively intact counterparts [3], despite a similar prevalence of pain problems. A Canadian study suggests that patients with pain who have cognitive impairments are often likely to be prescribed psychotropic rather than analgesic medications [4].

Clinical Pain Management: A Practical Guide, 1st edition.
Edited by Mary E. Lynch, Kenneth D. Craig and Philip W.H. Peng.
© 2011 Blackwell Publishing Ltd.

Age-related change in pain sensitivity and nociceptive processing

Experimental studies have shown a modest, although somewhat inconsistent, increase in pain threshold with advancing age (i.e. a reduced sensitivity to faint pain) [5]. Clinical case reviews suggest that pain becomes a less frequent presenting symptom in a variety of visceral and somatic medical complaints. There is also evidence of an age-related impairment in the structure and function of peripheral and central nervous system pain pathways [6]. Collectively, these changes may compromise the early warning functions of pain and contribute to a greater risk of delayed diagnosis of injury or disease. In marked contrast, there is also convincing evidence that older persons may be more vulnerable to strong or severe pain [5–7].

Dementia may exacerbate age-related impairments in pain processing and there is growing international debate as to whether persons with a dementing illness actually feel less pain than aged-matched peers. However, a recent neuroimaging study of central nervous system processing revealed significantly greater pain-related activations in patients with Alzheimer's disease (i.e. dorsolateral prefrontal cortex, mid cingulate cortex and insula

[8]). It is somewhat difficult to reconcile these disparate findings and the severity of dementia of those included in different studies may help to explain this inconsistency. At present, it appears that dementia may impair pain perception at least in more severe cases, but the extent of change in pain perception with the progression of dementia remains unclear and further research is needed in order to answer this important question.

Clinical pain assessment of the cognitively intact older adult

As reviewed in Chapter 7, the first step in pain assessment in a cognitively intact adult should be by patient self-report [9]. Older persons should be given every opportunity to provide their history and the person taking the history should be a skilled assessor. Sufficient time, adequate proximity, lighting and sensory assistive devices (e.g. glasses, hearing aid) should be utilized when required. The diagnostic formulation for the cause of pain may be more difficult in older persons as they often have pathology involving several systems. In addition, it is important to evaluate all medications that the patient is taking, especially in the context of renal or hepatic disease, cognitive impairment, issues with balance and general frailty, because these problems may restrict available pharmacological options.

The use of psychometric tools can help to provide a standardized assessment of pain and related suffering. As reviewed in Chapters 7, 8 and 10, numerous self-report measures of pain have been developed. In general, tools with demonstrated merit in younger adult populations are also thought to be useful with older adults. Several studies directly compare different self-report tools and suggest that the verbal descriptor scales are most preferred by older persons and have the strongest evidence of utility, reliability and validity [10]. Other acceptable measures include numeric rating scales, pictorial pain scales (i.e. pain thermometer), the multidimensional McGill Pain Questionnaire and Brief Pain Inventory (for a review see Gagliese & Melzack [11]). There is less uniform support for visual analog scales and

several authors raise concerns when using this measure with older adults (for a discussion of this issue see Gagliese & Melzack [11]). The longer the pain persists, the greater the probability that the older person will become depressed, socially withdrawn and somatically preoccupied. Anger, frustration, loss of ability to cope and increased anxiety also occur as the person tries and fails with a variety of medical and non-medical therapies. As reviewed in Chapter 7, a full biopsychosocial evaluation is an integral component of any comprehensive clinical evaluation and should be incorporated as a routine part of the assessment plan in the older adult as well.

There are a number of standardized tools that have demonstrated reliability and validity for use in older adults (e.g. Geriatric Depression Scale, Spielberger State-Trait Anxiety Inventory). The initial assessment can also include evaluation of other common psychological associations and mediators of pain, including, anger, cognitive and behavioral coping strategy use, beliefs and attitudes, stoicism, sleep, spousal bereavement and suicide risk. Developing a better understanding of the persons' social situation, beliefs, attitudes and current coping strategies in relation to their pain provides an important starting point toward individualizing the eventual management plan and should be considered as a routine part of the clinical assessment.

Chronic pain has a major impact on function and is likely to interfere with many of the activities of daily life. A number of options exist for the measurement of activity levels or disability, ranging from objective measures of uptime/movement and direct observation of activity task performance, through to self-report psychometric questionnaires and activity diaries. The psychometric scales typically used to measure function in geriatric populations, such as the Katz ADL scale [12], may be useful to monitor the personal and instrumental activities of daily living in the older person with chronic pain, although they tend to lack sensitivity and fail to measure the more discretionary activities that are affected by chronic pain (i.e. leisure and pastimes, home maintenance and social interactions). One must also exercise some care with the interpretation of activity measures because activity restriction can also occur as a consequence of a change in social circumstances, medical factors or other concurrent disease states rather than as a consequence of pain. Moreover, regardless of whether measures are via self-report or objective markers, activity performance is highly dependent upon motivational factors and the context in which measurement is undertaken. As a result, studies of chronic pain populations have tended to focus on measures of perceived pain-related interference in activity or self-rated measures of perceived disability (e.g. SF-36, Pain Disability Index, Oswestry Disability Questionnaire, Sickness Impact Profile) rather than documenting the actual levels of activity performance. Older persons with chronic pain often respond more dramatically with respect to improvements in function than in pain intensity and value improvements in function as most important. For this reason, the measurement of disability and perceived interference should become an essential component of any routine comprehensive assessment.

Clinical approach to pain assessment in persons with dementia

In recent years, we have seen a proliferation of research focusing on the development and validation of observational tools designed to assess pain in persons with cognitive impairment. A detailed review of these is beyond the scope of this chapter but some of the most researched and recommended scales include the Pain Assessment Checklist for Seniors with Limited Ability to Communicate (PACSLAC) [13], the DOLOPLUS-II [14] and the Pain Assessment in Advanced Dementia (PAINAD) [15]. The DOLOPLUS-II has the disadvantage that a considerable portion of its items require knowledge of the patient which may make it more difficult to use in acute situations. The PACSLAC, which is a checklist of 60 behaviors, takes less than 5 minutes to complete and, to our knowledge, is the only tool that fully covers all of the assessment domains that have been recommended by the American Geriatrics Society (AGS)

as being useful in the assessment of older persons. With this in mind, we recommend several practical steps in the assessment of older adults with dementia. These steps are adaptations of earlier recommendations by a variety of groups [9,16].

General guidelines

In addition to taking into account patient history and physical examination results, we recommend the Mini Mental Status Examination (MMSE) when possible [17]. While no cognitive measure can provide a definitive determination about the validity of self-report, examination of MMSE scores could be of assistance because research suggests that patients with scores of 13 or lower are unlikely to be able to provide valid self-report, whereas patients with scores of 18 or higher are most likely to be able to respond to basic self-report scales such as verbal rating scales [18,19]. Despite this rule of thumb, it is always prudent to attempt self-report (as a first step in the assessment process) with all patients as there are some individuals with low MMSE scores who are able to provide an accurate report of their pain. The pain assessment can also be supplemented with information from knowledgeable informants who are aware of changes in activity patterns as well as pain behaviors.

Under ideal circumstances, the clinician should collect baseline observational pain assessment scores on each patient on a regular basis. This would allow for the examination of unusual changes in a patient's usual pattern of scores. However, if assessments are to be repeated over time, it would be important to keep assessment conditions constant. That is, the assessment should be conducted under similar circumstances (e.g. during a routine program of physiotherapy or during a discomforting but necessary transfer), using the same assessment tool. In terms of the sequencing of the assessment process, we recommend that clinicians commence by attempting assessment of self-reported pain, followed by necessary physical examinations (including necessary laboratory and other investigations) and use of observational scales and proxy reports.

Using self-report scales

There are several self-report tools that have been shown to be valid among seniors with mild to moderate cognitive impairment. These tools include Numeric Rating Scales [18,19], Behavioral Rating Scales [18,19] and the 21-point Box Scale [19,20]. Some clinicians may choose to check the ability of the patient to understand the scale prior to the assessment (e.g. by asking the patient to point to the parts of the scale that represent the lowest or the highest level of pain). Given that some investigators have reported unusually high numbers of unscorable responses when horizontal visual analog scales are used among seniors, we would recommend against the use of this tool (for a discussion of this issue see Gagliese & Melzack [11]). As others have suggested [16], certain adaptations (e.g. using larger print) may be needed with seniors who present with sensory deficits and the use of synonyms such as "aching" and "hurt" may facilitate self-report among some patients with limited ability to communicate verbally.

Using observational scales

Reliable and valid tools for use with people who have severe dementia have been reviewed extensively [9]. None the less, clinicians should always exercise caution when using such measures because they are relatively new and research is continuing. When assessing pain in acute-care settings, tools that primarily focus on evaluation of change over time (e.g. the items have the format of "changes in behavior" or "changes in sleep pattern") should be avoided. Observational assessments during movement-based tasks would be more likely to lead to the identification of underlying pain problems than assessments during rest [16].

Clinicians frequently ask about cutoff scores to determine pain. Some pain assessment tools, such as the PACSLAC, do not have specific cutoff scores because of recognition of tremendous individual differences among people with severe dementia. Moreover, the typical scores on an assessment tool will vary depending on situational factors and duration of observation. Instead, for patients who require long-term care it is recommended that pain be assessed on a regular basis (establishing baseline scores for each patient) with the clinician observing changes over time. This will also allow more accurate assessment of response to treatment.

Some of the symptoms of delirium (which is seen frequently in long-term care) overlap with certain behavioral manifestations of uncontrolled pain (e.g. behavioral disturbance). Clinicians assessing patients with delirium should be aware of this. On the positive side, delirium tends to be a transient state and pain assessment, repeated or conducted when the patient is not delirious, is more likely to lead to valid results. It is important to note also that pain can cause delirium and clinicians should be astute in order to avoid missing pain problems among patients with delirium.

As a word of caution, clinicians are advised that observational pain assessment tools are only screening instruments and their use should be part of a more comprehensive clinical assessment.

Psychosocial interventions

Several psychosocial interventions have shown considerable initial promise with older adults. With some inconsistencies across studies, cognitive behavioral therapy is effective in older adults as well, with the benefits linked to specific areas of functioning such as pain beliefs, physical role functioning and pain intensity [21]. Self-management books [22], specifically tailored to older adults with pain, are also available but require empirical evaluation.

Research with seniors with dementia who reside in long-term care facilities has supported the view that the use of regular and routine pain assessment leads to improved pain management practices [23]. Moreover, the success of behavioral mood management interventions, focusing on pleasant activity scheduling, environmental manipulation and other behavioral procedures, in improving patient mood [24] suggests that these types of interventions have the potential of improving quality of life in pain patients with dementia.

Table 37.1 Non-pharmacological management of pain in older persons.

Category	Examples
Patient/ caregiver education	Nature of pain
	Use of pain assessment instruments
	Product and dosing information
Cognitive behavioral therapy	Distraction/mindfulness methods
	Relaxation
	Activity pacing
	Involvement in pleasurable activities
Supervised physical therapy	Flexibility
	Strength
	Endurance
	Range of motion
	Enhance postural and gait stability
Assistive devices	Canes/walkers
	Raised chairs/toilet seats
	Carpo-metacarpal braces
Adjunctive therapies	Heat
	Cold
	Massage
	Liniments
	Chiropractic
	Acupuncture/acupressure
	Transcutaneous electrical nerve stimulation

Other non-pharmacological approaches to pain management

Whenever possible, pain management should be mechanism-based, choosing the most cost-effective and safest approach to the problem in order to optimize health-related outcomes and minimize treatment-related morbidity. Non-pharmacological approaches often suffice for mild or mild to moderate pain (Table 37.1). The care setting may dictate which modalities are available, but every effort should be made to integrate these approaches into the care plan, because they may offer appreciable benefits with negligible potential harms.

Pharmacological therapies

Pharmacological therapies for pain control are indicated in cases of moderate to severe pain. The AGS has recently completed an evidence-based review of pharmacotherapies for this population, and recommendations are summarized in the Appendix at the end of the chapter. Dosing guidelines and other details related to analgesic pharmacotherapy can be found in the AGS document [25] and other primary sources.

References

1 Gibson SG, Chambers CT. (2004) Pain over the life span: a developmental perspective. In: Hadjistavropoulos T, Craig KD, eds. *Pain: Psychological Perspectives*. Lawrence Erlbaum Associates, Mahwah, NJ. pp. 113–54.

2 Charlton JE. (2005) *Core Curriculum for Professional Education in Pain*, 3rd edn. IASP Press, Seattle, WA.

3 Morrison RS, Sui AL. (2000) A comparison of pain and its treatment in advanced dementia and cognitively impaired patients with hip fracture. *J Pain Symptom Manage* **19**:240–8.

4 Balfour JE, O'Rourke N. (2003) Older adults with Alzheimer disease, comorbid arthritis and prescription of psychotropic medications. *Pain Res Manag* **8**:198–204.

5 Gibson SJ. (2003) Pain and aging: the pain experience over the adult life span. In: Dostrovsky JO, Carr DB, Koltzenburg M, eds. *Proceedings of the 10th World Congress on Pain*. IASP Press, Seattle, WA. pp. 767–90.

6 Gibson SJ, Farrell M. (2004) A review of age differences in the neurophysiology of nociception and the perceptual experience of pain. *Clin J Pain* **20(4)**:227–39.

7 Farrell M, Gibson S. (2007) Age interacts with stimulus frequency in the temporal summation of pain. *Pain Med* **8(6)**:514–20.

8 Cole LJ, Farrell MJ, Duff EP *et al.* (2006) Pain sensitivity and fMRI pain-related brain activity in Alzheimer's disease. *Brain* **129(11)**: 2957–65.

9 Hadjistavropoulos T, Herr K, Turk DC *et al.* (2007) An interdisciplinary expert consensus statement on assessment of pain in older persons. *Clin J Pain* **23(1 Suppl)**:S1–43.

10 Herr KA, Spratt K, Mobily PR *et al.* (2004) Pain intensity assessment in older adults: use of

experimental pain to compare psychometric properties and usability of selected pain scales with younger adults. *Clin J Pain* **20(4)**:207–19.

11 Gagliese L, Melzack R. (2003) Age-related differences in the qualities but not the intensity of chronic pain. *Pain* **104(3)**:597–608.

12 Katz S, Ford AB, Moskowitz RW *et al.* (1963) Studies of illness in the aged. The index of ADL: a standardized measure of biological and psychosocial function. *JAMA* **185**:914–19.

13 Fuchs-Lacelle S, Hadjistavropoulos T. (2004) Development and preliminary validation of the Pain Assessment Checklist for Seniors with Limited Ability to Communicate (PACSLAC). *Pain Manag Nurs* **5(1)**:37–49.

14 Wary B, Collectif Doloplus. (1999) DOLOPLUS 2, une échelle pour évaluer la douleur. *Soins Gérontol* **19**:25–7.

15 Warden V, Hurley AC, Volicer L. (2003) Development and psychometric evaluation of the Pain Assessment in Advanced Dementia (PAINAD) scale. *J Am Med Dir Assoc* **4(1)**:9–15.

16 Herr K, Coyne PJ, Key T *et al.* (2006) Pain assessment in the nonverbal patient: position statement with clinical practice recommendations. *Pain Manag Nurs* **7(2)**:44–52.

17 Folstein MF, Folstein SE, McHugh PR. (1975) "Mini-mental state": a practical method for grading the cognitive state of patients for the clinician. *J Psychiatr Res* **12(3)**:189–98.

18 Weiner DK, Peterson BL, Logue P *et al.* (1998) Predictors of pain self-report in nursing home residents. *Aging* **10(5)**:411–20.

19 Chibnall JT, Tait RC. (2001) Pain assessment in cognitively impaired and unimpaired older adults: a comparison of four scales. *Pain* **92 (1–2)**:173–86.

20 Jensen MP, Miller L, Fisher LD. (1998) Assessment of pain during medical procedures: a comparison of three scales. *Clin J Pain* **14(4)**: 343–9.

21 Waters S, Woodward JP, Keefe F. (2005) Cognitive behavioral therapy for pain in older adults. In: Gibson S, Weiner D, eds. *Pain in Older Persons*. IASP Press, Seattle, WA. pp. 239–61.

22 Hadjistavropoulos T, Hadjistavropoulos HD, eds. (2008) *Pain Management for Older Adults: A Self-Help Guide*. IASP Press, Seattle, WA.

23 Fuchs-Lacelle S, Hadjistavropoulos T, Lix L. (2008) Pain assessment as intervention: a study of older adults with severe dementia. *Clin J Pain* **24(8)**:697–707.

24 Teri L, Logsdon RG, Uomoto J *et al.* (1997) Behavioral treatment of depression in dementia patients: a controlled clinical trial. *J Gerontol B Psychol Sci Soc Sc* **52(4)**:P159–66.

25 American Geriatrics Society (AGS). (2009) Pharmacological management of pain: recommendations from the American Geriatrics Society guidelines on the management of persistent pain in older persons. *J Am Geriatr Soc* **57**:1331–6.

Acknowledgments

Thomas Hadjistavropoulos acknowledges the support of the RBC Foundation in the preparation of this work.

Appendix Pharmacological management of pain. Recommendations from the American Geriatrics Society guideline on the management of persistent pain in older persons (Used with permission from the American Geriatrics Society for "Pharmacological Management of Pain: Recommendations from the American Geriatrics Society Guideline on the Management of Persistent Pain in Older Persons" from the *Journal of the American Geriatrics Society*, 2009, Vol. 57, pp. 1341–3. For more information visit the AGS online at www.americangeriatrics.org).

Non-opioid analgesics

I   Acetaminophen should be considered as initial and ongoing pharmacotherapy in the treatment of persistent pain, particularly musculoskeletal pain, owing to its demonstrated effectiveness and good safety profile (high quality of evidence; strong recommendation)

     A Absolute contraindications: liver failure (high quality of evidence, strong recommendation)

     B Relative contraindications and cautions: hepatic insufficiency, chronic alcohol abuse/dependence (moderate quality of evidence, strong recommendation)

     C Maximum daily recommended dosages should not be exceeded and must include "hidden sources" such as from combination pills (moderate quality of evidence, strong recommendation)

II   Non-selective NSAIDs and COX-2 selective inhibitors may be considered rarely, and with extreme caution, in highly selected individuals (high quality of evidence, strong recommendation)

     A Patient selection: other (safer) therapies have failed; evidence of continuing therapeutic goals not met; ongoing assessment of risks/complications outweighed by therapeutic benefits (low quality of evidence, strong recommendation)

     B Absolute contraindications: current active peptic ulcer disease (low quality of evidence, strong recommendation), chronic kidney disease (moderate level of evidence, strong recommendation), heart failure (moderate level of evidence, weak recommendation)

     C Relative contraindications and cautions: hypertension, *Helicobacter pylori*, history of peptic ulcer disease, concomitant use of corticosteroids or SSRIs (moderate quality of evidence, strong recommendation)

III   Older persons taking non-selective NSAIDs should use a proton pump inhibitor or misoprostol for gastrointestinal protection (high quality of evidence, strong recommendation)

IV   Patients taking a COX-2 selective inhibitor with aspirin should use a proton pump inhibitor or misoprostol for gastrointestinal protection (high quality of evidence, strong recommendation)

V   Patients should not take more than one non-selective NSAID/COX-2 selective inhibitor for pain control (low quality of evidence, strong recommendation)

VI   Patients taking aspirin for cardioprophylaxis should not use ibuprofen (moderate quality of evidence, weak recommendation)

VII   All patients taking non-selective NSAIDs and COX-2 selective inhibitors should be routinely assessed for gastrointestinal and renal toxicity, hypertension, heart failure and other drug–drug and drug–disease interactions (weak quality of evidence, strong recommendation)

Opioid analgesics

VIII   All patients with moderate–severe pain, pain-related functional impairment or diminished quality of life due to pain should be considered for opioid therapy (low quality of evidence, strong recommendation)

IX   Patients with frequent or continuous pain on a daily basis may be treated with around-the-clock time-contingent dosing aimed at achieving steady state opioid therapy (low quality of evidence, weak recommendation)

X   Clinicians should anticipate, assess for and identify potential opioid-associated adverse effects (moderate quality of evidence, strong recommendation)

XI   Maximal safe doses of acetaminophen or NSAIDs should not be exceeded when using fixed-dose opioid combination agents as part of an analgesic regimen (moderate quality of evidence, strong recommendation)

XII   When long-acting opioid preparations are prescribed, breakthrough pain should be anticipated, assessed, prevented and/or treated using short-acting immediate-release opioid medications (moderate quality of evidence, strong recommendation)

XIII   Only clinicians well versed in the use and risks of methadone should initiate it and titrate it cautiously (moderate quality of evidence, strong recommendation)

XIV   Patients taking opioid analgesics should be reassessed for ongoing attainment of therapeutic goals, adverse effects, and safe and responsible medication use (moderate quality of evidence, strong recommendation)

Appendix *continued*

Adjuvant analgesics
XV   All patients with neuropathic pain are candidates for adjuvant analgesics (strong quality of evidence, strong recommendation)
XVI   Patients with fibromyalgia are candidates for a trial of approved adjuvant analgesics (moderate quality of evidence, strong recommendation)
XVII   Patients with other types of refractory persistent pain may be candidates for certain adjuvant analgesics (e.g. back pain, headache, diffuse bone pain, temporomandibular disorder) (low quality of evidence, weak recommendation)
XVIII   Tertiary tricyclic antidepressants (amitriptyline, imipramine, doxepin) should be avoided because of higher risk for adverse effects (e.g. anticholinergic effects, cognitive impairment) (moderate quality of evidence, strong recommendation)
XIX   Agents may be used alone, but often the effects are enhanced when used in combination with other pain analgesics and non-drug strategies (moderate quality of evidence, strong recommendation)
XX   Therapy should begin with the lowest possible dose and increase slowly based on response and side effects, with the caveat that some agents have a delayed onset of action and therapeutic benefits are slow to develop. For example, gabapentin may require 2–3 weeks for onset of efficacy (moderate quality of evidence, strong recommendation)
XXI   An adequate therapeutic trial should be conducted before discontinuation of a seemingly ineffective treatment (weak quality of evidence, strong recommendation)
Other drugs
XXII   Long-term systemic corticosteroids should be reserved only for patients with pain-associated inflammatory disorders or metastatic bone pain. Osteoarthritis should not be considered an inflammatory disorder (moderate quality of evidence, strong recommendation)
XXIII   All patients with localized neuropathic pain are candidates for topical lidocaine (moderate quality of evidence, strong recommendation)
XXIV   Patients with localized non-neuropathic pain may be candidates for topical lidocaine (low quality of evidence, weak recommendation)
XXV   All patients with other localized non-neuropathic persistent pain may be candidates for topical NSAIDs (moderate quality of evidence, weak recommendation)
XXVI   Other topical agents, including capsaicin or menthol may be considered for regional pain syndromes (moderate quality of evidence, weak recommendation)
XXVII   Many other agents for specific pain syndromes may require caution in older persons and merit further research (e.g. glucosamine, chondroitin, cannabinoids, botulinum toxin, α_2-adrenergic agonists, calcitonin, vitamin D, bisphosphonates, ketamine) (low quality of evidence, weak recommendation)

COX, cyclo-oxygenase; NSAID, non-steroidal anti-inflammatory drug; SSRI, selective serotonin reuptake inhibitor.

Chapter 38

Pain in children

Tonya M. Palermo[1], Jeffrey L. Koh[2] & Lonnie K. Zeltzer[3]

[1] *Anesthesiology, Pediatrics, and Psychiatry, Seattle Children's Hospital, University of Washington School of Medicine, Seattle, USA*
[2] *Anesthesiology & Perioperative Medicine, Oregon Health & Science University, Portland, USA*
[3] *Pediatric Pain Program, Mattel Children's Hospital at UCLA, Los Angeles, USA; Pediatric Anesthesiology, Psychiatry and Biobehavioral Sciences, David Geffen School of Medicine at UCLA, Los Angeles, USA*

Introduction

Children and adolescents have unique needs that should be considered in assessment and management of pain, given their neurophysiology associated with development, the influence and involvement of their parents and families, and differences in their methods and abilities in communication. Evaluation and management of recurrent and chronic pain in children can present challenges for the treating clinician. In this chapter, we review the special considerations in managing chronic pain in children, including discussion of the significance of recurrent and chronic pain for children, adolescents and their families; basic mechanisms of chronic pain; and evaluation and evidence-based management approaches.

In pediatric populations, chronic or recurrent pain may be associated with ongoing underlying chronic or recurrent medical conditions, such as arthritis, cancer, nerve damage, Crohn's disease or sickle cell disease. Cancer-related pain and pain associated with life-limiting and life-threatening

medical conditions, as in end-stage diseases, are other forms of serious chronic pain. However, the most frequent form of chronic pain in children is when chronic and recurrent pain is the problem itself, without underlying clearly identifiable etiology, as in pain associated with irritable bowel syndrome, headaches, musculoskeletal pain or complex regional pain syndrome (CRPS). All forms of chronic pain irrespective of etiology can hinder the body's ability to heal itself and can impact on children's quality of life, and so the pain itself becomes an additional or primary chronic problem.

Significance of recurrent and chronic pain in children

Recent epidemiological studies provide prevalence estimates of recurring or persisting pains in 15–30% of children and adolescents [1]. The most common bodily locations for persistent pain in children are the head, limbs, abdomen and back. Recurrent and chronic pain can lead to significant interference with daily functioning for some children and adolescents and may increase their risk of having a chronic pain syndrome in adulthood. Although the overall base of knowledge of the natural history and course of pain in children and adolescents is limited, the data that are available suggest that early exposure to pain may alter later

Clinical Pain Management: A Practical Guide, 1st edition.
Edited by Mary E. Lynch, Kenneth D. Craig and Philip W.H. Peng.
© 2011 Blackwell Publishing Ltd.

pain response and that initial pain complaints often are maintained over time and may occur in another part of the body, or other somatic symptoms may develop in the child.

Of concern for many children with recurrent and chronic pain is the potential for associated decrements in their ability to function in important life roles. Children may experience limitations in their ability to attend school and complete academic work as well as in their participation in physical, social, recreational and peer activities [2]. Chronic pain can also have a negative impact on family life, including increased stress and financial implications for parents.

Basic mechanisms

A number of models have been developed over the years to understand children's recurrent and chronic pain. Many of these theories focus on factors that explain the considerable interindividual variability in pain perception, and the chronicity and impairment experienced from pain. Central to contemporary models are interrelationships among physical, cognitive, affective and social factors that influence children's pain and disability – commonly referred to as biopsychosocial models of pain [3]. Current conceptualizations of pain in children recognize the importance of age, sex, psychosocial stressors and central nervous system mechanisms for understanding the etiology of pain problems.

The incidence of most pain complaints increases dramatically with age and pubertal development for girls but not for boys [4]. Sex and age differences have also emerged in children's symptom reporting where girls generally report higher pain intensity, longer lasting pain and more frequent pain than do boys.

There are also a variety of central nervous system pain mechanisms that are implicated in the persistence of pain [5]. As one example in understanding functional bowel disorders, current theories suggest that the pain or symptoms are caused by abnormal brain–intestinal neural (neuroenteric) signaling that creates visceral hypersensitivity. Abdominal pain may be caused by alterations in the sensory

receptors of the gastrointestinal tract, abnormal modulation of sensory transmission in the peripheral or central nervous systems or changes in the cortical perception of afferent signals.

Psychological factors, in particular children's anxiety and depressive symptoms, have been found in a number of studies to have a strong association with functional disability related to chronic pain. Parent factors have also been recognized as important in explaining the interindividual variability in children's response to pain [6]. Much of the research on specific parent factors has focused on the role of parent behaviors, such as providing excessive attention to pain complaints. A number of researchers have noted a family aggregation of pain complaints, finding that children with chronic pain often live in households where other family members also have chronic pain.

Clinical practice: evaluation and management

Evaluation

Basic understanding of the biological, social and psychological factors that impact on children's experience of pain helps to inform and guide clinical practice with pediatric patients. Most notably, in the management of children with chronic pain, clinicians are advised to use an approach that considers multiple rather than single etiologies and that de-emphasizes complete symptom resolution or cure. In general, clinical guidance starts with the principle that all children with chronic pain that is interfering with functioning in everyday life can benefit from attention to the psychosocial as well as the biomedical aspects of their pain.

A focused interview can be used for gathering a pain history from the child and parents (for an excellent overview see Chapter 8). Medical evaluation of the child with chronic pain is covered extensively in other texts (for a review of the physical examination see for example Zeltzer & Schlank [7]). Comprehensive evaluation focused on multiple etiologies such as identification of any comorbidity, such as anxiety, depression or psychosocial or family contributors is needed. Additional resources on psychological assessment of the child with chronic pain can be found in a recent review [8].

A productive way to initiate the history is to elicit the patient's and parents' narrative about the pain, rather than beginning with targeted questions. Further prompts about the pain can then be provided. Throughout the initial evaluation, communication that establishes reassurance, rapport and a belief in the significance of the pain problem will enhance the receptivity of the parents and child to the treatment approach.

Treatment approach

It is essential that a team approach be used in treating a child with chronic pain. The clinical team may consist of any combination of pediatrician, anesthesiologist, nurse practitioner, pediatric psychologist, child psychiatrist and physical or occupational therapist to assist in both diagnosis and management of the pain. Communication among the team should occur on a consistent basis as providers may not be physically proximate. In fact, there are few dedicated pediatric pain treatment facilities and most centers are located in major urban cities. Even when adequately trained clinicians and resources are available, time, expense and insurance barriers may also prevent children from accessing appropriate services, and may compromise the optimal team approach. Primary care physicians should be kept informed of management plans, as they may be able to provide important support and coordination for the families.

If experts in chronic pain cannot be located, the primary care physician can assemble a team of knowledgeable professionals and serve as a coordinator to help to educate the team on chronic pain treatment. Psychologists and rehabilitation therapists can have a useful role in treatment even when they do not have expertise in pain management, provided an overarching treatment plan is in place with specific assessments and interventions outlined.

Once the treatment team is assembled, a variety of intervention options are available. A complete review of treatment strategies for pediatric chronic pain is beyond the scope of this chapter. The reader

is referred to clinical practice guidelines available from the American Pain Society for the management of pain conditions in children (see http://www.association-office.com/APS/etools/products/products.cfm).

Pharmacological strategies, psychological treatments, physical therapy, complementary and alternative treatments, and their combination, have been used to reduce pain sensations, increase comfort and/or reduce associated disability and dysfunction in children with pain conditions. In the sections below, we review the evidence base associated with each type of intervention strategy in children with chronic pain.

Evidence base for pharmacological treatments

Medications have been used for children with recurrent and chronic pain conditions for the purpose of treating acute exacerbations of their underlying chronic pain, reducing inflammation, helping with sleep problems, treating comorbid psychological disorders including anxiety and/or depression, and reducing spontaneous neural transmission that may be contributing to their pain. For some conditions, treatments can be specific and mechanism-driven. For example, for children with juvenile idiopathic arthritis, pharmacological treatment is largely directed at underlying inflammatory processes, which may in turn reduce pain. Similarly, pharmacotherapy for migraine and for specific types of chronic abdominal pain may be directed at underlying mechanisms. However, for most other types of childhood chronic pain there is a very limited evidence base for any class of medication. Treatment is largely based on anecdotal evidence or derived from the adult literature rather than controlled clinical studies in the pediatric population. We review below the available evidence base for pharmacotherapy for specific pain conditions in children.

Most of the evidence from randomized controlled trials concerns the treatment of pediatric headache including the efficacy and safety of migraine prophylactic agents as well as acute abortive migraine treatment in children and adolescents. In general, findings are favorable although there remains a limited amount of pediatric specific information in the literature. Several review articles of pharmacotherapy for pediatric migraine are available (see for example Eiland [9]). Cyclic vomiting syndrome, which some clinicians believe to be similar in pathophysiology to migraine headaches, has also been treated using migraine prophylactic medication with some success.

A Cochrane review of the evidence base for pharmacological interventions for recurrent abdominal pain (RAP) and irritable bowel syndrome (IBS) was recently published [10]. It included three small randomized controlled trials evaluating pizotifen, peppermint oil capsules and famotidine. There was significant improvement in children with RAP and IBS treated with peppermint oil capsules. Similarly, in the trial comparing famotidine with placebo, significant improvement was found in children with RAP and dyspepsia treated with famotidine. Several recent controlled trials evaluating amitriptyline for functional abdominal pain and IBS have produced equivocal findings for pain relief in children. Overall, the evidence base is quite small and there is no clear indication of effectiveness for any particular pharmacological intervention for recurrent abdominal pain.

Other common chronic pain conditions seen in children include musculoskeletal pain, neuropathic pain syndromes and pain related to underlying medical conditions such as cancer. For adults with many forms of chronic pain, especially neuropathic pain disorders, there is evidence for efficacy of several anticonvulsant and antidepressant medications. In pediatrics, there have been multiple case reports and case series reporting success in treating children with CRPS and other neuropathic pain conditions with anticonvulsants including gabapentin, oxcarbazepine and pregabalin. Unfortunately, there have been no controlled studies of anticonvulsants in children with CRPS or any other neuropathic pain syndrome.

Opioids have been extensively studied for pediatric acute pain management and for pain in children with life-limiting conditions. However, there is no consensus regarding which children with chronic non-malignant pain have a favorable risk–

benefit ratio for long-term opioid analgesia. To date, there are no controlled trials of opioids for the management of chronic pain in children.

Because of the lack of evidence-based pediatric research for most medications used in chronic pain, dosing is usually based on clinical experience or derived from pediatric dosing guidelines for the approved use of the medication (e.g. seizures for gabapentin). Dosing range guidelines are beyond the scope of this chapter but can be found in several published textbooks (see for example Schechter et al. [11]).

Evidence base for psychological treatments

Psychological treatments have had an important role in reducing pain sensations and modifying situational, emotional, familial and behavioral factors that contribute to pain-related disability in children. Behavioral strategies include relaxation training, biofeedback and behavioral management programs (e.g. teaching operant strategies to parents to reinforce adaptive behaviors such as school attendance). For example, thermal biofeedback involves teaching patients how to increase their peripheral temperature using electronic instruments such as a temperature probe on the finger to measure temperature and a computer monitor to display reinforcing information back to the patient (biofeedback usually incorporates instruction in relaxation strategies).

Cognitive strategies include hypnosis, stress management, guided imagery and cognitive coping skills. Cognitive behavioral therapy (CBT) programs incorporate elements of both behavioral and cognitive strategies. The goals of CBT are typically to enhance children's coping skills by instructing them in behavioral and cognitive skills that allow them to think and behave differently to reduce the negative effects of having chronic pain. In addition, specific areas of concern such as school avoidance, difficulties in social relationships or significant anxiety or depressive symptoms can be therapeutic targets. CBT interventions often involve considerable work with parents to teach them ways to support their children and to implement behavioral plans, such as rewarding the child for participation in therapies or attendance at school.

Several meta-analytic reviews have documented the efficacy of psychological therapies for children with chronic pain. In a meta-analysis of therapies for pediatric migraine [12], biofeedback and relaxation were found to be more effective than placebo treatments and prophylactic drug treatments in controlling headache. Most recently, an updated systematic review and meta-analysis including 29 studies of psychological therapies for management of chronic pain in children found that across pain conditions, biofeedback, relaxation training and CBT were effective at reducing pain intensity in youth [13].

On the basis of this evidence, psychological interventions are considered appropriate for children and adolescents with any chronic pain condition, including youth with disease-related pain. At this time, the only psychological intervention that has been developed and evaluated for youth with a specific pain condition is biofeedback. Biofeedback has undergone empirical evaluation only in children with migraine and tension headache although in clinical practice biofeedback may be applied in other pain conditions.

Some new developments in psychological treatments for chronic pain that have received promising initial support include the use of acceptance and commitment strategies [14], and the application of technology to deliver treatment such as the delivery of psychological treatment strategies via the Internet.

Evidence base for physical therapy interventions

Physical therapy (PT) and maintaining a regular exercise program are important aspects of pain treatment in children with chronic pain. Most commonly, PT interventions are targeted toward deconditioning and restricted range of motion or desensitization of painful body parts. The majority of studies describing PT-based interventions in children with chronic pain have focused on exercise programs in youth with widespread mus-

culoskeletal pain and in youth with localized musculoskeletal pain such as in CRPS.

Exercise-based programs have significantly reduced pain in clinical samples of youth with fibromyalgia and CRPS. The frequency and intensity of exercise necessary to accomplish symptom reduction is unclear at this time; both inpatient intense rehabilitation as well as outpatient PT has been effective in the management of pain related to CRPS. Within community-based samples of adolescents with low back pain, exercise interventions have produced significant reductions in pain [15]. Currently, data on other physical therapy interventions such as trigger release or massage are limited to case series.

Evidence base for complementary and alternative medicine therapies

Many parents of children with chronic pain seek out complementary and alternative medicine (CAM) therapies such as acupuncture, yoga and herbal remedies. All of these therapies require further study in order to recommend their use in children. Studies of CAM modalities for chronic pain in adult populations are increasing (Chapter 26). The reader is referred for a general review of CAM studies for pain treatment in children [16].

Putting it all together: a treatment algorithm

As shown in Figure 38.1, a basic treatment algorithm for pediatric chronic pain management begins with assembling a treatment team and providing education to the child and family that will engage their participation in a comprehensive evaluation and management plan for the child's pain condition. The clinical team develops and sets goals for the child's treatment plan which will generally include pain management, enhancing the child's coping skills, improving the child's functioning (physical, social, recreational) and enhancing the child's sleep quality and quantity. Throughout the evaluation and management period, the team provides critical support to parents through emphasizing the normalcy of

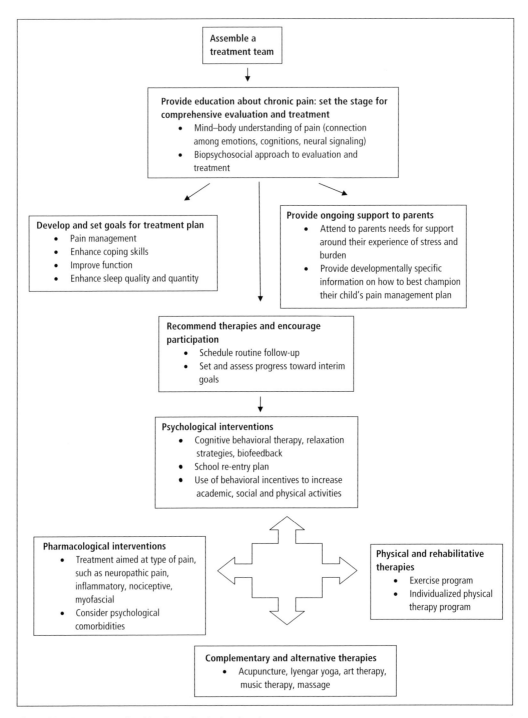

Figure 38.1 A treatment algorithm for pediatric chronic pain.

their experience of stress and burden, providing developmentally specific information on how to best champion the child's pain management plan and through referral of parent(s) or family for additional therapeutic support. Specific therapies are recommended which generally involve a multimodal approach including some combination of psychological interventions, pharmacological interventions, physical and rehabilitative therapies or complementary and alternative therapies. Routine follow-up is useful for encouraging the child's participation in therapies and providing feedback on progress toward interim goals.

References

1 Stanford EA, Chambers CT, Biesanz JC *et al.* (2008) The frequency, trajectories and predictors of adolescent recurrent pain: a population-based approach. *Pain* **138**:11–21.

2 Palermo TM.(2000) Impact of recurrent and chronic pain on child and family daily functioning: a critical review of the literature. *J Dev Behav Pediatr* **21**:58–69.

3 Meyer MJ, Goldschneider KR, Bielefeldt K *et al.* (2008) Functional abdominal pain in adolescence: a biopsychosocial phenomenon. *J Pain* **9**:984–90.

4 LeResche L, Mancl LA, Drangsholt MT *et al.* (2005) Relationship of pain and symptoms to pubertal development in adolescents. *Pain* **118**:201–9.

5 Aguggia M.(2003) Neurophysiology of pain. *Neurol Sci* **24(Suppl 2)**:S57–60.

6 Palermo TM, Chambers CT.(2005) Parent and family factors in pediatric chronic pain and disability: an integrative approach. *Pain* **119**:1–4.

7 Zeltzer L, Schlank C.(2005) *Conquering your Child's Chronic Pain: A Pediatrician's Guide for Reclaiming a Normal Childhood.* Harper Collins, New York.

8 Palermo TM.(2009) Assessment of chronic pain in children: current status and emerging topics. *Pain Res Manag* **14**:21–6.

9 Eiland LS.(2007) Anticonvulsant use for prophylaxis of the pediatric migraine. *J Pediatr Health Care* **21**:392–5.

10 Huertas-Ceballos A, Logan S, Bennett C *et al.* (2008) Psychosocial interventions for recurrent abdominal pain (RAP) and irritable bowel syndrome (IBS) in childhood. *Cochrane Database Syst Rev* **1**:CD003014.

11 Schechter N, Berde C, Yaster M.(2003) *Pain in Infants, Children and Adolescents.* Lippincott Williams & Wilkins, Philadelphia, PA.

12 Hermann C, Kim M, Blanchard E.B.(1995) Behavioral and prophylactic pharmacological intervention studies of pediatric migraine: an exploratory meta-analysis. *Pain* **60**:239–55.

13 Eccleston C, Palermo T, Williams A *et al.* (2009) Psychological therapies for the management of chronic and recurrent pain in children and adolescents. *Cochrane Database Syst Rev* **2**: CD003968.

14 Wicksell RK, Melin L, Lekander M *et al.* (2009) Evaluating the effectiveness of exposure and acceptance strategies to improve functioning and quality of life in longstanding pediatric pain: a randomized controlled trial. *Pain* **141**:248–57.

15 Fanucchi GL, Stewart A, Jordaan R *et al.* (2009) Exercise reduces the intensity and prevalence of low back pain in 12–13 year old children: a randomised trial. *Aust J Physiother* **55**: 97–104.

16 Tsao JC.(2006) CAM for pediatric pain: what is state-of-the-research? *Evid Based Complement Alternat Med* **3**:143–4.

Chapter 39

Pain in individuals with intellectual disabilities

Tim F. Oberlander[1], Chantel C. Burkitt[2] & Frank J. Symons[2]

[1] Pediatrics, University of British Columbia; BC Children's Hospital, Vancouver, Canada
[2] Department of Educational Psychology, University of Minnesota, Minneapolis, USA

Introduction and overview

Expression of pain by individuals with intellectual and related development disabilities (e.g. cerebral palsy) and disorders (e.g. autism) is frequently ambiguous and its recognition by caregivers and healthcare providers can be highly subjective. This presents a tremendous challenge for clinicians, researchers, individuals with disabilities and their families. Even when pain-specific behaviors are present, such behaviors may be regarded as altered, blunted or confused with other sources of generalized stress, arousal or in the extreme, misinterpreted as a reflection of a behavior disorder of psychological origin. However, there is no reason to believe that pain is any less frequent in the lives of someone with an intellectual or related developmental disability that alters the way they communicate, or that such an individual would be insensitive or indifferent to pain.

Until recently pain in people with intellectual disability (ID) received little scientific attention,

and as study participants individuals with ID have been systematically excluded from pain and related research. This is starting to change [1]. The International Association for the Study of Pain (IASP) originally defined pain as "an unpleasant sensory and emotional experience associated with actual or potential tissue damage, or described in terms of such damage" [2] but, because the emphasis on self-report assumed a capacity for verbal communication, the IASP clarified the definition of pain to recognize that "the inability to verbally communicate in no way negates the possibility that an individual is experiencing pain and is in need of appropriate pain relieving treatment" [3]. In this sense our goal is to recognize and assess features of an individual's behavioral and physiologic repertoire as legitimate indices of pain expression and experience and develop strategies to manage this universal, but highly individual, human condition.

The purpose of this chapter is to provide an overview of a number of issues inherent to assessing and managing pain among children and adults with intellectual and developmental disabilities. Wherever possible, our focus is specific to intellectual disability as distinct from but related to the concept of developmental disability (e.g. cerebral palsy is a developmental disability in which some

Clinical Pain Management: A Practical Guide, 1st edition.
Edited by Mary E. Lynch, Kenneth D. Craig and
Philip W.H. Peng.
© 2011 Blackwell Publishing Ltd.

children also have intellectual disability but some do not). It is beyond the scope of the chapter to provide an exhaustive review; for more information, readers are directed to Oberlander & Symons [1] or Siden & Oberlander [4]. The chapter begins by defining ID to clarify the clinical population and then reviews briefly the scope of the problem of pain among individuals with ID. Recent developments in assessment approaches are discussed and specific tools are described. Issues and approaches to management are then presented. Readers will note that the chapter and its citation pattern reflects the current reality of our knowledge in this area – the majority of the research addressing issues in pain and ID has focused on the scope of the problem and assessment in pediatric populations with very little work specific to management.[1]

Defining ID and conceptual issues

The World Health Organization (WHO) defines ID as:

A disorder defined by the presence of incomplete or arrested mental development, principally characterized by the deterioration of concrete functions at each stage of development and that contribute to the overall level of intelligence, such as cognitive, language, motor and socialization functions; in this anomaly, adaptation to the environment is always affected. For ID, scores for intellectual development levels must be determined based on all of the available information, including clinical signs, adaptive behavior in the cultural medium of the individual and psychometric findings.

However, the American Association on Intellectual and Developmental Disabilities (AAIDD) indicates

[1] Note on terminology: there are many terms in use professionally and scientifically with respect to individuals with significant intellectual impairments including mental retardation, intellectual disability, severe neurological impairment, and cognitive impairment. For the purposes of this chapter, the term "intellectual disability" will be used.

that in addition to a significantly subaverage intellectual functioning, concomitant limitations are observed in two or more areas of adaptive skills, and the disorder presents itself before the age of 18.

Regardless of the degree of ID and the underlying neurological condition, functional limitations frequently confound the presentation of pain in individuals with intellectual and developmental disabilities [5]. In the absence of easily recognized verbal or motor-dependent forms of communication, it remains uncertain if the pain experience itself is different or whether only the expressive manifestations are altered. Indeed, without recognizable means of communication or functional motor skills, pain may remain under-recognized and under-treated. In spite of the potential for altered nociception and pain expression, there is no evidence that cognitively or motor impaired individuals are spared any of the miseries of a noxious experience [6].

Scope of the problem of pain in individuals with ID

Epidemiology

Whether from a single or multifactorial cause (e.g. genetic and/or metabolic disorders or traumatic brain injury), ID can be associated with multiple sources of acute and chronic pain. There is a limited but emerging database regarding the epidemiology of pain among children and adults with ID [7], examples of which include the following. Based on a 4-week window during a longitudinal study (N = 94), Breau et al. [8] reported that 78% of children with ID experienced some type of pain and 62% experienced non-accidental pain (pain type varied by motor ability). The pain reported was of a significant severity to be disturbing and was long-lasting and frequent. Stallard et al. [9], using a diary study (N = 34), reported that 74% of the sample of children with ID experienced some form of pain over a 2-week period (for 68% it was rated as moderate to severe). Most troubling was that none of the children were reported to be receiving any type of pain management. Although less is known about adults, studies with adults with cerebral palsy (some with ID) have produced similar results in relation to chronic conditions that are most likely associated with pain [10]. Minihan [11] found that 99% of residents in a New York State facility had at least one chronic medical condition that required continued monitoring. Research has noted that adults with ID often have multiple medical conditions [12]. Many of these medical conditions (e.g. fractures, dental problems, arthritis) result in pain and some are associated with chronic pain.

Pain sources and risk factors

The activities of daily living associated with an intellectual and co-occurring developmental disability may involve the use of assistive devices for positioning and mobility and are associated with new and different sources of pain [13]. Dislocated hips, pressure sores from skin breakdown and repetitive use injuries occur and must be considered. Splinting and casting may be required for the prevention and treatment of contractures and can be associated with pain. Feeding tubes can result in gastric distention and as well tugging on the tube, or skin breakdown at the insertion site are all potential sources for everyday pain.

Motor impairments may be characterized by increased tone, spasms, increased deep tendon reflexes and clonus, coupled with weakness and loss of dexterity (cerebral palsy). Spasticity and spasms can cause significant discomfort through waking and sleeping hours. Treatment of spasticity frequently involves invasive procedures; high tone/spasticity may be treated through surgical intervention (selective dorsal rhizotomy) or by surgical implantation of an intrathecal baclofen pump, while pharmacologic management of tone may include intramuscular injection of botulinum toxin A. Non-invasive therapies can also contribute heavily to frequent pain; adult patients with cerebral palsy report that their memories of pain in childhood center around regular physical therapy sessions and stretching [14].

There are times when repeated surgery, or direct trauma to a nerve, results in long-lasting pain that may be similar to neuropathic pain. Neuropathic

pain can be difficult to identify and treat, but should be considered in individuals with severe neurological impairments associated with ID with prolonged pain after an intervention. Another potential source of pain is central in origin, where the pain afferents appear to be activated without an ongoing input either from tissue damage or peripheral nerve injury. The major evidence for such an entity comes from the observation of pain behavior in children with advancing neuro-degenerative diseases such as Krabbe's disease, children with severe neurological impairments, adults with thalamic strokes and Alzheimer's disease [15,16] but the pain mechanisms associated with these conditions remain to be demonstrated. However, even with a determined search for an underlying cause, one is frequently faced with the considerable probability that the final diagnosis becomes a "medically unexplainable pain" [17], leading to clinical dead-end – "I can't diagnose, therefore I can't treat" (C. Montgomery, personal communication).

Pain assessment tools

In this section, we briefly outline a number of pain assessment scales (Table 39.1) designed to evaluate pain specifically among children and adults with ID (for more detailed reviews specific to scale development see Bodfish et al. [18] and Breau et al. [19]). It should be noted that although existing scales for other vulnerable populations (neonates, elderly) also have been adapted for use with children with ID (e.g. revised FLACC) [20], the scales reviewed in Table 39.1 were designed and developed specifically for individuals with ID. The measures developed to date focus on identifying a variety of possible pain signs in children and adults with intellectual impairment [21–23,31]. These include vocalizations (e.g. cry, scream, moan), facial expression, movement (both increased and decreased), change in muscle tone (increased and decreased), guarding/protection and changes in every day activity (social interaction, eating and sleeping). Most often the scales are completed by proxy report, vary somewhat in their administration time, may be used for initial assessment and, in

Table 39.1 Pain assessment tools for children and adults with intellectual disabilities (ID).

Pain scale	Brief description	Items	Psychometric properties	Recommendations
Child pain scales				
Pain Indicator for Communicatively Impaired Children (PICIC) Stallard *et al.* (2002) [9]	200 pain cues derived from caregiver interview narrowed to 6 main cues	6	Showed accuracy Not retested for validity or reliability	Short and simple Possible preliminary measure of pain
Pediatric Pain Profile (PPP) Hunt *et al.* (2002) [23]	Semi-individualized measure providing predetermined categories of behaviors which are then added to by the parent/caregiver	20	Valid, reliable and sensitive measure for each individual child Does not provide generalizable measures across children	May distinguish individual child's good days from bad days May be well suited for monitoring pain for an individual across long time scales
Non-Communicative Children's Pain Checklist Revised (NCCPC-R Breau *et al.* (2002) [21]	Observational assessment tool quantifies pain responses observed by parents and caregivers and postoperative versions are available	30	Reliable and valid in detecting pain	Useful across populations and settings Consistently accurate with short observation times and by those unfamiliar with the child
Adult pain scales				
Pain and Discomfort Scale (PADS) Bodfish *et al.* (2001) [29] Phan *et al.* (2005) [31]	Measures pain and discomfort during a standardized physical examination (pain examination procedure)	18	High inter-rater reliability Sensitivity to pain	Useful in isolating the location/source of pain
Chronic Pain Scale for Non-verbal Adults with Intellectual Disabilities (CPS-NAID) Burkitt *et al.* (2009) [26]	Adapted the NCCPC-R for adults with ID during chronic or recurring pain	24	Strong internal consistency, inter-rater reliability and construct validity and sensitive to pain Cutoff score was established	CPS-NAID is best suited for assessing chronic pain
Non-Communicating Adult Pain Checklist (NCAPC) Lotan *et al.* (2009) [27]	Adapted the NCCPC-R to assess acute pain in adults with ID	21	High internal consistency Sensitive to pain	NCAPC is recommended currently for assessing acute or procedural pain in adults with ID

some applications, for repeated evaluation for acute, postoperative and chronic pain. Measurement approaches focused on establishing sensitive and specific measures of non-verbal facial pain displays (e.g. facial action unit activity) [24] and biobehavioral reactivity (heart rate variability) [25] have been studied, but the clinical utility of these approaches remains to be established.

Pain management

Where to begin?

The pain history can be guided by the use of an established, symptom cluster assessment tool, such as those offered by several studies [21,26–28]. This approach might provide a profile of typical everyday behaviors, how they have changed during this period of "pain" and other associated changes in everyday function and activities (Table 39.2). An alternative but complementary approach was developed by Bodfish *et al.* [29] based on pairing assessment with an examination.

In using these approaches, understanding changes from an agreed upon baseline set of behaviors observed by experienced caregivers, compiled to reflect a longitudinal perspective, may be the most reliable measure of pain and distress available. A detailed history should include an account of known baseline behaviors or physical conditions, temporal sequences, known stressors and an understanding of the typical repertoire of verbal and non-verbal cues used to communicate pain and a variety of affective states. One helpful technique is to ask the family to make a brief home video recording of the behavior; watching the video with the parents develops understanding and agreement about the exact nature of the complaint. The influence of the caregiver's perceptions, social setting and the individual's tolerance

Table 39.2 Key questions to consider in assessing pain in an individual with intellectual disabilities (ID).

What is the underlying neurological condition/process? How might this influence pain system function and the expression of distress/pain? What is the developmental level? What is the usual behavioral and health condition, baseline condition and nature of everyday function? Usual means of communication Caregivers' views and understanding of what is happening Role of intercurrent illness Differential diagnosis: what else is going on?

to change or stress are keys to understanding the child's current situation. Context of the pain behavior is crucial. Pain on changing a diaper suggests hip subluxation or sacral decubitus ulcers; pain after eating or upon lying down suggests gastroesophageal reflux, for instance. Beyond a pain history, a detailed review of all systems, medications, allergies, diet and recent procedures remains essential. Finally, during the physical examination, careful observation, with guidance by experienced caregivers looking for specific areas of discomfort or injury is essential. Throughout the examination, one should observe the individual's facial and vocal reactions to manipulations, as well as the reaction of the parent or caregiver (as a proxy for self-report; a "gut-reaction" or intuition can sometimes help more than asking them for a more complex evaluation of pain behaviors). In the search for the source of irritability of unknown origin (IUO), one should consider a broad differential diagnoses as illustrated in Figure 39.1.

Moving forward

Typical pain management focuses on identifying the underlying pathology leading to a diagnosis and treatment plan, reducing distress and facilitating a return to baseline function. However, even with a careful history and thoughtful approaches investigating irritability, sources of pain frequently remain uncertain. A diagnosis in this setting may not always be possible, and even after a careful empiric evaluation, identification of exacerbating and mediating factors, an empiric medication trial and careful ongoing evaluation may be the only available management options. The success of pain management in this setting requires three key elements:

1 A clearly identified plan including pharmacologic and non-pharmacologic options;

2 Coordinated communication and decision making among the individual (to the greatest extent possible), caregivers and clinicians alike; and

3 A process for ongoing evaluation to keep this management plan on track especially when the pain has not resolved.

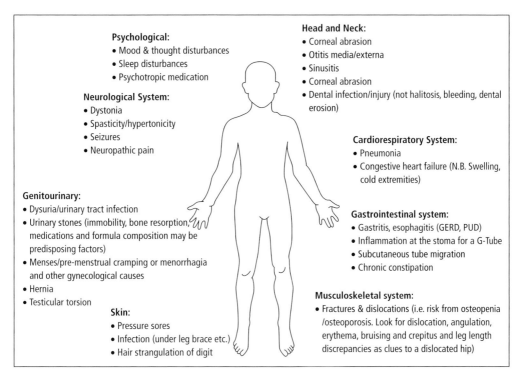

Psychological:
- Mood & thought disturbances
- Sleep disturbances
- Psychotropic medication

Neurological System:
- Dystonia
- Spasticity/hypertonicity
- Seizures
- Neuropathic pain

Genitourinary:
- Dysuria/urinary tract infection
- Urinary stones (immobility, bone resorption, medications and formula composition may be predisposing factors)
- Menses/pre-menstrual cramping or menorrhagia and other gynecological causes
- Hernia
- Testicular torsion

Skin:
- Pressure sores
- Infection (under leg brace etc.)
- Hair strangulation of digit

Head and Neck:
- Corneal abrasion
- Otitis media/externa
- Sinusitis
- Corneal abrasion
- Dental infection/injury (not halitosis, bleeding, dental erosion)

Cardiorespiratory System:
- Pneumonia
- Congestive heart failure (N.B. Swelling, cold extremities)

Gastrointestinal system:
- Gastritis, esophagitis (GERD, PUD)
- Inflammation at the stoma for a G-Tube
- Subcutaneous tube migration
- Chronic constipation

Musculoskeletal system:
- Fractures & dislocations (i.e. risk from osteopenia /osteoporosis. Look for dislocation, angulation, erythema, bruising and crepitus and leg length discrepancies as clues to a dislocated hip)

Figure 39.1 IUO: Possible differential diagnoses for Irritability of Unknown Origin (IUO).

Analgesics

In general, one follows the same principles for pharmacotherapy in the cognitively impaired that are used in other populations with chronic pain (Chapters 11 and 14–18). In this population, route of administration and assessment of response may be more complex. The route of medication administration should be the least invasive and appropriate for the patient's condition and sources of pain. Oral or G-tube route is preferable. Subcutaneous medications delivered via indwelling catheters may be an appropriate way to administer opioids for selected, severe pain states; thus, with the added pain of multiple injections and reduced muscle mass, intramuscular injections can be avoided. Topical anesthetic creams or other topical agents should be considered prior to injections, venipuncture, refills of intrathecal baclofen pumps and other cutaneous procedures. Silver nitrate and sulcrate in zinc oxide can be very effective topical agents for controlling local irritation at gastric tube sites. In this setting, an "n-of-1" trial to determine therapeutic efficacy may be helpful, comparing the patient's response on a medication against their own response to a placebo. This requires the use of a blinding procedure, often by a pharmacist, to use placebos and medication interventions in a randomized fashion. This can also be helpful in eliminating an expectation bias.

Non-pharmacological management approaches

Acute procedural or postoperative pain management requires the same imaginative approach used in other healthcare settings. Simple non-pharmacological approaches may be helpful. At the outset, keeping primary caregivers at hand may help in assessment and allow differentiation of non-specific arousal behavior from pain behavior. Similarly, maintaining communication with the inpatient treating team will avail them of the accumulated knowledge of how the individual reacts to pain and prior treatments, and improve the management of ongoing or pre-existing problems. Depending on the individual's ability to communicate or responsiveness to external stimulation, behavioral interventions such as distraction, guided imagery and hypnosis may be used in individuals with ID, depending on the cognitive level [30]. Physical measures such as massage, touch, heat or cold therapy may be helpful, although to date there have been no published studies evaluating these measures for this population. Effective coordinated team work, including a case manager, an understanding of where the pain fits into the individual's life (i.e. drawing a "pain map") and the elements that comprise an individual's pain (the "clinical topography" of pain), may be helpful in avoiding "therapeutic failure" (Table 39.3).

Therapeutic failure and drug interactions

In the individual where multiple medications are needed to manage a diverse number of conditions it is especially important to be aware of potential drug interactions and the potential for genetic variation in drug response and metabolism (Chapters 14–18).

Table 39.3 Factors that might underlie therapeutic failure.

1	Limited knowledge and bias about pain in individuals with ID
2	Impact of an altered neurological system: a. What do we know about the underlying neurological disorder that influences function of the pain system?
3	Limited access to pain experience: a. Is an assessment of pain possible using a standard tool? b. Have we targeted the right symptom endpoint?
4	Diagnosis in doubt: a. Have we searched for the "irritability of unknown origin"? b. Multiple candidate diagnoses and conditions (e.g. sleep disturbances, nutrition, intercurrent infection)
5	Right drug, ….but still not effective a. Pharmacokinetic, pharmacodynamic and genetic factors b. Drug–drug interactions c. Drug–environment interactions (e.g. smoke, grapefruit juice)
6	Contextual factors: a. Lack of an understanding of elements that comprise the clinical topography of the pain or a "pain map" b. Presence of multiple caregivers but poorly coordinated healthcare team c. Lack of a case manager

Conclusions

In the past decade tremendous strides have been taken in recognizing the problem of pain among individuals with ID. Problems with the definition of pain are readily recognized as is the fact that conventional approaches to assessment are limited. A great deal of effort has led to improved assessment techniques which include a broader range of possible pain indicators beyond verbal self-report. Despite this, caution should be exercised when using any of the tools described in this chapter because in most instances their development and use has been under very specific circumstances. Regardless of the instruments used, however, it is clear that systematic pain assessments should be routinely undertaken, regardless of the disability, particularly when extraordinary

behavior or context dictates the possibility that pain is present. The development of pain assessment tools for adults with ID is in its infancy; thus, a multifaceted approach to pain assessment and its management is necessary. Although efforts to understand the nature of pain in the context of a neurological injury leading to an ID are underway, we need to focus on the individual, his/her typical behavior and their own experience as an individual living with pain.

References

1 Oberlander TF, Symon FJ. (2006) *Pain in Children and Adults with Developmental Disabilities*. Paul H. Brookes, Baltimore, MD.

2 Merskey HE. (1986) Classification of chronic pain: descriptions of chronic pain syndromes and definitions of pain terms. *Pain Suppl* **3**:51.

3 http: and www.iasp-pain.org/terms-p.html. http://www.iasp-pain.org/terms-p.html. http://www.iasp-pain.org. (2001)

4 Siden H, Oberlander TF. (2008) Pain management for children with a developmental disability in a primary care setting. In: Walco GA, Goldschneider KR, eds. *Pain in Children: A Practical Guide for Primary Care*. Humana Press, Totowa, NJ. pp. 29–37.

5 Abu-Saad HH. (2000) Challenge of pain in the cognitively impaired. *Lancet* **356**:1867–8.

6 Sobsey D. (2006) Pain and disability in an ethical and social context. In: Oberlander TF, Symons FJ, eds. *Pain in Children and Adults with Developmental Disabilities*. Paul H. Brookes, Baltimore, MD. pp. 19–39.

7 Bottos S, Chambers CT. (2006) The epidemiology of pain in developmental disabilities. In: Oberlander TF, Symons FJ, eds. *Pain in Children and Adults with Developmental Disabilities*. Brookes, Baltimore, MD. pp. 67–87.

8 Breau LM, Camfield CS, McGrath PJ *et al.* (2003) The incidence of pain in children with severe cognitive impairments. *Arch Pediatr Adolesc Med* **157**:1219–26.

9 Stallard P, Williams L, Velleman R *et al.* (2002) The development and evaluation of the Pain Indicator for Communicatively Impaired Children (PICIC). *Pain* **98**:145–9.

10 Jensen MP, Engel JM, Hoffman AJ *et al.* (2004) Natural history of chronic pain and pain treatment in adults with cerebral palsy. *Am J Phys Med Rehabil* **83**:439–45.

11 Minihan PM. (1986) Planning for community physician services prior to deinstitutionalization of mentally retarded persons. *Am J Public Health* **76**:1202–6.

12 Beange H, McElduff A, Baker W. (1995) Medical disorders of adults with mental retardation: a population study. *Am J Ment Retard* **99**: 595–604.

13 Ehde DM, Jensen MP, Engel JM *et al.* (2003) Chronic pain secondary to disability: a review. *Clin J Pain* **19**:3–17.

14 Kibele A. (1989) Occupational therapy role in improving the quality of life for persons with cerebral palsy. *Am J Occup Ther* **43**:371–7.

15 Appelros P. (2006) Prevalence and predictors of pain and fatigue after stroke: a population-based study. *Int J Rehabil Res* **29**:329–33.

16 Cole LJ, Farrell MJ, Duff EP *et al.* (2006) Pain sensitivity and fMRI pain-related brain activity in Alzheimer's disease. *Brain* **129**:2957–65.

17 Mayer EA, Bushnell MC. (2009) *Functional Pain Syndromes: Presentation and Pathophysiology*. IASP Press, Seattle, WA.

18 Bodfish JW, Harper VN, Deacon JM *et al.* (2006) Issues in pain assessment for adults with severe to profound mental retardation: from research to practice. In: Oberlander TF, Symons FJ, eds. *Pain in Children and Adults with Developmental Disabilities*. Paul H. Brookes, Baltimore, MD. pp. 173–92.

19 Breau LM, Stevens B, Eckstein Grunau R. (2006) Developmental issues in acute and chronic pain in developmental disabilities. In: Oberlander TF, Symons FJ, eds. *Pain in Children and Adults with Developmental Disabilities*. Paul Brookes, Baltimore, MD. pp. 89–107.

20 Malviya S, Voepel-Lewis T, Burke C *et al.* (2006) The revised FLACC observational pain tool: improved reliability and validity for pain assessment in children with cognitive impairment. *Paediatr Anaesth* **16**:258–65.

21 Breau LM, McGrath PJ, Camfield CS *et al.* (2002) Psychometric properties of the non-communicating children's pain checklist-revised. *Pain* **99**:349–57.

22 Collignon P, Giusiano B. (2001) Validation of a pain evaluation scale for patients with severe cerebral palsy. *Eur J Pain* **5**:433–42.

23 Hunt A, Goldman A, Seers K *et al.* (2002) Validation of the paediatric pain profile, a behavioural rating scale to assess pain in children with severe neurological impairment. In: *10th World Congress on Pain*. International Association for the Study of Pain, San Diego, CA. p. 251.

24 Nader R, Oberlander TF, Chambers CT *et al.* (2004) Expression of pain in children with autism. *Clin J Pain* **20**:88–97.

25 Oberlander TF, O'Donnell ME, Montgomery CJ. (1999) Pain in children with significant neurological impairment. *J Dev Behav Pediatr* **20**:235–43.

26 Burkitt C, Breau LM, Salaman S *et al.* (2009) Pilot study of the feasibility of the Non-communication Children's Pain Checklist Revised for pain assessment for adults with interlectual disabilities. *J Pain Manage* **2**(**1**): 37–50.

27 Lotan M, Moe-Nilssen R, Ljunggren AE *et al.* (2009) Reliability of the Non-Communicating Adult Pain Checklist (NCAPC), assessed by different groups of health workers. *Res Dev Disabil* **30**:735–45.

28 Hunt A, Goldman A, Seers K *et al.* (2004) Clinical validation of the paediatric pain profile. *Dev Med Child Neurol* **46**:9–18.

29 Bodfish JW, Harper VN, Deacon JR *et al.* (2001) Identifying and measuring pain in persons with developmental disabilities: a manual for the Pain and Discomfort Scale (PADS). Available from Western Carolina Center Research Reports, Western Carolina Center, 300 Enola Road, Morganton, NC, 28655.

30 Fanurik D, Koh JL, Harrison RD *et al.* (1998) Pain assessment in children with cognitive impairment: an exploration of self-report skills. *Clin Nurs Res* **8**:103–19.

31 Phan A, Edwards CL, Robinson E. (2005) The assessment of pain and discomfort in individuals with mental retardation. *Res Dev Disabil* **26**:433–8.

Acknowledgments

T.F.O. is supported by a HELP Senior Career Award and is the R. Howard Webster Professorship in Child Development (College of Interdisciplinary Studies, UBC). F.S. and C.B. are supported, in part, from NIH/NICHD Grant Nos. 44763 and 47201 to the University of Minnesota. We are very grateful to Ursula Brain for her thoughtful contributions in preparing this chapter.

Chapter 40

Pain and addiction

Roman D. Jovey

Credit Valley Hospital, Addictions and Concurrent Disorders Center; CPM Centers for Pain Management, Mississauga, Canada

Introduction

Pain clinicians need to understand the basic principles of addiction medicine in order to reduce the risks of addiction associated with some of the medications used in the management of pain. It is also important to know when to refer to colleagues in addiction medicine.

Prevalence, neurobiology and definitions

Recent results from the US National Survey on Drug Use and Health (NSDUH), the largest anonymous annual population survey in the world, estimated that 9.2% of the population aged 12 or older, met DSM-IV criteria for substance dependence or abuse in the past year. The survey reported a prevalence rate of 8.3% for illicit drug use in the past month and a 2.0% prevalence rate for misuse of prescription opioids in the past month [1].

Surveys from chronic pain clinics quote prevalence rates of addiction among patients from a low of 3% up to a high of 27%. However, many older studies used non-standardized definitions or relied

Clinical Pain Management: A Practical Guide, 1st edition.
Edited by Mary E. Lynch, Kenneth D. Craig and Philip W.H. Peng.
© 2011 Blackwell Publishing Ltd.

on physiologic criteria to diagnose addiction. Studies were not explicit in separating iatrogenic opioid dependence from pre-existing substance use disorders and did not account for medication behaviors related to inadequately treated pain.

Surveys of patients attending outpatient methadone maintenance treatment programs (MMTP) or inpatient addiction treatment programs report that 61–80% complained of a chronic pain problem with severe pain experienced by 37% of MMTP patients and 24% of inpatients. Among those with chronic severe pain, 65% of MMTP patients and 48% of inpatients reported high levels of pain-related interference in physical and psychosocial functioning. Compared with addicted patients without pain, those with pain reported significantly more health problems, more psychiatric disturbance, more use of illicit drugs, as well as alcohol, to treat their pain, and more prescription and non-prescription medication use [2].

Neurobiology of addiction

Addiction is a chronic biopsychosocial illness involving brain reward centers (Figure 40.1). These brain circuits are involved in arousal, motivation and compulsion towards survival even in the presence of danger. Eating, sexual activity, social interaction and unexpected novel stimuli activate these reward circuits. Drugs associated with abuse have an ability to turn on reward circuits to a much

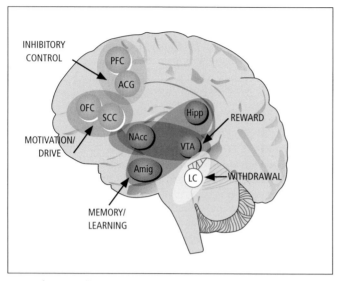

Figure 40.1 Brain centers involved in addiction.

After Nora Volkow, Director NIDA, 2004 Locus Ceruleus added, after Koob

greater extent and for a longer period of time than natural stimuli. By activating endogenous reward circuits, addictive drugs override behavior leading to progressive loss of control over drug intake in spite of medical, emotional, interpersonal, occupational and legal consequences. The compulsion to use drugs is compounded by deficits in impulse control and decision-making. Certain individuals are born with a greater or lesser sensitivity in these reward pathways making them biogenetically more or less at risk for developing an addictive disorder [3].

The development of addiction requires not only repeated exposure to a potentially addicting substance or behavior, but also an individual with a particular biopsychogenetic vulnerability living in a particular social milieu. Without the presence of these risk factors, it is unlikely that an opioid-naïve patient will become an addict by the prescription of opioids for pain [4]. Because of sensitized reward pathways in the brain, there is a high risk of cross-addiction to opioids in patients with previous addiction to other substances. Therefore it is important to screen patients for risk factors associated with addiction before prescribing opioids.

Defining opioid addiction in a patient with pain

It is important to use appropriate terminology when discussing patients with pain on therapeutic opioids in order clarify communication among health professionals and reduce stigma for patients.

Under the current classification system for psychiatric illness, DSM-IV(TR), the term "substance dependence" continues to be used instead of the term "addiction." This definition was intended to decrease the stigma associated with the term "addict" but unfortunately has resulted in a less precise definition, especially when referring to substances with a therapeutic use such as opioids. The DSM-IV criteria for "opioid dependence" may be appropriate for diagnosing addiction to alcohol or illicit heroin use, but are not appropriate when the drug in question is an opioid prescribed for a therapeutic purpose [5].

The Liason Committee on Pain and Addiction was formed in order to facilitate collaboration between pain and addiction specialists and has clarified the importance of clear unambiguous terminology [6]. It was identified that three fundamental concepts must inform terminology related to addictions:

Table 40.1 Definitions developed by the Liaison Committee on Pain and Addiction. The Liaison Commmittee was made up of representatives from the American Pain Society, the American Academy of Pain Medicine and the American Society of Addiction Medicine.

Addiction	A primary chronic neurobiological disease with genetic, psychosocial and environmental factors influencing its development and manifestations. It is characterized by behaviors that include one or more of the following: **IMPAIRED *CONTROL* OVER DRUG USE** **COMPULSIVE USE** **CONTINUED USE DESPITE HARM** **CRAVING** These phenomena may be accompanied by distortions in thought, chiefly denial, and a tendency to relapse once in recovery. Physical dependence and/or tolerance may, or may not, be present in addiction
Physical dependence	A state of adaptation manifested by a drug class specific withdrawal syndrome that can be produced upon abrupt cessation, rapid dose reduction, decreasing blood level of the drug and/ or administration of an antagonist
Tolerance	A state of adaptation in which exposure to the drug results in changes that result in diminution of one or more drug effects over time

Source: After Savage *et al.* [6].

1 Although some drugs produce pleasurable reward, critical determinants of addiction rest with the user.
2 Addiction is a multidimensional disease with neurobiological and psychosocial dimensions.
3 Addiction is a phenomenon distinct from physical dependence and tolerance.
Table 40.1 presents currently recommended definitions of tolerance, physical dependence and addiction.

Physical dependence is an expected physiological response in most individuals in the presence of continuous opioid use for therapeutic or nontherapeutic purposes. It is not, by itself, diagnostic

of addiction. Tolerance to unwanted opioid side effects, such as respiratory depression, sedation and nausea, occurs readily and is a welcome phenomenon. Some patients also develop tolerance to the analgesic effects of opioids, indicated by the need for increasing or more frequent doses of the medication to maintain analgesic effect. Tolerance to opioids, by itself, is also not diagnostic of addiction.

Pseudoaddiction

Some people with severe unrelieved pain may become intensely focused on finding pain relief and may appear to be preoccupied with obtaining opioids, but the preoccupation is with finding pain relief, rather than with the use of opioids per se. Such therapeutic preoccupation can be distinguished from true addiction by observing that when effective analgesia is obtained, by whatever means, the previous behaviors, which may have suggested addiction, resolve. Controversy continues over the use of this term. There is a risk that clinicians can misinterpret true addictive behaviors as pseudoaddiction.

Screening and risk stratification

There is now an evolving consensus that safe opioid prescribing requires individualization of a pain treatment plan that incorporates risk stratification. Thus, pain clinicians need to become proficient in performing and documenting a risk assessment. The use of time-efficient validated screening tools can improve both the quality and efficiency of documentation to meet regulatory requirements. [7]

The Opioid Risk Tool (ORT) is a five-item questionnaire designed to predict the probability of aberrant drug behaviors when prescribed opioids for chronic pain (Figure 40.2). Because of its brevity and ease of scoring, the ORT is clearly the simplest way to perform and document a risk assessment. It stratifies patients into low, moderate and high risk categories. Its only drawback is its higher susceptibility to deception. The SOAPP-R is a somewhat longer tool but is less susceptible to deception

	Mark each box that applies	
1 Family history of substance abuse	**Female***	**Male**
Alcohol	☐ 1	☐ 3
Illegal drugs	☐ 2	☐ 3
Prescription drugs	☐ 4	☐ 4
2 Personal history of substance abuse:		
Alcohol	☐ 3	☐ 3
Illegal drugs	☐ 4	☐ 4
Prescription drugs	☐ 5	☐ 5
3 Age (mark box if between 16 and 45)	☐ 1	☐ 1
4 History of pre-adolescent sexual abuse	☐ 3	☐ 0
5 Psychological disease		
Attention deficit disorder, obsessive-compulsive disorder, bipolar disorder, schizophrenia	☐ 2	☐ 2
Depression	☐ 1	☐ 1

Scoring totals: Low risk = 0–3; Moderate risk = 4–7; High risk = > 7
* Note that Female or Male refers to the gender of the patient, not the relative.

Figure 40.2 Opioid Risk Tool (ORT) (with scoring). Reproduced from Webster LR, Webster RM. (2005) Predicting aberrant behaviors in opioid-treated patients: preliminary validation of the Opioid Risk Tool. *Pain Med* **6(6)**: 432–42, with permission from Wiley-Blackwell.

(Figure 40.3). It stratifies patients into lower risk or higher risk categories.

The purpose of screening and risk stratification is to determine the intensity of follow-up and monitoring required, not to deny opioid therapy.

Universal Precautions in pain management

In order to strike a balance between optimum individual patient care and safety, the concept of Universal Precautions in pain management was coined in a seminal paper by Gourlay & Heit in 2005 (Table 40.2).

All patients require adequate documentation of the initial assessment, diagnosis, differential diagnosis, a treatment plan and the five A's of pain outcome assessment. In addition, all controlled substance prescriptions must have appropriate documentation according to local regulations.

Utilizing a written prescribing agreement when starting a trial of long-term opioid therapy is one way to document informed consent. It helps to clarify treatment expectations and boundaries

with the patient [8]. Although the use of treatment agreements is recommended in most guidelines for the prescribing of opioids for pain, not all clinicians are in agreement that they are ethical and accomplish the goal of reducing the misuse of opioids [9]. Agreements typically cover such issues as the risk of developing addiction, the use of one prescriber and one pharmacy, the requirement to take medication as directed, agreed participation in multimodal treatment modalities and consent to communicate with family and other health professionals. It is important to adapt written agreements to the language and reading level of the local population.

Random urine drug testing is one method of assessing which drugs the patient is taking, but is of limited use in detecting a patient who is diverting part of their prescription. If urine screening is to be used it is important to check with the local laboratory regarding methodology, detection limits and cross-reacting substances. Because urine is very susceptible to tampering, research into other methods of body fluid monitoring (e.g. saliva testing) is ongoing [10].

1	How often do you have mood swings?	0 Never	1	2	3	4 Very often
2	How often have you felt a need for higher doses of medication to treat your pain?	0 Never	1	2	3	4 Very often
3	How often have you felt impatient with your doctor?	0 Never	1	2	3	4 Very often
4	How often have you felt that things were just too overwhelming that you can't handle them?	0 Never	1	2	3	4 Very often
5	How often is there tension in the home?	0 Never	1	2	3	4 Very often
6	How often have you counted pain pills to see how many are remaining?	0 Never	1	2	3	4 Very often
7	How often have you been concerned that people will judge you for taking pain medication?	0 Never	1	2	3	4 Very often
8	How often do you feel bored?	0 Never	1	2	3	4 Very often
9	How often do you take more medication than you are supposed to?	0 Never	1	2	3	4 Very often
10	How often have you worried about being left alone?	0 Never	1	2	3	4 Very often
11	How often have you felt a craving for medication?	0 Never	1	2	3	4 Very often
12	How often have others expressed concern over your use of medication?	0 Never	1	2	3	4 Very often
13	How often have any of your close friends had a problem with alcohol or drugs?	0 Never	1	2	3	4 Very often
14	How often have others told you that you had a bad temper?	0 Never	1	2	3	4 Very often
15	How often have you felt consumed by the need to get pain medication?	0 Never	1	2	3	4 Very often
16	How often have you run out of pain medication early?	0 Never	1	2	3	4 Very often
17	How often have others kept you from getting what you deserve?	0 Never	1	2	3	4 Very often
18	How often, in your lifetime, have you had legal problems or been arrested?	0 Never	1	2	3	4 Very often
19	How often have you attended an AA or NA meeting?	0 Never	1	2	3	4 Very often
20	How often have you been in an argument that was so out of control that someone got hurt?	0 Never	1	2	3	4 Very often
21	How often have you been sexually abused?	0 Never	1	2	3	4 Very often
22	How often have others suggested that you have a drug or alcohol problem?	0 Never	1	2	3	4 Very often
23	How often have you had to borrow pain medications from your family or friends?	0 Never	1	2	3	4 Very often
24	How often have you been treated for an alcohol or drug problem?	0 Never	1	2	3	4 Very often

Total SOAPP-R Score: (Positive = a score of 18 or above)

Figure 40.3 Screener and Opioid Assessment for Patients with Pain Revised (SOAPP-R). Reproduced from Butler SF, Fernandez K, Benoit C *et al.* (2008) Validation of the revised Screener and Opioid Assessment for Patients with Pain (SOAPP-R). *J Pain* **9(4)**: 360–72, with permission from Elsevier.

Table 40.2 Summary of Universal Precautions for Pain Management. Adapted with permission from [12].

1	Make a diagnosis with appropriate differential diagnosis
2	Provide a psychological assessment including screening for risk of addictive disorders
3	Provide informed consent for the use of opioids (verbal or written)
4	Document a treatment agreement (verbal or written)
5	Assess and document pain level and function before the start of treatment
6	Provide an appropriate trial of opioid therapy +/– adjunctive medication
7	Regularly reassess pain scores and level of function
8	Regularly assess the "four A's" of pain medicine outcome:
	(This concept has since evolved into the "five A's" of pain treatment outcome:
	Analgesia – pain relief using an NRS, VAS, the percentage pain relief or other tool
	Affect – current mood and any changes since treatment
	Adverse effects – and recommended solutions
	Activity level – physical and social functioning
	Ambiguous drug behaviors with resulting actions by the clinician
9	Periodically review the pain diagnosis and comorbid conditions, including risk for opioid misuse/addiction
10	Document appropriately

NRS, numeric rating scale; VAS, visual analog scale.

Opioid therapy is not a panacea for all pains in all patients. When the use of opioid therapy is not resulting in significantly reduced pain and improved function, or in fact is doing more harm than good, clinicians need to have an "exit strategy" and feel comfortable in tapering patients off of opioids in favor of other therapies. In the case of a developing opioid addiction, referral to an addiction specialist for consideration of opioid therapy with methadone or buprenorphine is recommended.

If clinicians follow Universal Precautions in all patients taking controlled substances for pain, no one patient needs to feel stigmatized. This process can optimize outcomes for the patient and reduce risks for the prescribing clinician and society.

Strategies for treating the high risk patient

Patients who misuse substances experience pain just as acutely and probably more so than "normal" patients. They often have concurrent mental health problems with lives that tend to be chaotic and stressful. Their coping mechanisms are heavily biased towards use of chemicals and they

may be sceptical regarding non-pharmaceutical treatments.

Addicted patients often expect to be treated poorly by healthcare professionals resulting in apparent manipulative behaviors. To address this concern, clinicians need to use an open respectful approach, with clear direct communication as the key. It is helpful to discuss realistic expectations – aiming for good analgesia rather than a pain-free state but also to set appropriate but firm boundaries on acceptable behaviors. Mental health professionals with experience working in addictions are a valuable asset to the treatment team.

In high risk patients, the use of a biopsychosocial multimodal treatment plan is especially important [11]. Many high risk patients who present with problematic medication behaviors often have not had the benefit of a trial of non-pharmacological and non-opioid treatment options. With very high risk patients, co-management with an addiction professional, where available, is recommended.

Controlled release and/or long-acting opioids in a fixed dosing regimen are generally preferred over immediate release and/or short-acting drugs in order to try to disconnect the drug taking from the stimulus and reduce the risk of interdose withdrawal-mediated pain. Other modalities (drug or non-drug) should be utilized to manage transient increases in pain. Methadone can be a good treatment option when dealing with both nociceptive and neuropathic pain but must be carefully titrated and dispensed. Buprenorphine has a similar half-life to methadone with an enhanced safety profile but has a limit to dosing range, because it is a partial μ agonist. Various drug technologies are evolving to reduce the ability of patients to disable the controlled release mechanism of opioids, by crushing, snorting or injecting. One example is a tamper-resistant coating making it difficult to crush and inject the tablet; another is mixing naloxone and an opioid in the same tablet to dissuade crushing and snorting or intravenous injection.

Similar to patients without addiction, tolerance to therapeutic opioids can develop and dosage needs to be adjusted accordingly. Clinicians need to maintain awareness of opioid hyperalgesia and be prepared to switch or taper opioids when indicated.

The high risk patient on opioids requires a more structured treatment approach including more frequent follow-up, closer monitoring, including urine drug testing, and dispensing of smaller amounts of medication on a more frequent basis – even daily if required. Involving family members or significant others in the treatment plan can provide a collateral source of information and can help bolster social support and functioning.

High risk patients on appropriate opioid therapy can benefit from participation in a structured addiction treatment program to learn psychosocial coping strategies and reduce the risk of relapse. The pain clinician may have to negotiate the continued use of therapeutic opioids with a program that uses an abstinence-based model. The patient with both pain and addiction needs to commit to an ongoing program of recovery to optimize the benefit and increase the safety of long-term opioid therapy.

By learning some fundamentals of addiction medicine and utilizing the principles of Universal Precautions, pain clinicians can optimize benefits and reduce the risks of opioid therapy for pain.

References

1 Office of Applied Studies. (2007) *Results from the 2006 National Survey on Drug Use and Health: National findings*. Substance Abuse and Mental Health Services Administration, Office of Applied Studies, Rockville, MD. NSDUH Series H-32, DHHS Publication No. SMA 07-4293.
2 Rosenblum A, Joseph H, Fong C *et al.* (2003) Prevalence and characteristics of chronic pain among chemically dependent patients in methadone maintenance and residential treatment facilities. *JAMA* **289(18)**:2370–8.
3 Koob GF. (2006) The neurobiology of addiction: a neuroadaptational view relevant for diagnosis. *Addiction* **101(Suppl 1)**:23–30.
4 Fishbain DA, Cole B, Lewis J *et al.* (2008) What percentage of chronic nonmalignant pain patients exposed to chronic opioid analgesic therapy develop abuse/addiction and/or aberrant drug-related behaviors? A structured evidence-based review. *Pain Med* **9(4)**:444–59.
5 Heit HA, Gourlay DL. (2009) DSM-V and the definitions: time to get it right. *Pain Med* **10(5)**:784–6.
6 Savage SR, Joranson DE, Covington EC *et al.* (2003) Definitions related to the medical use of opioids: evolution towards universal agreement. *J Pain Symptom Manage* **26(1)**:655–67.
7 Passik SD, Kirsh KL, Casper D. (2009) Addiction-related tools and pain management: instruments for screening, treatment planning and monitoring compliance. *Pain Med* **9(Suppl 2)**:S145–66.
8 Fishman SM, Mahajan G, Jung SW *et al.* (2002) The trilateral opioid contract: bridging the pain clinic and the primary care physician through the opioid contract. *J Pain Symptom Manage* **24(3)**:335–44.
9 Arnold RM, Han PK, Seltzer D. (2006) Opioid contracts in chronic nonmalignant pain management: objectives and uncertainties. *Am J Med* **119(4)**:292–6.
10 Jaffee WB, Trucco E, Levy S *et al.* (2007) Is this urine really negative? A systematic review of tampering methods in urine drug screening and testing. *J Subst Abuse Treat* **33(1)**:33–42.

11 Savage SR, Kirsh KL, Passik SD. (2008) Challenges in using opioids to treat pain in persons with substance use disorders. *Addict Sci Clin Pract* **4(2)**:4–25.

12 Gourlay DL, Heit HA, Almahrezi A. (2005) Universal precautions in pain medicine: a rational approach to the treatment of chronic pain. *Pain Med* **6(2)**:107–12.

Further reading

British Pain Society. (2007) Pain and substance misuse: improving the patient experience. A consensus statement prepared by The British Pain Society in collaboration with The Royal College of Psychiatrists, The Royal College of General Practitioners and The Advisory Council on the Misuse of Drugs. Available from: http://www.britishpainsociety.org/book_drug_misuse_main.pdf. Accessed August 31, 2009.

Chou R, Fanciullo GJ, Fine PG *et al*.; American Pain Society/American Academy of Pain Medicine Opioids Guidelines Panel. (2009) Clinical guidelines for the use of chronic opioid therapy in chronic noncancer pain. *J Pain* **10(2)**: 113–30.

Chapter 41

Pain and psychiatric illness

Harold Merskey

Professor Emeritus of Psychiatry, University of Western Ontario, London, Canada

Introduction

Theories and facts about the relationship between pain and psychiatric illness have fluctuated considerably during the previous century and the present one. The issues of the relationship between pain and psychological factors receive much attention at the beginning of this volume and psychiatrists and psychologists have contributed substantially to discussion and ideas concerning how to understand pain, particularly in the last 40–50 years. The purpose of this chapter is more limited. It is to identify and describe the relationships between pain and psychiatric illness strictly defined. Within the range of what is called psychiatric illness as found for example in the DSM-IV, and the DSM-V now in preparation, does pain emerge as a state that results from mental processes, and, if so, is it made worse or relieved by them?

Pain may also be seen as a cause of psychological change – which undoubtedly it is. In medical affairs dealing with psychological phenomena, major, intermediate and minor contributions of one to the other are almost always to be found. Severe pain from a major physical cause may

Clinical Pain Management: A Practical Guide, 1st edition.
Edited by Mary E. Lynch, Kenneth D. Craig and
Philip W.H. Peng.
© 2011 Blackwell Publishing Ltd.

produce a variety of psychological responses. However, psychological causes, rarely, if at all, produce severe pain. The mind is more often blamed for causing pain than can be proven to be the case. In this chapter discussion is confined to major psychiatric illness such as psychoses, dementia and severe depressive illness, and the major features of psychological states in patients who have pain for physical reasons.

There is little to support the view that severe pain is caused by the psyche. The highly popular notion that pain is produced by the mind through a process of "somatization" is no longer logically tenable [1]. That is unfortunate because the concept of "somatization" was originally part of a well-intentioned attempt to get away from the diagnosis of "hysteria."

Pain occurs quite often in psychiatric patients [2], as it does in the rest of the general population [3]. However, pain is less common as a complaint [2] among patients with major psychiatric illness overall, and particularly so with schizophrenia.

With dementia (e.g. Alzheimer's disease, atherosclerotic dementia) pain usually occurs at the same rate among psychiatric patients as among the rest of the general population of similar ages, except that patients with moderately severe or severe dementia are less likely to be able to describe their experiences and may have to be observed quite closely to see if they are affected. Intellectually impaired patients also complain of pain less than others, whereas patients with an anxiety disorder or a depressive disorder complain of pain to a variable extent.

Dementia

Dementia is the most common major psychiatric illness. It affects the elderly population increasingly, so that from the age of 60 to 80 there is a gradual increase in dementia in both sexes and all populations. Twenty to thirty percent of patients over 80 years are recognized to have some degree of dementia but some remain untouched past the age of 90. If one is considering normal standards for individuals in their eighties, and certainly those past 90 it might be more appropriate to consider that intellectually impaired is the normal while intact intellectual capacity is less common. Although the ability to read may remain for some while in dementia, the ability to write consecutive intact logical sentences falls away, memory and spelling decline and the product of grammatical verbal material becomes patchy. Impairment of orientation begins with loss of recognition of dates and progresses, or perhaps one should say regresses, to the days of the week, followed by loss of awareness of months, seasons and the year.

In these circumstances individuals with lesions who report the experience of pain do not seem to be more frequent than those who do not, but physicians treating the elderly all recognize that in patients who have lost all verbal skills, or are somewhat sedated, restlessness – when it occurs – may be a fairly frequent indicator of physical change that in the verbally competent would give rise to the expression or complaint of pain.

Such painful conditions as osteoarthritis, neuropathic pain from stroke (nasty but relatively rare), will ordinarily be treated by the regular medical practitioner of a patient and often do not come to the attention of pain specialists except for those who are neurologists.

Occasional cases may arise where, in 80- and 90-year-old patients, the need for control of pain raises the question whether they should have opioids and, apart from adjusting for differences in the metabolic disposal of medication, and also the need to recognize the more frequent occurrence of conditions that can be affected by opioids (e.g. constipation, infarct, impaired attention), patients who are elderly and afflicted with such painful conditions as osteoarthritis, rheumatoid arthritis or neuropathic pain can still be effectively treated by pain medications including opioids. In such circumstances, it is often necessary to adjust treatment for the many more medications that the elderly are liable to be taking compared with younger persons.

Schizophrenia

Schizophrenia is the most severe and prolonged mental disorder of late youth and adult life. However, a proportion of patients with schizophrenia remit or return to relative normality under the influence of regular treatment with neuroleptic medication such as the phenothiazines and now, more often, the newer antipsychotic drugs including risperidone, quetiapine, olanzapine, aripiprazole and ziprasidone. In fact, if anything, schizophrenic patients complain less than others about pain. Because of the relatively sedentary nature of their lives there is a tendency for them to have less illnesses of certain types e.g. back pain which is not well documented, or rheumatoid arthritis, which is quite well documented [4].

Severe depression

Severe depression is occasionally accompanied by pain which starts with the depression and ends when the depression is over [5]. This usually means headache. Severe depression has occasionally been found to be accompanied by severe pain, especially in the face, that has been attributed clinically to the depression. There do not appear to be any good systematic studies that confirm this viewpoint. Post-herpetic neuralgia has commonly been accompanied by depression and can be exacerbated by severe depressive illness.

The literature that deals with this topic of pain and depression is related in large measure to a time prior to the widespread use of DSM-III, and DSM-IV criteria for major depressive disorder. The latter is not necessarily as severe a condition as the types of depression that were previously considered. Most of the severe cases of pain due to depression date from the early literature when antidepressants were not available and electroconvulsive therapy (ECT) was the only effective common remedy for severe depression (short of leucotomy) and anecdotal reports were common. The relief of pain – with fluctuation in the associated depression – is well recognized whatever the cause, whether the pain be caused by depression or the depression be caused by pain. Suicide in relation to severe chronic pain does not appear to be common in patients with otherwise normal expectation of life but may occur, perhaps more often, with terminal illness. These few, and rather sparse, items of information reflect the essentials of the relationship between pain and severe depression.

Moderately severe depression

Moderately severe depression is generally characterized by the criteria of major affective disorder as identified currently in DSM-IV and in the World Health Organization criteria for major depressive disorder [6]. In patients with depression, without a history of injury or other cause of pain, headache may occur as one of the features of depression and, as Bradley [5] found, usually departs when the patient is treated.

It is important to know that amitriptyline is not only an antidepressant and a good hypnotic, but also provides considerable analgesic benefit for patients with pain who are not depressed. This was first noted in 1972 [7] and established in double-blind controlled trials by Watson et al. [8], and has subsequently been confirmed by numerous investigators using similar double-blind controlled trials, measuring the presence of depression with the Beck Depression Inventory and monitoring the change in pain [8–10]. Watson et al. [8] used amitriptyline with benefit in patients who were not depressed at an average dose of 75 mg/day.

The clinical application of this information is important in that very small doses of amitriptyline may work for some patients and large doses may work for others. Physicians treating patients with

amitriptyline or similar antidepressants may find that some patients tolerate large doses while others only tolerate tiny ones (Chapter 14). There is a wide range of variation in individual metabolism and ability to tolerate various drugs acting on the central nervous system although, as indicated, antidepressants have been reportedly beneficial for pain with depression [8–10].

Obsessional neurosis

Obsessional neurosis (DSM-IV Obsessive-Compulsive Disorder) has no particular association with chronic pain.

Anxiety conditions

Of the anxiety conditions, various sorts are associated with chronic pain. In general, the anxiety found is proportional to the patient's distress because of pain. If it is related to post-traumatic stress disorder it also tends to be proportional to the severity of the troublesome event that precipitated the injury. However, individuals vary and anxious individuals are liable to have more anxiety, while individuals who were not previously anxious are likely to have less anxiety, albeit some may develop anxiety because of pain or because of stressful recollections of the injury.

In brief, post-traumatic stress disorder is associated with actual threatening or damaging events, troublesome recollections of the event, dreams or "flashbacks," intense distress at reminders of the event, persistent avoidance of stimuli associated with the trauma and numbing of general responsiveness with persistent de novo symptoms of increased arousal and clinically significant distress or impairment in functioning.

In general, if it is found in patients with chronic pain it most often appears to be because of the association with injury. Patients who are injured in traffic accidents and subsequently develop chronic musculoskeletal pain are liable to experience some symptoms relating to the stress of the accident in addition to those from pain itself. Thus, they may become uneasy in traffic in general, particularly fearful as passengers ("backseat drivers"), and are most uneasy at the site of the accident. Usually, the disorder presents several months after a traffic accident, is accompanied by nightmares, often but not always focusing on injury, and is marked during the day by jumpiness in the presence of anything reminiscent of the injury. The full criteria for posttraumatic stress disorder are most often not satisfied but some related symptoms in vehicles are fairly common.

As a rule, patients with moderately severe whiplash injuries and those with low back sprains who develop pain of sufficient severity to cause continuing complaints after 3 months also tend to develop stress symptoms in relation to driving, including fearfulness on highways, fearfulness near the site of the accident and dreams of collisions or other violent events. In many instances they make bad passengers because of anxiety as well as because of discomfort related to their posture in a car seat. The symptoms of posttraumatic stress tend to decline for the most part over months or years in patients subject to whiplash injuries. Patients who have more severe injuries, such as head injuries with loss of consciousness or disturbance of consciousness exceeding more than a few minutes, are also liable to have increased difficulties in concentration and attention as well as chronic pain.

"Somatoform disorders"

This topic is an issue at the present time [1,11]. "Somatization" and "somatoform disorders" originated in an attempt to provide a systematic method of describing individuals who were thought to have what traditionally had been called "hysteria", i.e. a disorder in which a patient thought she or he had a disability, experienced or produced the symptoms of the disability, but had no physical basis for it. Historically, this was explained in various ways but ultimately the most popular one became the Freudian notion of repression of a conflict into the unconscious mind with solution of the conflict by the production of the symptom. Thus, a soldier might want to run away from danger. He might want not to seem a coward or to be a coward. The problem was solved by

acting upon the unconscious wish to be ill (e.g. with a paralysis, deafness or other "hysterical" symptom that would enable him to escape the obligations of duty on the basis of a medical label). Recognition of this pattern became particularly apparent in the First World War internationally and the popularity of Freudian concepts between the two World Wars was sufficient to establish in the medical mind the notion that "hysteria" was a valid disorder with a proven mechanism. It appears that similar or related symptoms occurred in the Allied Armies but did not reappear in the Wehrmacht where they led to execution. Instead, the Nazi Army had a special battalion or two of soldiers with stomach complaints.

The diagnosis of hysteria was never a popular one with patients nor with physicians who gave it, nor with other physicians who disapproved of it. Nevertheless, it had a widespread degree of acceptance and provided a partial solution for many years. In the 1950s and 1960s a group of Boston psychiatrists [12–14] endeavored to establish a method of characterizing patients with "hysteria" in such a way that there would be agreement on the diagnosis but without relying upon theoretical notions like the idea that the symptom served the purpose, had a symbolic value and reflected an attempt at problem-solving. Their concern was how to rediagnose individuals with multiple bodily complaints who were considered not to have a physical cause for their complaints. Today it seems likely that at least some of the patients they diagnosed had fibromyalgia which does have a strong physical basis. However, a serious scientific attempt was made to provide for this situation and criteria were set up based upon multiple insufficiently substantiated physical complaints and called Somatization Disorders.

This did not take account of the single hysterical symptom (e.g. a paralysis or a loss of hearing) which remained to be diagnosed on the basis of the physical examination and neurological or other physical proof that the patient had capacity that he or she appeared not to be able to use. In any case two major factors have entered into the decay of these diagnoses. In the first place, with regard to the multisymptomatic patient, diagnoses have subsequently become feasible (e.g. fibromyalgia) that provide a good pathophysiological explanation for the disorder. Second, some so-called "hysterical" symptoms on an individual basis turned out to be attributable to the development of brain disease [15,16].

Competent physicians could still see the "conversion disorder" or hysterical symptom as a convenient means of escape for patients, which needed to be given consideration but not to be misunderstood as an unconscious process [17,18]. When it seemed necessary to postulate an unconscious process it remained necessary to rely on Freudian notions.

Following a series of publications in social history, the publication by Masson of Freud's correspondence with his friend Fliess [19] and examination of Freudian claims, it became evident that there was a considerable mass of information that made the Freudian theories untenable [19–21] and Freud's claims untrue. Thus, the atheoretical approach of Guze and colleagues seemed more desirable than ever and was encapsulated in the DSM-III and DSM-IV descriptions of "somatization disorder." But the notion of active repression persisted.

Another serious blow to the diagnosis of hysteria came from the unraveling of the concept of "dissociative disorders." Dissociative disorders are types of illness in which the hysterical mechanisms of repression and loss of material from consciousness are postulated but held to produce psychological symptoms rather than physical ones. The leading symptoms of this type were loss of memory, fugues and multiple personality disorder. Starting with the latter and reaching back to the others, dissociative disorders became increasingly suspect and a significant number of psychiatrists have rejected the concept of dissociative identity disorder [16]. Along with this it is implied and accepted by some, including this writer, that dissociative symptoms and physical conversion symptoms are all equally suspect along with dissociative identity disorder [16,20,22].

In consequence, the diagnosis of "pain disorder" in DSM-IV, which was originally intended to be a more sophisticated version of hysteria, has strict criteria so that it ought not to be made in patients with severe depression or anxiety or physiological illness, and is now redundant and should be discarded.

Conclusions

Chronic pain that is clinically important rarely has psychological causes. Depression is often found with chronic pain – and anxiety with acute pain. These conditions are mostly a consequence of pain and its attendant circumstances, rather than its cause. However, they may interact with the physical disorder to increase pain. Headache is increasingly recognized as having pathophysiological rather than psychological mechanisms of production. If anything, pain in schizophrenia is usually less than in the population at large. Similar considerations apply to anxiety as to depression. The disorder is often, or usually, the result of a physical change and the emotional changes tend to be secondary. Somatization and pain disorder are diagnoses to avoid.

References

1 Merskey H. (2009) Somatization: or another God that failed. *Pain* **145**:4–5.
2 Delaplaine R, Ifabumuyi OI, Merskey H *et al.* (1978) Significance of pain in psychiatric hospital patients. *Pain* **4**:361–6.
3 Magni G, Caldieron C, Rigatti-Luchini S *et al.* (1990) Chronic musculoskeletal pain and depressive symptoms in the general population: an analysis of the 1st National Health and Nutrition Examination Survey data. *Pain* **43**:299–307.
4 Mohamed SN, Merskey H, Kazarian S *et al.* (1982) An investigation of the possible inverse relationships between the occurrence of rheumatoid arthritis, osteoarthritis and schizophrenia. *Can J Psychiatry* **27**:381–3.
5 Bradley JJ. (1963) Severe localized pain associated with the depressive syndrome. *Br J Psychiatry* **109**:701–45.
6 World Health Organization. (1992) *The ICD-10 Classification of Mental and Behavioural Disorders.* World Health Organization, Geneva.

7 Merskey H, Hester RN. (1972) The treatment of chronic pain with psychotropic drugs. *Postgrad Med J* **48**:594–8.

8 Watson CP, Evans RJ, Reed K *et al.* (1982) Amitriptyline versus placebo in postherpetic neuralgia. *Neurology* **32**:671–3.

9 Max MB, Culnane M, Schafer SC *et al.* (1987) Amitriptyline relieves diabetic neuropathy pain in patients with pain and depressed mood. *Neurology* **37**:589–96.

10 Sharav Y, Singer E, Schmidt E *et al.* (1987) The analgesic effects of amitriptyline on chronic facial pain. *Pain* **31**:199–209.

11 Crombez G, Beirens K, Van Damme S *et al.* (2009) The unbearable lightness of somatization. *Pain* **145**:131–5.

12 Purtell J, Robins E, Cohen ME. (1951) Observations on clinical aspects of hysteria: a quantitative study of 150 hysterical patients and 156 control subjects. *JAMA* **145**:902–9.

13 Perley JM, Guze SB. (1962) Hysteria: the stability and usefulness of clinical criteria. *N Engl J Med* **266**:421–6.

14 Guze SB. (1967) The diagnosis of hysteria: what are we trying to do? *Am J Psychiatry* **124**:77–84.

15 Slavney P. (1990) *Perspectives on "Hysteria".* Johns Hopkins University Press, Baltimore, MD.

16 McHugh PR. (2008) *Try to Remember.* Dana Press, New York.

17 Slater E. (1965) Diagnosis of "hysteria". *Br Med J* **1**:1395–9.

18 Gould R, Miller BI, Goldberg MA *et al.* (1986) The validity of hysterical signs and symptoms. *J Nerv Ment Dis* **174**:593–8.

19 Masson G. (1985) *The Complete Letters of Sigmund Freud to Wilhelm Fliess, 1887–1904.* Belknap Press, Harvard, Cambridge, MA.

20 Crews F. (1998) *Unauthorized Freud: Doubters Confront a Legend.* Viking, New York.

21 Esterson A. (1993) *Seductive Mirage: An Exploration of the Work of Sigmund Freud.* Open Court, Chicago, IL.

22 Merskey H. (1992) The manufacture of personalities: the production of multiple personality disorder. *Br J Psychiatry* **160**:327–40.

Subject Index

Notes

Page numbers in *italics* represent figures, those in **bold** represent tables.

To save space in the index, the following abbreviations have been used:

CPSP – chronic post surgical pain

CRPS – complex regional pain syndrome

NSAIDs – non-steroidal anti-inflammatory drugs

Clinical Pain Management: A Practical Guide, 1st edition.
Edited by Mary E. Lynch, Kenneth D. Craig and Philip W.H. Peng.
© 2011 Blackwell Publishing Ltd.